Navigating Childhood Stuttering

Ramandeep Kaur

Navigating Childhood Stuttering

A Guide to Management of Stuttering at Home and School

Springer

MANIPAL
UNIVERSAL PRESS

Ramandeep Kaur
Department of Speech and Language Therapy
Father Muller Charitable Institution
Mangalore, Karnataka, India

Jointly published with Manipal Universal Press
Copyright page of International Edition: This edition is not for sale in India. Customers from India should order the print book from Manipal Universal Press (MUP).
ISBN of the India edition: 978-81-977592-5-3.

Copyright page of India Edition: This edition is not for sale outside India. Customers outside India should order the print and electronic book from Springer Nature.
ISBN of the International edition (outside India): 978-981-96-6205-0

ISBN 978-981-96-6205-0 ISBN 978-981-96-6206-7 (eBook)
https://doi.org/10.1007/978-981-96-6206-7

This Springer imprint is published by the registered company Springer Nature Singapore Pte Ltd.
The registered company address is: 152 Beach Road, #21-01/04 Gateway East, Singapore 189721, Singapore

Preface

It always seems impossible until it's done.
Nelson Mandela

Stuttering is one of the most undefeatable obstacles in speech, not only for children but for their families as well. Stuttering hinders most of the activities, which involve fluent speech, thereby making speech overwhelming and filled with setbacks and challenges. However, as quoted by Nelson Mandela, "Even the most formidable challenges can be overcome with determination and effort." Stuttering too can be conquered with conscious efforts, persistence, patience, and the right support.

Stuttering is a complex speech disorder which not only affects a child's speech and communication but also impacts their self-confidence, social interactions, life quality, and overall perspective on life. This book aims to demystify stuttering and provide an elaborative resource for all individuals who wish to dedicate themselves to supporting children with stuttering.

This book is a result of various interactions and experiences with children who stutter. It is consistently seen that these children find it difficult to implement stuttering management techniques learnt in therapy centers to their home and school environments. This was the primary motivational factor in preparation of this book, to help children to be able to transition from therapy to real life with help of parents and teachers.

The book highlights comprehensive strategies that aim to bridge professional insights with real-life therapy strategies to provide effective support for these children at home and school. Filling this gap intends to reduce the chances of recurrence (or relapse) of stuttering and thus improve the overall quality of life for children who stutter.

The book provides home- and school-based practical tips and exercises, which can help children integrate therapy techniques into everyday lives. The book explains the rationale behind each technique, which in turn makes therapeutic strategies more accessible and understandable by the readers. The overall aim is to provide real-life solutions to common issues and challenges faced by a child with their speech, even after receiving speech therapy.

The book also incorporates a chapter on the use of artificial intelligence and various applications that can be used by individuals who stutter, especially children. Such innovative technologies and advanced approaches enhance the use of traditional methods, making therapy techniques fun and easier to adapt.

The book highlights the key role of educators, apart from parents, in the life of children especially to shape communication skills, promote social interaction, develop better confidence skills, and thereby develop better self-esteem. For this, the book includes exclusive classroom-based practical strategies and tips to help foster better fluency in classroom environment. By integrating these strategies into teaching practices, a substantial difference can be made in the lives of these children.

The book completes with an additional chapter on inspiring stories of individuals who have successfully overcome stuttering by being strong, determined, and positive in their thoughts. These individuals have not only successfully overcome their stuttering but have also reached remarkable success in their lives. Their journey surely inspires and motivates millions proving that perseverance with sheer determination along with positive thoughts can help readers achieve any heights.

One of the fascinating facts of stuttering is the "Chameleon Effect" due to which individuals who stutter can speak fluently in certain situations such as when singing or speaking in groups and so on. This feature of stuttering highlights that the pathways of speech production are not universally impaired. Instead, they can be trained to achieve better fluency. This book intends to inspire hope and reinforce such ideas through right techniques and environment, to achieve better fluency. Additionally, the book highlights facts like brain's neuroplasticity—the remarkable ability to reorganize and develop novel neural connections. This further demonstrates that with consistent practice and intervention significant improvements in fluency can be achieved.

The book also includes mindfulness practices, which have consistently shown improvements in reducing anxiety issues and implement overall relaxation, thereby enhancing speech fluency.

This book stands as a guiding light not only for children who stutter but also their parents and teachers, helping them illuminate the strengths and capabilities within every child who stutters. By integrating scientific insights with practical applications, a clear framework is provided to help children succeed in achieving better fluency.

Therefore, stuttering management is not about finding a quick solution to the speech problems but is instead about developing a child's ability to communicate effectively by choosing the right mindset and being positive throughout the process. To achieve this successfully, patience, understanding, and a commitment to ongoing learning and adaptation are required. We hope that this book will serve as a valuable resource in the journey to achieve a better speech, providing insights and tools necessary to make a positive impact on everyone's lives.

Happy Reading!

Mangalore, Karnataka, India Ramandeep Kaur

Contents

List of Tables

The First Words: Nurturing Communication with Care

1

Abstract

The chapter explores the emotional and developmental journey of children who stutter, highlighting its profound impact on both the child and their family. While early speech milestones bring immense joy to parents, the onset of stuttering often turns communication into a source of anxiety and frustration. The chapter highlights the effects of stuttering on the overall quality of life of the entire family.

The chapter underlines the shift from a deficit-focused perspective to a more acceptance-driven approach, emphasizing the importance of viewing stuttering as a unique communication style rather than a defect. It highlights the crucial roles of parents, educators, and peers in fostering resilience, self-confidence, and supportive communication environments.

Keywords

Stuttering impact · Speech development · Child communication · Parental support · Acceptance

1.1 Stumbling Speech: The Bitter Truth of Stuttering

As a child is born, a parent eagerly anticipates every step the child takes while achieving the developmental milestones. From first foods to first steps, from first coos to first words, and from first birthday to first day at school, everything is a new and exciting experience for a parent. Every coo and babble of an infant, though unintelligible and confusing, is celebrated as a huge herald of growth and development. These signs of growing

R. Kaur, *Navigating Childhood Stuttering*, https://doi.org/10.1007/978-981-96-6206-7_1

interactions then mark the child's first words, which eventually turn into a rich world of communication.

For parents, a child's first words are not just signs of development but are a deep, emotional connection with the child. It is those memorable moments when thoughts and feelings, previously guessed at, now become more pronounced through words like "I love you," "Mommy I want to be with you," and so on.

As words turn into phrases and phrases into complete sentences, the child's voice turns into a soothing melody that parents and family members wait to listen to, unless the notes of this melody *begin to falter*. For some children, speaking smoothly is not so easy. The whole task of speaking and communicating with others suddenly starts becoming tougher with every sentence these children speak. Their speech, which was once fluent, slowly starts becoming bumpy at times with pauses, repetitions, and frustrations. Tragically, they may now find themselves labelled not by their beautiful names but as children who stutter, a label that shadows their true identities. This speech problem, known as "stuttering," now starts casting a shadow over the pleasure that communication once brought, slowly turning it into a source of anxiety and concern.

As the stuttering worsens, the conversations become more effortful and the child who was once proud of their speech now starts getting conscious and nervous with every word spoken (or stuttered). This anxiety gets worse with parental reactions and concerns toward the child's stuttering. The parents, once proud of the child's speech, now look with fear and sympathy. The smiles now turn into helpless faces with their brows furrowing, eyes filled with worry, tightened voices, and stiffened smiles. Each repetition or block, even though minor, now starts building a wall of worry. Slowly, this worry starts turning into signs of blame when parents may wonder silently, burdened by guilt, about the origin of their child's stuttering.

"Did I miss something, or could I have done something differently?" "Why my child, what wrong did I do to anyone?"
"Can it be my brother as he stutters too?"
"Is this due to my child's dad who is extremely strict?"

All these are the confusions that arise with every blocked word the child demonstrates.

The child, who was once enjoying their speech with delight and discovery, now begins to develop a new burden and anxiety toward what they are about to say. Home, once a shelter of unconditional acceptance, subtly shifts as now conversations no longer flow freely. The home atmosphere now haunts the child with silent expectations and the echoes of unspoken words, teaching the child that speaking is no longer just sharing—it is a constant trial to be faced.

School, which is one of the most rewarding experiences for most children, becomes another warzone for these children. When the school bell rings, the child develops a fear of speaking in class and facing nasty remarks about their stutter, rather than enjoying the lessons in math and science. Classmates who once paid little attention to how words are spoken now look puzzled or, worse, speak words that mock and mimic, making the child's life experiences worse. The classroom now transforms from a place of learning to a stage of scrutiny, not only making communication a challenge but also ruining the child's self-esteem.

If this mocking was not enough, then sometimes there are overly concerned and well-meaning friends and relatives, who are all well-armed with advice as easy and ineffective as it can be. "Just slow down," they say, or "Take a deep breath," as if these simple phrases would unlock the stuttering puzzle effortlessly. Each suggestion they bring intensifies the problem rather than erasing it, thereby making the child more troubled and painfully aware of their stuttering. With every failed advice and suggestion, the child's grief gets heavier, and the child learns to withdraw into silence. Thereby, the child begins to choose the grief of unspoken thoughts, which sound more soothing than the struggle of stuttered words.

To be precise, the condition called "stuttering," which is just a speech problem, becomes grave with every minute as it completely shatters the expectations of the child and their family in terms of societally accepted forms of speech and communication. Thereby, it subtly alters every interaction along with the overall self-perception and self-esteem of the child. Moreover, the constant desire to "fix" the speech further overshadows the child's need for acceptance and understanding.

On the other hand, the scenario changes when we use a different approach to look at a child who stutters, an approach that supports resilience and acceptance over worry and corrections. Instead of looking at stuttering as a defect that needs to be eradicated, it is important to look at it as a child's unique way to communicate. All of us go dysfluent at times, and thus, achieving complete fluency is just an ideal situation impossible to achieve. Children who stutter may become dysfluent more often than those who do not stutter, and the best way to address this includes redefining a child's thoughts, emotions, and experiences, along with the therapeutic strategies they need to use. *This reframing is subtle but powerful.* It allows an individual to look at stuttering just the way it is and not as a challenge impossible to overcome.

To make this possible, it is important to understand our role as a society where parents, family members, teachers, and peers play an important role in supporting and facilitating the right development of speech among children. This includes changing the perspective of parents from fixers to facilitators, where corrections are substituted by positive encouragement and the provision of spaces where children feel safe to make mistakes, correct themselves, and learn to speak with better fluency, i.e., a society where teachers practice active listening, encourage small achievements, and avoid passing unwanted judgements or negative comments in every situation. Such safe spaces are also ones where peers foster an understanding of diversity in communication, encourage inclusivity, and support each other instead of engaging in unhealthy competition, mockery, or mimicry, especially with respect to speech and communication. Embracing this perspective enables a child to not only manage stuttering better but also become successful in being able to elicit fluent communications most of the time. This "lookout" approach for stuttering provides a child with better tools to achieve smoother communication at their own pace, rather than rushing through the pressure of achieving all at once.

The acceptance and understanding offered by such a society can further enhance a child's ability to engage with therapeutic strategies more effectively. Being accepted and valued, rather than judged, naturally makes the child feel more relaxed in implementing the techniques they learnt in therapy sessions in various situations. This calm attitude further reduces the psychological and emotional struggle that is associated with stuttering, thereby reducing the frequency and severity of the problem. Moreover, this creates a positive self-image and encourages the child to participate actively with confidence in their therapy sessions and to practice their skills in everyday settings without fear of judgment or failure.

As we continue to explore each of these domains in future sections, it is important to highlight that parents, educators, and speech therapists should equip children with deep understanding and valuable tools to make them feel heard and encouraged for their unique voices, irrespective of the way they communicate.

1.2 Baby Steps: Babbling to Conversation

To understand the development of speech fluency among children, it is important to understand the way speech develops during the early years of child development. During infancy, the child starts vocalizing by using vegetative sounds (such as gurgling and burping), which slowly transition into cooing, babbling, and vocal gestures. These early vocalizations are the foundational blocks of language as they serve as important keys of communication.

With further development, children start babbling more consonants and sound combinations to form proper syllables and sounds, initially meaningless but later denoting specific meanings. This is a remarkable period where a child's articulators (lips, tongue, jaws, palate, and so on) develop complex movements and coordinate among each other for creating sophisticated verbal responses.

Around the first birthday, these babbling sounds start transitioning into the first actual words, which denote meanings. Parents get to hear specific words like "Mama," "Dada," "Caty," or "Dolly," which correspond to immediate people or things the child is familiar with. These words give the child the ability to transform their thoughts into words and thus equip them with the ability to alter their environment through language.

As the vocabulary further expands, the first words then start combining to form two-word combinations like "Daddy car" or "Mumma sleep" to denote further understanding of language rules and grammar. The two words then grow into longer phrases that slowly develop into complete sentences, indicating further language development.

As the child reaches the preschool level, the child's language becomes more complex, with reporting, narration, and storytelling skills becoming evident in language and communication. During this stage, children learn to explore their social role and share experiences, thereby further defining their social relationships.

Overall, speech and language development is a dynamic and complex process that helps children develop communication skills. This journey highlights the importance of each developmental phase in contributing to a child's communication needs (Hoff 2009).

During these stages of speech and language development, it is common for children to face dysfluencies in their speech. These dysfluencies typically manifest during the early stages of speech development. Typically, these disruptions might begin as children transition from babbling to word formation and the development of complex sentence structures. This is a stage of exponential growth in vocabulary and grammar. Since the development takes place rapidly at this stage, some moments of hesitation or repetitions are common. The child's limited cognitive and articulatory abilities add further to these developmental issues.

The dysfluencies during this stage might include repetitions of whole words or phrases, prolongations, and the use of filler words like "um" or "uh." These are generally normal dysfluencies that are transient and resolve with the child's developing linguistic skills. However, in some children, these disruptions may persist and eventually develop into stuttering. Stuttering can be distinguished from normal dysfluencies by its frequency, the types of dysfluencies, and the presence of physical tension (like facial grimacing or hand/leg movements, eye blinking, and so on).

It is important for parents and educators to understand the differences between typical (or normal) dysfluencies and stuttering. Recognizing these signs helps in preventing further development of stuttering by following the right approaches to deal with these children. It also helps in identifying stuttering early, thereby aiding in planning early intervention.

Reference

Hoff E. Language development. 4th ed. Wadsworth: Cengage Learning; 2009.

Demystifying Fluent Speech

2

Abstract

This chapter explores essential components of speech fluency and how it affects communication and daily interactions. It focuses on key elements of fluency—rate of speech, rhythm, automaticity, and strategic pausing—explaining the interaction of each of these to frame fluent speech.

Furthermore, the chapter introduces the speech mechanism, outlining coordination between the respiratory, phonatory, articulatory, resonatory, and neurological systems to produce fluent speech. It stresses the relationship between incoordination among these systems and how it leads to disfluent speech. The chapter discusses the demands and capacities model (DCM) to illustrate the relationship between environmental demands and a child's speech capacities.

Keywords

Fluency · Speech mechanism · Normal nonfluency · Disfluencies · Demands and capacities model

2.1 Fluency

Before delving deeper into the insights of stuttering and other speech dysfluencies, it is crucial to understand the aspects of fluency. Speech fluency refers to the flow, speed, and rhythm with which language is expressed. It allows speakers to convey their thoughts and emotions effectively, enabling listeners to grasp the intended message without undue effort.

R. Kaur, *Navigating Childhood Stuttering*,
https://doi.org/10.1007/978-981-96-6206-7_2

2.2 Definition

There are various definitions that explain fluency. Fillmore (1979) described fluency as an ability to produce written and/or spoken language readily. This definition highlights the ease and smooth flow of language, emphasizing that fluency is an important indicator of proficiency.

On a similar perspective, Lennon (1990) defines fluency as the rapid, smooth, and effortless flow of language in real-time interaction. This highlights the smoothness of speech exclusively in real-time communication.

Ratner (1997) talks of fluency as the ability to link units of speech together with ease and without strain or inappropriate slowness or undue hesitation. He highlights the linkage of speech units in a natural way through rhythm and continuity in spoken language.

2.3 Components of Fluency

Fluency is achieved through the interaction of various key components. Each of these components contributes efficiently to achieving a constant flow of speech:

1. *Rate of Speech*: This refers to the speed at which a person speaks. An optimum rate of speech is important to develop fluency. The rate of speech, undoubtedly, affects the listener's ability to understand the spoken language. For example, a fast talker may overwhelm the listener by making it difficult to follow and understand the narrative. Conversely, speaking too slowly may bore the listener or may give an impression of uncertainty or lack of confidence in the content being spoken. An optimum speech rate is crucial for maintaining listener engagement and conveying the message effectively.
2. *Rhythm and Intonation*: This includes stress and melody, which are important in speech. A proper rhythm and intonation in speech helps to convey emotion in speech. It also helps provide emphasis on the right elements of speech and thereby improvise the meaning of the spoken message. Rhythm and intonation thereby stand essential for effective communication. Consider the difference in perception for a statement, "Really appreciate that work" with a flat tone versus delivering the same statement with a warm and enthusiastic tone. The former might denote insincerity or sarcasm, while the latter clearly conveys gratitude. Similarly, when rhythm and intonation are varied appropriately in storytelling, a better meaning is conveyed with a better engagement of the audience as opposed to a poor rhythm and monotonous delivery, which can turn the most interesting story sound dull and boring.
3. *Automaticity*: This refers to the ability to speak without pausing to think about the mechanics of speech, like word pronunciation or grammar and so on. Good automaticity allows a speaker to focus more on the content of the message and less on the form.

4. *Pausing*: Strategic pausing during the speech helps the speaker to take necessary breaks and thus improves fluency. It helps the speaker to process information better during these pauses and thus maintain speech continuity. However, excessive pausing or pausing at inappropriate points can disrupt fluency and hinder comprehension.

2.4 Impact of Fluency on Speech

Fluency is important not only to understand speech clearly but also to elicit the right meaning from conversations. It has a significant impact on one's daily communication across both professional and personal domains. When the speaker is fluent, it is easier for the listener to comprehend and engage with the spoken message. Conversely, a non-fluent message can lead to misunderstandings and a lack of engagement from the listener.

Apart from the comprehension of the message, fluency clearly impacts the social image of an individual. A fluent speaker is often perceived to be more confident, credible, and intelligent compared to someone who is nonfluent. This perception can lead to greater social success, as fluent speakers are more likely to be viewed positively by their society. This social image also impacts a person's self-image and overall confidence level.

Research in social psychology suggests that people are more likely to judge a person as truthful if their speech is fluent. The fluent information is processed more easily, creating a sense of familiarity and comfort. Familiarity is often instinctively associated with truth. Similarly, a fluent message is more persuasive and convincing compared to a non-fluent one. Fluency undoubtedly increases the credibility and charm of the message being spoken, making it more impactful. Consider advertisements, speeches, or written communications; they all make the most impact when spoken fluently. Lev-Ari and Keysar (2010) conducted a study where it was seen that statements read fluently were more likely to be judged as true than those read with hesitations.

Fluency plays an equally important role in children as well. Fluent children are usually considered more confident and smarter in school and at home. In school, fluency affects a child's ability to participate in debates, class discussions, comprehension, and delivery of messages to teachers and peers, perform well in oral presentations, elocutions, and overall academics. Due to better confidence levels, fluent children are more inclined to take up active roles in their education. They are more likely to ask questions, engage in discussions, debates, and perform well in oral presentations and other exams.

At home as well, fluency helps a child form better connections with family members due to better interaction and facilitates their overall language development. Speech and language skills provide a foundation to bond and develop conversations at home. Fluent children are bound to be more engaged in family discussions, can express their needs and feelings better, and are more responsive toward communication from their parents and siblings. A better understanding and support system provided by family members at home boosts self-esteem, confidence, and resilience among children.

To sum up, fluency is undeniably critical in shaping the quality of our communication and social interaction with the outside world. It serves as the backbone of effective communication required to convey thoughts and intentions clearly and persuasively. However, it is equally important to recognize that perfect fluency is *NOT ALWAYS ATTAINABLE*. Even the most eloquent speakers may face moments of dysfluencies, days of emotional stress, nervousness or anger, loss of focus, some fatigue, unexpected distractions, and so on. Speech is related to the psychological status of an individual. There are situations that can evoke strong emotions, such as psychological pressure, which can disrupt even the smoothest flow of speech, thereby calling in for hesitations, repetitions, or prolongations in speech. These moments of dysfluency, though negative, do not diminish an individual's overall communicative competence; instead, they highlight something very important. They mark the human aspect of speech, according to which it is normal to be dysfluent in some instances. It is important to understand that speech fluency can ebb and flow depending on the context, content, and emotional state of the speaker. This reminds us that although it is important to strive for fluency, it is vital to be patient and compassionate with ourselves and others when disruptions occur. Accepting and embracing speech dysfluencies can lead to more genuine and empathetic communication.

Who Kills Fluency?

There are various factors that can interrupt the flow of our speech. These factors can cause breaks in the flow of speech, hinder communication, alter listener perceptions, and impact interpersonal interactions. The factors influencing fluency can be psychological, linguistic, physical, environmental, and social. It is important to address these factors to improve communication and elicit a smoother flow of speech. By managing psychological factors like anxiety, enhancing linguistic skills by preparing the message to be spoken, and adapting to environmental and social dynamics, individuals can better manage their speech fluency. This comprehensive approach can enhance fluency, making speech smoother, more effective, and positively impactful for both speakers and listeners.

These factors include:

1. *Psychological Factors*: Anxiety and stress are among the most significant factors that disrupt fluency in children. As anxiety and stress increase, so do the dysfluencies in speech. This could be evident in school performances or social interactions, where performance pressures are common (Eggers et al. 2010). These situations are when children are most likely to show repetitions or frequent pauses during conversation. For example, a child who is nervous about reading aloud in class may stumble over words or speak with more dysfluencies, which is not typical of their usual speech patterns at home. During periods of anxiety and stress, the cognitive load on a child consumes

more mental resources compared to a relaxed mental state, leading to noticeable dysfluencies. Studies by Eggers et al. (2010) have documented that children under stress exhibit higher rates of speech dysfluencies, such as stuttering. This can be particularly evident in school environments.

2. *Linguistic Factors*: Lack of preparation, complexity, and familiarity with topics also influence a child's fluency. When children are asked to talk about a subject they are not well-versed in, they may exhibit more dysfluencies. Children may use filler words like "um," "ah," or "like," or they may pause often as they search for words to express their thoughts. Dysfluencies like repetitions, hesitations, pauses, and so on can occur during debates, oral quizzes, classroom discussions, or when speaking on a new topic. The role of linguistic factors is well-documented in various research studies. Arnold et al. (2007) reported a significant increase in children's fluency when they speak on known or rehearsed linguistic content. It was observed that lack of preparation led to increased use of fillers, repetitions, and hesitations.
3. *Physical Factors*: Physical well-being is undoubtedly important for bodily functions. Speech and language are no different from this. Physical factors significantly affect a child's speech fluency. Physical fatigue can reduce cognitive functioning and slow down a child's speech, thereby increasing errors in their spoken language (O'Shea et al. 2016). Health conditions that affect neurological or muscular control (as seen in cerebral palsy or muscular dystrophy) can impair a child's ability to speak fluently (Ziegler and Ackermann 2013). For the same reason, these children show articulation difficulties with slurred and unclear speech.
4. *Environmental Factors*: The environment can play an indirect yet crucial role in determining speech fluency, especially among children. In environments with poor acoustics or background noise, such as busy classrooms or school playgrounds, children may find it difficult to hear themselves or their peers (Liu et al. 2019). This can lead to frequent repetitions or corrections in speech, thereby reducing overall fluency. Similarly, when visual or auditory distractors are present in a room, a child's train of thought may be affected, leading to reduced fluency. For example, if a child is trying to tell a story in a noisy school canteen with a TV playing and people chatting all around, their speech patterns may become broken and disrupted. A study by Dockrell and Shield (2006) found that auditory distractions in classroom environments can significantly reduce speech intelligibility and fluency, as children struggle to focus on their speech production.
5. *Social Factors*: Every child wants to be socially accepted. Most of the learning in childhood accelerates with constant rewards and encouragement given to the child. Similar to other developments, an audience can greatly influence a child's speech fluency (McCroskey 1977). A child may exhibit fewer dysfluencies with close friends and family members (like a mother or grandparents). However, the dysfluencies may increase with strangers or classmates who may not be close acquaintances. Similarly, a child, when asked to present a project in front of the class, may experience stage fright,

leading to more dysfluencies or disrupted speech, atypical of their usual speaking style. The social setting and perceived judgment can make children overly conscious about their speech, leading to fluency issues.

In conclusion, various factors may influence the fluency of speech, ranging from psychological stress to environmental conditions. Understanding these factors helps support children in different environments, both at school and at home, thereby enhancing their fluency and overall communication skills.

2.5 The Speech Mechanism

The speech mechanism refers to a complex system for producing speech sounds, involving various anatomical structures that work in synchrony. To understand speech production, it is important to explore physical components as well as neurological areas that control these actions.

The process of speech development is undoubtedly remarkable in the course of children's ontogenesis from the point of view of the organization and coordination of anatomical systems. In the process of development, children acquire the ability to regulate and coordinate these systems for speaking. However, this development does not always occur in a sequential, stair-like pattern for every child. Dysfluencies can be frequent, becoming noticeable quite early in childhood during the periods of language development. Such disruptions can interrupt the development, which, in turn, may affect the child's social relationships and self-esteem.

Knowledge of the speech mechanism is helpful not only to speech pathologists but also to parents and teachers, who play a pivotal role in a child's language development. Communication is an essential part of life that influences numerous aspects of a child's experience—from social interactions to academic success. Therefore, it becomes easier for parents and educators to understand whether a child is on track concerning speech development or if he or she is having a developmental disorder that needs to be addressed.

In addition, the knowledge of the speech mechanism enables parents and teachers to encourage the use of proper speaking skills, which further ensures the healthy development of speech and language. It helps provide correct feedback, promote practice in speaking, and, whenever necessary, seek professional advice and treatment. Therefore, knowledge about the biological mechanisms that underlie speech is useful for parents and teachers in helping children become better communicators who are fully capable of effortlessly speaking in well-formed sentences. This knowledge not only helps avoid possible speech dysfluencies but also strengthens the children's ability to communicate effectively with the surrounding environment.

2.6 How Speech Is Produced

When it comes to speech production, the intentional plan or framework for communication is created in the brain. The brain then fires neural signals to the respiratory muscles to initiate breath support. As air is forced out of the lungs, the vocal folds start to vibrate, releasing sound as voice.

This sound is further modulated into different phonemes by the articulatory system, which includes the tongue, jaws, nose, lips, and so on. For instance, to pronounce the letter "p," the lips must come together to momentarily obstruct the air and then release it in a burst. At the same time, the resonatory or nasal system modifies the quality of sound by varying the form and dimensions of the resonators.

The entire process depends on the timely action and integration of many muscles and structures with the help of the neurological system. If there is an improper coordination of any part of this system, possibly due to physical damages, diseases, or disorders affecting the nervous system, speech difficulties such as stuttering may arise. To understand this better, let us elaborate on each of these components in detail:

1. *Respiratory System*: This is called the powerhouse of breath. The lungs and diaphragm, as part of the respiratory system, are the engines that drive speech simply by supplying air pressure. While talking, air is forced out of the lungs, passing through the trachea and reaching the vocal cords. This airflow is necessary since, without it, producing any vocal sound would be impossible. For young children, learning to control this breath determines the loudness of the sounds as well as the steadiness with which these sounds are produced.
2. *Phonatory System*: The key components of the phonatory system are the vocal folds, commonly called vocal cords, which are located in the larynx or voice box. The vocal folds start to vibrate when air from the lungs passes through them. These vibrations determine the pitch and loudness of the voice. Depending on the tension of the cords as well as the distance between the two parts of the cords, the sounds of the voice may change. This system is significant in terms of how children begin to play with various sounds, which is an essential part of learning a language.
3. *Articulatory System*: The articulatory system consists of various parts, such as the tongue, lips, teeth, and the roof of the mouth—that may be the hard or soft palate. This system helps in molding the phonation that is set off by the vocal folds into comprehensible speech sounds and words. Every sound in a word needs the coordinated action of this system, and this totality of movements gradually becomes more precise as children advance in age.
4. *Resonatory System*: This system includes the throat, nasal passages, mouth, and sinus. It acts as a natural loudspeaker and sound quality booster. This alters the quality of sound emitted during speaking and singing, resulting in a more impactful and resonant

voice. Children learning to use this system must emphasize not only the loudness of their voice but also the tone and quality, which further enhances emotional communication.

5. *Neurological System*: The brain controls and coordinates the entire process of speech production by giving signals to all muscles involved in the speech mechanism. This integrated activity involves several brain areas responsible for planning what to say, how to say it, and executing these plans by controlling muscles. This system is crucial in understanding speech delays or difficulties like stuttering in children.

2.7 Disturbances in Speech Mechanism

Interferences in speech fluency and speech disorders (like stammering) occur when there is a disruption in the normal functioning of the speech mechanism. For children, these disruptions can dramatically interfere with the communicative process, decreasing their confidence and interactions. When dysfluencies arise, the normal speech process, which is supposed to occur in a smooth, fast, coordinated, and automatic manner, becomes slow, segmented, disordered, and lacking in smooth transitions. This disruption is not only on the phonological level but also has consequences on the child's psychological health. The social phobia and feelings of shame related to the inability to speak can aggravate the related physical signs, thus contributing to the development of speech impairments.

2.8 Impairments in the Speech Mechanism Include

1. *Respiratory System*: In children, dysfluencies are commonly accompanied by abnormalities in breathing, and since breathing is an important component in the process of speaking, the child may experience some problems in this area as well. For example, a child can breathe rather quickly and superficially or forget to breathe at all when expecting to speak. This creates low air pressure, which is required for producing continuous speech. Hence, they must pause or stop their speech due to the low air pressure. Such breathing abnormalities will force the child to stop breathing at some point or lead to a lack of adequate breath to complete a sentence, thus interrupting fluent speech.
2. *Phonatory System*: The phonatory system, which includes the vocal folds, is responsible for sound generation. During periods of dysfluency, it is possible that there is a pathology in the tension of the vocal cords, causing irregular vibrations. This can lead to a strained or harsh voice or breaks in phonation, where the voice cuts out unexpectedly. These difficulties can cause a child's speech to sound forced and broken, notably differing from the normal, smooth flow.
3. *Articulatory System*: Dysfluencies can also impact the articulatory system, which determines the manner in which sound is produced. Infants might say a part of a word like "ba-ba-ball," instead of "ball," or produce elongation of sounds like "sssssnake."

Indeed, it often includes observable struggle, like tensing the facial muscles when making certain phonemes or pronouncing certain words. Such difficulties are typically associated with dysphonia, which arises when an individual struggles to coordinate the motion of the tongue, lips, or jaw, which is necessary for proper pronunciation.

4. *Resonatory System*: Though the resonatory system is less directly involved, the incoordination and inconsistencies in the functioning of the soft palate and nasal cavity can also be a cause of dysfluencies. For instance, the inability to control the soft palate can cause the patient to develop a nasal voice quality, with either too much or too little nasal resonance. This can further affect speech clarity and contribute to dysfluency.
5. *Neurological System*: The neurological system plays a key role in the management of the whole process of speaking, and thus, dysfluencies may be signs of neurological issues. At times, the brain might provide erratic or mistimed signals to the muscles used in speech. This, in coordination with other factors, can lead to speech blocks, where the child has the thought and knows what to speak but cannot pronounce the desired sounds at that time. This causes various degrees of pauses and breaks in speech.

2.9 Role of Language in Fluency

Language development among children is essential for developing speech fluency. The first stage of cooing and babbling slowly progresses into the stage of forming words, phrases, and, later, sentences. This progression is not just about developing vocabulary; it encompasses adequate mastery of the rules of language usage and syntax, all of which form the foundation of communication. Gradually, children develop new abilities and acquire better cognitive capabilities that allow them to process and express ideas in more dynamic and complex ways.

Nevertheless, the general fluency of speech depends crucially on the environment, the experiences, and the interactions done by the child.

Thus, fluency development in children is an interesting process that presupposes the child's linguistic experience and environmental expansion. As children acquire language and refine their thinking, the ability to express their thoughts improves. For instance, a child who is learning to narrate a story may simply string together a series of events, like "I went to the school. I saw a cat. It meowed." Over time, the process of language acquisition and personal linguistic development progresses to more complex ones as the child grows and obtains skills of language and thought. Now, the same sentence may be produced as "I went to the school and saw a huge fat cat. It was fiercely looking at me, then I threw a ball to chase it away, but the cat meowed loudly chasing after me. Somehow, I saved myself and reached home." This example demonstrates how the child's developing language skills enable him or her to produce longer and more connected narrations, thus illustrating the active and developmental nature of language and its effects on fluency.

2.10 The Demands and Capacities Model

Starkweather (1987) presented the demands and capacities model (DCM), which defines how the child's language development system matches with the demands and capacities of the environment. This model suggests that fluency is optimally obtained whenever the demands made on the child's speech and language are reasonable and within the child's capacity to handle. Starkweather (1987) aimed at observing how children in the process of their growth and development enhance their speech and language skills. At the same time, the pressures from the social environment, school, and the individual goals to successfully convey information tend to increase.

The DCM therefore provides valuable information on the relationship of a child's language abilities with the demands made upon them. This model helps to explain the interplay between a child's growing speech and communication skills with obstacles that can be present in an environment, including expectations from parents and other children, as well as the child's own wish to express himself or herself properly. The relationship of these personal and societal needs with the child's language development is vital in determining the trajectory of the child to achieve fluent speech.

Let us understand this model through a case study of Raj, a young child who moves from India to Britain. In India, Raj's nonnative language, English, was limited to simple words and phrases that he learned in school or picked up as he went along in his day-to-day life. However, when he gets to Britain, the pressure is stepped up, and he is expected to speak and comprehend English fluently. Raj will be expected to learn the other variant of English—British English—and this is not only about using a broader glossary of terms and syntactically more complex phrases but also about learning the subtleties of British culture and colloquialisms. At school, Raj has to deal with the aspects of listening and adhering to directives, engaging in deeper conversations, and using a higher level of language to articulate his ideas. These demands greatly surpass the child's linguistic skills, thus creating a substantial amount of stress. This significant change can lead to situations where the child may pause often, stutter, or use words and phrases over and over because they do not have a better word to use, or they may resort to using very simple language as a way of dealing with challenging situations. These difficulties are observed as a child's attempts to match the child's prior linguistic abilities with the increased linguistic demands of the new school setting.

Consequently, the emergence of fluent speech in children depends on the interplay between the child's language competence and the language demands and requirements that exist in their environment. Capacities are related to a child's language and speech development, which include the ability to comprehend and use language, the ability to produce sounds and words, and construct sentences. These functions enhance over the years as the child interacts with the language. The demands include the social norms and the child's own interactions and perceptions regarding communication. External pressures may consist of the ability to communicate in a given environment, while internal pressures may be the child's desire to convey themselves in a proper manner. When the child's speaking abilities are greater than the challenges they encounter, the child can express himself or herself easily and naturally. In such a situation, the skills they possess are sufficient or even more than enough to tackle the issues encountered, leading to natural fluency. On the other hand, when the task requirements are beyond a child's speech production, then the child may experience some problems. For example, one can demand a child to use compound and complex sentences even when he or she has not yet developed the skill, and this may lead to fluency breakdowns like stammering. This inconsistency can cause the child's speech development to stagnate if they are unable to meet the high standards.

Harmful Effects of Raising Demands Over a Child's Capacities

Based on the above explanation of DCM, it is clear that dysfluencies, which are pauses and other disruptions of speech, appear when the child's communicative load is more than his/her language development allows. These dysfluencies are not just stuttering errors during interaction; they are evidence of the child's attempts at handling the disparity between her or his abilities and the demands of the environment.

This can be clearly observed in the case of Raj shifting from India to Britain, as the expectations of employing elaborated language may challenge a child's communication skills. Sometimes, these pressures may lead to the transformation of some of the common dysfluencies into more chronic ones like stuttering.

This shift from the temporary dysfluencies to stuttering shows the pressure that is put on Raj to speak. It is a disorder that is characterized by the repetition of words, sounds, and syllables and can also involve facial movements that indicate the subject's difficulty, such as grimacing. These characteristics show the child's struggle to coordinate the verbal output with the cognitive and linguistic requirements of the task. The shift from dysfluencies to stuttering takes place when these interruptions do not just remain as brief interludes in speech but are more frequent, severe, and persistent forms of disruptions that greatly interfere with the speaker's communication. This can be seen as a problem of fluency in speech development and shows that there is no surefire way of managing capacities and demands in this regard.

In the case of Raj, a child who was overwhelmed by high linguistic expectations, the stress and anxiety that come with speaking may entrench the child's stuttering. It is likely that Raj may begin to anticipate that he will have problems with some words or conditions, and hence, the anxiety and carrying out avoidance behaviors as well may lead to a higher level of effect on his confidence and willingness to communicate. In such cases, the dysfluencies that become chronic and transform into stuttering are not just a manifestation of a child's inability to speak without glitches but are very much linked to the social context they find themselves in.

Therefore, the case of the emergence of stuttering from dysfluencies in children is a perfect example of the capabilities of DCM. However, this equilibrium is not fixed and has to be constantly renegotiated based on the child's language progress and the environment's challenges. It is important for practitioners, teachers, parents, and everyone around the child to understand these dynamics in order to facilitate children's communication competence and self-esteem.

2.11 Normal Dysfluencies

Language development in children is a dynamic process that is accompanied by fast learning and skill building as well as by certain deviations that are considered to be normal. These dysfluencies are normative and are observable in the child's language development and may manifest when children attempt to use language in new and complex ways. Knowing these dysfluencies will aid parents, teachers, and clinicians in knowing the difference between children's normal language development and those with language impairments such as stuttering.

2.12 The Nature of Normal Dysfluencies

Normal dysfluencies are interruptions in the child's speech, which are common and expected as the child is learning how to speak. These dysfluencies are often manifested as hesitations, repetitions, and revisions, which are quite common when a person is learning how to communicate effectively using language and speech. They are typical for children while they practice new words, phrases, and more intricate structures of speech.

2.13 Developmental Progression of Dysfluencies

Stuttering and other dysfluencies are usually observed during the significant linguistic growth, which typically includes the ages of 2–5 years old. At this stage, the frequency and types of dysfluencies may be quite diverse and depend on the child's age, level of stress, excitement, or even fatigue.

1. *Early Stage*: In toddlers and preschoolers, the normal dysfluencies are most readily observable. As children's vocabulary and sentence structures grow more complex, they may temporarily exhibit increased dysfluencies. These disruptions are not entirely new and are partly because of the cognitive load or mental effort that goes into choosing the right words and constructing proper sentences. When children start to join words into phrases, the use of repetition and pausing is observed as they try to sort and search through their rapidly expanding vocabulary.

2. *Peak Dysfluency*: Around 2.5–3.5 years old, children begin to use more complex and longer sentences, which leads to a rise in the rate of dysfluencies. This is quite typical and can be explained by the child's efforts to acquire the rules of the language.
3. *Decline in Dysfluencies*: By the time children reach school age (around 5–12 years old), they usually acquire a more fluent and precise mode of speech. It does not completely cease, but the instances and types of dysfluencies gradually reduce and begin to resemble those of typical adult speech. However, sometimes when faced with new challenges such as the introduction of formal education, reading, and writing, dysfluencies may temporarily increase as children adapt to advanced use of language.

2.14 Causes and Contributing Factors for Normal Dysfluencies

Let us understand the possible reasons that may lead to normal dysfluencies and factors that may exacerbate the condition.

1. *Cognitive Development*: With the development of children's brains, they get new cognitive abilities that affect their language. It should be stated that the incorporation of new words and structures in spoken discourse may result in a temporary growth of dysfluencies.
2. *Social Interaction*: While peers and adults are good at providing an opportunity to practice communication skills, there is an inherent societal pressure that may lead to more dysfluencies. Children usually deal with the pressure by using various fillers or rephrasing what they want to say.
3. *Emotional Factors*: Feelings like excitement, anxiety, or shyness may influence a person's ability to articulate their thoughts Craig et al. (2003). For instance, it could be noted that a child is more likely to speak more fluently when in a relaxed state than when in a state of anxiety.
4. *Language Development Stages*: As discussed above, in some phases of language development, it is quite normal for children to have an increase in their normal dysfluencies. For instance, as children move from saying one word to two and then to sentences, their speech cannot always be smooth. This is a normal process of language development where the need for the production of certain aspects of the language temporarily outstrips the child's capacities.
5. *Attention and focus*: Another factor that can influence the child's ability to speak without dysfluencies is the child's capacity to sustain attention. The above-listed factors are likely to result in higher rates of dysfluencies, including factors such as distractions, lack of interest, or divided attention. The results of this research also indicate that when children are fully engaged or are in a concentrative state, their speech seems to have a fluidity that is absent in other conditions where they are not fully focused.
6. *Rapid Speech Development*: At those moments when children learn new words and communicate actively, their brains work intensively and must process a lot of information. At times, it may result in overloading the speech production system, hence

causing dysfluencies. Due to the inability of children to properly express themselves or even when they are thinking at a fast rate, they can have dysfluencies in their speech.

7. *Genetic and Hereditary Factors*: Some studies show that genetic factors may be involved in some way in the dysfluencies of speech. Therefore, children who have other family members with a history of stuttering or any other speech problems are likely to have the same problem. However, genetics is not the sole factor that determines a person's ability to speak fluently. It can be a factor that influences it in combination with other factors.
8. *Environmental influences*: It is possible to analyze the effect of the surrounding environment on communication in children. Positive approaches toward the speakers have been shown to reduce dysfluencies, while negative pressures may lead to an increase in dysfluencies. The behavior of parents and caregivers toward a child's attempts to speak can either build their confidence and fluency or break it.

Knowing all these factors will help us to be able to assist children as they navigate through their stuttering, knowing that it is a normal part of their development. Hence, reducing the effects of these factors helps to create a comfortable environment, enabling the child to speak more fluently and with confidence.

2.15 Normal Nonfluency

Normal nonfluency is defined as the breaks in the flow of speech that are characteristic of most children as they develop speech and language. These dysfluencies are typical for the child's language development and do not usually continue or hinder the child's ability to communicate. The concept of "normal nonfluency" is like normal dysfluencies but emphasizes more on the acceptability and typicality of the speech irregularities in everyday communication. It is defined by the presence of dysfluencies that do not significantly hinder communication and are commonly observed in the speech of most children and even adults.

2.16 Characteristics of Normal Nonfluency

1. *Frequency and type*: Normal nonfluencies are typical and include hesitations, repetitions, and revisions as discussed earlier. They are usually short and not very severe; they do not cause the listener or the speaker much concern.
2. *Impact on communication*: Normal nonfluencies are, therefore, different from the ones that occur because of stuttering or any other form of speech disorder as they do not have a negative impact on the communication process to a great extent. This usually means that the listeners have no problems in comprehending the speaker, and the speaker's message is conveyed fluently.

3. *Lack of awareness and concern*: Normally, children who have nonfluencies do not even realize that they have such problems with their speech. They seem to have no concern, frustration, or even embarrassment as to how they speak.
4. *Natural resolution*: It is usually advised that normal nonfluencies are self-limiting and will reduce as the child's language develops and he or she gets more exposure to different contexts of spoken language.

2.17 Features of Normal Nonfluencies

1. *Repetitions*: This is the most frequent type of stuttering in children, which is the repetition of syllables, words, or phrases, like *ba-ba-ball*, *can I can I go*, and *I want I want cookie*. These repetitions generally take place because the child's language planning skills are not yet fully developed.
2. *Hesitations and pauses*: Sometimes, children stop words in the middle of their conversation while they try to find the right word or how to say something. These pauses may be filled with filler words such as "uh" or "um."
3. *Revisions*: It is common for a child to start a sentence and then decide to say something else in the middle of the sentence. This results in the correction and editing, which is a good sign of the development of thinking and statement organization.
4. *Interjections*: The use of filler words like "um," "uh," "like," and "you know," which give children extra time to think.
5. *Whole word repetitions*: Incomplete words or whole words being said once or twice, for example, "Can can I go outside?"
6. *Phrase repetitions*: Repeating multi-word phrases, commonly used to extend time to formulate thoughts.

Nonfluencies are a part of the normal speech and language development that is characterized by minor dysfluencies that do not hinder communication. It is vital to be able to identify these patterns as part of the normal language development to foster children's communication development and to be able to decide when it might be appropriate to seek help for the child.

In the sphere of language acquisition, normal nonfluency is of paramount importance. There are certain stages in the development of the child's speech when they may use more incorrect or strange words and sentences. These are usually minor errors and tend to reduce as children and young people gain more confidence in their language skills. At this stage, parents and teachers should ensure that they create free practice conditions for a child without putting pressure on him/her.

Understanding what is considered normal nonfluency also enables one to differentiate the same from stuttering or other fluency disorders, given that the latter involves more frequent and severe disruptions that interfere with communication. It is essential to notice the distinctions after which many a time a speech-language pathologist's help is needed.

In this case, educators and parents need to be aware of normal nonfluency, to be able to effectively support the child's development. It enables educators to cope with parents' concerns, use appropriate communication techniques in the classroom, and determine when the speech-language pathologist should be consulted.

2.18 "Dys"-Fluencies Versus "Dis"-Fluencies

The terms "dysfluency" and "disfluencies" are connected to the ways of speech production but are utilized to denote certain peculiarities of speech disturbances.

Dysfluency: The term "dysfluency" can be defined in a very general sense as any kind of disruption or deviation from the normal flow of speech. It is commonly employed in a clinical setting to explain a speech that deviates from the fluent, smooth, and uninterrupted delivery of speech. It is mainly linked to stuttering, which entails the repetition of sounds, syllables, or words and the prolongation of sounds or the occurrence of stoppages (blocks). It encompasses two components: both the observable speech behaviors and the underlying cognitive, emotional, and neurological factors that contribute to these patterns.

Dysfluency refers to a situation where such hesitations and repetitions are part of the normal pattern of an individual's speech. This term stresses the ongoing nature of such speech and frequently indicates the requirement for assessment by speech-language pathologists. It considers speech production as a multifaceted process that entails cognitive, neurological, and motor mechanisms.

Disfluencies: On the other hand, disfluencies are specific types of speech deviations that are also evident in both typical and atypical speech patterns. Some of the features include hesitations, revisions, and filler words, such as "um," "uh," "you know," and other variations that people use in everyday speech. Disfluencies are normal phenomena in spoken language that occur when the speaker is planning what to say next, experiencing uncertainty, or needing to correct or revise spoken content on the whole.

In daily use, these disfluencies are generally not very severe and thus do not greatly affect the speaking process. They can also function as a communicative aid, for instance, to allow the speaker to ponder on his or her next statement, to stress on a certain issue, or to express doubt. But in the case of speech disorders such as stuttering, disfluencies are seen more often and are more severe and affect communication more.

2.19 Comparison and Clinical Relevance

While both terms describe the disruption of speech, "dysfluency" is a more general and more chronic term, which is associated with a specific speech disorder. "Disfluencies," at the same time, denote single episodes of speech disruption that are a normal part of speech and the communication process that may become a symptom of a speech disorder depending on the frequency, type, and impact they have on communication.

This is a very important distinction for speech-language pathologists when diagnosing and treating speech disorders. It helps differentiate between typical speech variations and those with a speech pathology. For educators and parents, this knowledge assists in recognizing when a child might benefit from further evaluation or intervention to address potential speech issues.

To summarize, both dysfluency and disfluencies relate to the idea of a pause in speech, though they focus on different aspects of it, dysfluency as a type of disorder and disfluencies as specific instances of that condition or as part of normal speech variability. This distinction between the two is crucial in the assessment and management of the child's communication.

2.20 Facing Reality: Is My Child Stuttering?

To many parents, the development of a child's speech and any dysfluencies that come with it are a source of worry. A frequent concern is if such interruptions are natural for children of a certain age or if they may point at stuttering—a speech issue that calls for the help of a professional. Therefore, to distinguish between children's normal nonfluency and stuttering, one must pay attention to the certain patterns and characteristics of their speech. Such differences help the parents determine if their child needs to see a speech-language pathologist. The following are some key points that can help distinguish stuttering from normal speech dysfluencies:

1. *Multiple Repetitions*

   In normal nonfluency, between the ages of 18 months to 7 years, children are likely to experience phases of stuttering as they learn to speak. During this stage, children may present features such as repeating sounds, syllables, and words primarily at the beginning of the sentence. These usually occur about once in every ten sentences.

   At 3 years of age and beyond, children with normal nonfluency are less likely to stutter or stumble over single sounds or syllables but instead begin to substitute entire words or phrases (*I-I-I can't,* or *I want, I want, I want to go*). They also often use fillers like "uh" or "um" and sometimes may also shift from one topic to another, revising and leaving sentences unfinished.

   Normal children can have dysfluencies at any time but are likely to increase their dysfluencies when they are tired, excited, or upset or if someone is rushing them to speak. These types of children may also be more dysfluent when they ask questions or are being questioned.

   On the other hand, *children with stuttering* may develop stuttering at any time between 18 months and 7 years, although the most common time is between 3 and 5 years, when the child's language development is rapid. In some children, stuttering first appears even under conditions of normal stress, such as when a new sibling is born or when the family moves to a new home, and so on.

Children who stutter may make the same sound, syllable, and word repetitions as children with normal dysfluencies, but the children who stutter tend to repeat more frequently and more intensively than those with typical dysfluencies Carlson (2013). For example, instead of one or two repetitions of a syllable, they may repeat it four or five times, as in "di-di-di-did I do that?"

They may also sometimes prolong the stressed syllable or the whole word, as in "MMMMMMMommy, it's mmmmmy ball." Further, children with mild stuttering may demonstrate signs of awareness of their stuttering.

2. *Use of Schwa Vowel*

   Sometimes, the child may use a schwa vowel or "uh" in between the repetitions as in "b-uh-b-uh-ball." This insertion can be a strategy for disentangling oneself from a block or stutter. The schwa insertion is not typically seen in normal nonfluency and can indicate more profound speech planning and production difficulties. *For example,* when a child is struggling to say "basketball" he or she may attempt to say, "b-uh-b-uh-basketball." The use of the schwa sound "uh" is not usual in instances of typical speech dysfluencies. This is usually done to help the affected individual bypass the stuttering moment, indicating more significant speech planning and execution challenges.

3. *Awareness of Problem and Physical Signs of Struggle*

   Typically, children with normal nonfluency may not have any idea of the pauses and do not show any signs of discomfort or frustration toward the dysfluencies. Instead, the parents' reactions to normal dysfluencies are more kind as compared to that of the stuttering children.

   On the other hand, a child with stuttering may feel a little shy or upset with his/her dysfluencies, though this too will not be a deep concern. Children in this stage of the disorder may even ask their parents questions as to why they cannot speak fluently. It is for this reason that children who stutter may display some physical signs of struggle when they speak. These could be facial grimacing, eye blinking, tension in the jaw, or head movement. All these behaviors imply that it is hard to regulate the muscles for speech in a smooth way and are not typical of most children's normal speech errors.

   For example, when the child is discussing a favorite movie, their face becomes tense, they blink a lot, and their head moves slightly. These are the physical indications of the struggle to produce sounds that would help in communication. In normal speech development, there are no such visible signs of struggle that can be pointed out, and this is why it is a clear indicator that the child might be dealing with stuttering.

4. *Blocks*

   Speech blocks are instances where the child seems to be unable to produce any sound for a certain period, which could be in seconds. Within a block, the child may open his or her mouth to speak, but no sound will come out, signifying a more profound disruption of the flow of speech.

   Stuttering is usually characterized by blocks, and such blocks are not typical of the normal development of speech. For example, during a discussion of the child's school day, the child may freeze in the middle of a sentence, his or her mouth open but saying nothing for a few seconds. These are those phases where the child seems to be stuck and does not make any sound at all, which can be somewhat alarming. While other types of pauses are smooth and brief, these blocks are characterized by a clear break in speech.

5. *Avoidance Behaviors*

   Drawing from the earlier discussion, children with stuttering may consequently avoid certain situations or use strategies to deal with their speaking dysfluency. They may avoid certain words or sounds that they find challenging, or they may become hesitant to speak in certain situations that bring out their stutter. These types of behaviors may influence their social relations and are not often prevalent in normal nonfluency.

   For example, during the class reading activity, the child may consistently attempt to avoid reading. Probably, when it is their turn, they may read very few words or use short sentences that they believe are easier to read. Rarely using words or avoiding being in situations where one must speak is a result of the fear of stuttering. It is a coping strategy related to the prospect of stammering rather than a characteristic feature of children who exhibit normal nonfluency.

6. *Consistency and Frequency*

   Stuttering is consistent and frequent, thus impacting a large part of the speech of the child. On the other hand, normal nonfluency is characterized by occasional stuttering, and the child's fluency improves with age due to language development. Persistent speech patterns that do not change or even get worse might be a sign of stuttering.

   It may also be observed that normal nonfluency becomes frequent for several days or weeks and then may become almost imperceptible for some time and then may return again. For example, for a few weeks, a parent realizes that the child has repeated the same sounds or words while speaking to parents, friends, teachers, or when answering questions at school. The persistence and regular occurrence of stuttering traits, regardless of the situation, suggest an ongoing issue rather than occasional developmental dysfluencies, which tend to decrease as language skills improve.

2.21 Warning Signs of Stuttering

It is crucial to differentiate between normal childhood disorders, which are part of a child's development, and more concerning behaviors that may suggest stuttering. Recognizing the early signs of stuttering is crucial for timely intervention, which can significantly ease the pathway to smoother communication. The following are signs that, if recognized in time, can assist in identifying stuttering and therefore do an early intervention if needed.

1. *Family and genetic factors*: As for hereditary components if someone in the family has stuttering, there is a higher chance for the child to inherit it. It is recommended to pay attention to the child's speech if there is a family history of stuttering as it is genetic.
2. *Age of onset*: Stuttering generally has an onset in childhood, especially between 2 and 5 years, a time when children are learning language. It is very important to pay

attention to stuttering that begins or continues at this age or even after it and may require a referral.

3. *Duration since onset*: While many children go through phases of stuttering during early speech development, persistent stuttering lasting more than 6 months might indicate a more prevailing form of stuttering. Thus, the duration of such speech disruptions is important in determining whether these are temporary and just a part of a child's development or if they may be a persistent dysfluency.
4. *Gender differences*: Boys are the most affected compared to girls, and this makes boys two or three times more vulnerable to developing a stuttering disorder. This disparity highlights the need for parents and teachers to be more concerned with the speech development of boys while still ensuring girls who stutter are given adequate care.
5. *Speech production and clarity*: Some of the risk factors that may increase a child's likelihood of developing stuttering include difficulties in the articulation of words or having speech that is not easy to comprehend. These difficulties should not be overlooked, especially when they are accompanied by stuttering signs. The earlier the child is referred to, the better.
6. *Language development*: A child's language complexity can influence stuttering. Children who can construct compound sentences are likely to stutter more as they try to put into words their more elaborate ideas. Likewise, children with delayed speech might stutter due to the extra effort needed to communicate.
7. *Behavioral and emotional responses*: Children's feelings and behaviors when speaking can help to understand the influence stuttering has on the child Gagnon & Ladouceur (1992). A child's signs of frustration or avoidance of speaking situations are evidence of their difficulties in speaking, thus necessitating the need for intervention.
8. *Environmental factors*: There are several factors that have been identified to influence the occurrence and persistence of stuttering, and one of these is the environment. Certain contexts that can be stressful, like high parental expectations or negative peer interaction, can worsen the condition. Establishing favorable and tolerant conditions for communication at home and at school is also vital.

References

Arnold HS, Conture EG, Ohde RN. Phonological neighborhood density in the picture naming of young children who stutter: preliminary study. J Fluen Disord. 2007;32(1):31–42.

Carlson NR. Physiology of behavior. 11th ed. Boston: Pearson; 2013.

Craig A, Hancock K, Tran Y, Craig M. Anxiety levels in children and adolescents who stutter. J Speech Lang Hear Res. 2003;46(5):1197–206.

Dockrell JE, Shield BM. Acoustical barriers in classrooms: the impact of noise on performance in the classroom. Br Educ Res J. 2006;32(3):509–25.

Eggers K, Van Eerdenbrugh S, Van den Bergh BRH. Temperament dimensions in stuttering and typically developing children. J Fluen Disord. 2010;35(4):355–372.

Fillmore CJ. On fluency. In: Fillmore CJ, Kempler D, Wang WS-Y, editors. Individual differences in language ability and language behavior. New York: Academic Press; 1979. p. 85–101.

Gagnon M, Ladouceur R. Behavioral treatment of child stutterers: replication and extension. Behav Ther. 1992;23(1):113–29.

Lennon P. Investigating fluency in EFL: a quantitative approach. Lang Learn. 1990;40(3):387–417.

Lev-Ari S, Keysar B. Why don't we believe non-native speakers? The influence of accent on credibility. J Exp Soc Psychol. 2010;46(6):1093–6.

Liu C, Chen C, Luo Y, Huang H. The effect of transcranial direct current stimulation on stuttering: a systematic review. J Fluen Disord. 2019;60:1–12.

McCroskey JC. Oral communication apprehension: a summary of recent theory and research. Hum Commun Res. 1977;4(1):78–96.

O'Shea G, De Wit L, Szymkowicz SM, McLaren ME, Talty R, Dotson VM. Effects of transcranial direct current stimulation on cognition and mood in older adults: a systematic review and meta-analysis. Neuropsychol Rev. 2016;26(3):216–28.

Ratner NB. Linguistic behaviors at the onset of stuttering. In: Hulstijn W, Peters HFM, van Lieshout PHHM, editors. Speech production: motor control, brain research, and fluency disorders. Amsterdam: Elsevier; 1997. p. 585–94.

Starkweather CW. Fluency and stuttering. Prentice Hall. 1987.

Ziegler W, Ackermann H. Neurological aspects of dysfluency. In: Howell P, Van Borsel J, editors. Multilingual aspects of fluency disorders. Bristol: Multilingual Matters; 2013. p. 23–56.

Insights to Stuttering

3

Abstract

The chapter explores the nature, causes, and development of stuttering. It covers definitions, stages of stuttering in children, and behaviors associated with the disorder. This chapter discusses various stages of stuttering along with their specific characteristics. It emphasizes the emotional and psychological impacts of stuttering through models like Sheehan's Iceberg Analogy and the ICF framework. Finally, the chapter sheds light on living with stuttering and highlights the struggles a stutterer faces in every domain of life. It also examines the variability of stuttering across different situations, people, contexts, languages, and so on. Furthermore, the chapter explores the role of various professionals in supporting individuals who stutter and improving the quality of life for children with stuttering. It concludes by discussing stuttering and its status in India.

Keywords

Development of stuttering · ICF framework · Variability effect · Core behaviors · Secondaries

3.1 Unfolding Stuttering

Stuttering, or stammering, is a fluency disorder defined clinically as dysfluent speech and is a problem that occurs in people worldwide. Stuttering is a disorder that is characterized by involuntary repetitions and prolongations of sounds, syllables, words, phrases, involuntary silent pauses, or blocks which affect the fluency of speech and can greatly affect overall communication and quality of life (National Institute on Deafness and Other Communication Disorders 2010).

R. Kaur, *Navigating Childhood Stuttering*,
https://doi.org/10.1007/978-981-96-6206-7_3

The American Speech-Language-Hearing Association (ASHA) defines stuttering as a fluency disorder that entails disruptions in the production of speech sounds, also referred to as dysfluencies. It could be the repetition of sounds or parts of sounds, the prolongation of sounds, or entire silences of sounds and syllables. ASHA also pointed out that stuttering includes affective aspects such as anxiety and feelings of discomfort when speaking. Stuttering is accompanied by fear of speaking, leading to avoidance of certain words or social situations, such as speaking on the telephone, which may exacerbate their stuttering.

The World Health Organization (WHO) in the International Classification of Diseases, 10th revision (ICD-10), groups stuttering under "childhood onset fluency disorder," pointing out that the condition usually begins in childhood during speech and language development (WHO 1992). According to Wingate (1964), stuttering is defined as a disorder in speech where there are unwanted, audible or silent, repetitions or prolongations of any part of speech, including sounds, syllables, and words with one syllable. These disturbances are usually frequent or rather prominent and are generally not easily regulated by the speaker. According to Wingate, stuttering is a complex of symptoms that result in disruptions of fluency in the patient's speech, which are involuntary and recurrent, including prolongation of phonemes and repetitions of syllables and sounds.

Bloodstein and Ratner (2008) defined stuttering as a dynamic process of speech production that is characterized by involuntariness in the form of repetitions, prolongations, and blocks which hinder the continuity of speech fluency. Such disruptions may differ in the level of severity and the rate of occurrence, which is why the process of stuttering is considered multifaceted.

According to Guitar (2013), stuttering can be described as an evident and involuntary abnormality in the rhythm and pattern of speech, which may include physical pressure and hesitation. He stresses that stuttering is not just a speech disorder but also affects the psychosocial and emotional aspects of communication.

Yairi and Seery (2015), in their research on stuttering, described it as a type of speech disorder characterized by involuntary repetitions or prolongations of sounds, syllables, or words with involuntary blocks or pauses that occur in an individual's speech and prevent him or her from speaking fluently. These disturbances can be observed mainly in speech output and are influenced by different linguistic, cognitive, and emotional levels.

Tichenor and Yaruss (2019) elaborated more on the perception of stuttering by the people who go through it. They defined stuttering as a "phenomenon of experience" which comprises not only the overt speech dysfluencies but also the covert phenomena which are not perceptible to the audience. These experiences are often characterized by anticipatory anxiety about stuttering on specific words and the sensation of losing control over speech.

Carlson (2013) also offers a discussion on the biological factors as well as the behavioral factors that are involved in the development of stuttering in individuals. His work shows that stuttering is a multifaceted phenomenon determined by the interconnection of neurogenic factors, environmental conditions, and the subject's behaviors, thus pointing out the necessity of integrated treatment strategies.

In conclusion, stuttering is a type of communication disorder that is defined as an involuntary disruption in the flow of speech. These disruptions can be in the form of repetitions of sounds, syllables, or words, and prolongations of sounds, or even no output at all which is known as a block. Dysfluencies of this nature can greatly affect the normal flow of communication of an individual.

3.2 Causes of Stuttering

Stuttering is one of the most intriguing disorders in the field of speech disorders, with its causes and management still under extensive study. The disorder is not only restricted to physical manifestations but also by the emotional and psychological aspects. It is often seen that people who stutter tend to be very fearful of speaking out, which consecutively amplifies their stuttering problem. This anxiety often results in the development of avoidance behaviors, whereby people may avoid particular words, other individuals, or speaking situations such as telephoning or speaking in front of other people. Specific causes of stuttering are:

1. *Genetic Factors*: Several research studies have suggested that stuttering is genetic in nature. Research has pointed out certain genetic factors that are associated with the development of stuttering. For instance, there are some genes that relate to the metabolism of cells and neural function, and their alteration is linked with stuttering. Smith and Weber (2017a) pointed out that N-acetylglucosamine-1- phosphate transferase subunits alpha and beta (GNPTAB) is one of the genes in which mutations can be associated with stuttering, thus underlining genetic factors. These genetic predispositions suggest that stuttering can run in families and is not merely a result of environmental factors or learned behaviors.
2. *Neurophysiological Factors*: Recent developments in the field of neuroimaging have shown that there are differences in the brains of people who have a fluency disorder and those who do not. These differences are seen mainly in the areas of the brain that are primarily for speech production, such as the motor cortex and Broca's area. Abnormalities in brain circuits that coordinate speech timing and speech processing could, therefore, be attributed to neurophysiological dysregulation in patients with stuttering. Some of the functional magnetic resonance imaging (fMRI) studies indicate that persons with stutter may have alterations in the connectivity of the speech and motor-related areas of the brain (Chang et al. 2008).
3. *The Role of Neurotransmitters*: Dopamine, a chemical that is responsible for controlling movement and speech, has been associated with stuttering. It is hypothesized that people who stutter might be experiencing asymmetry in the dopamine system, which in turn impacts their speech. It was discovered that the use of drugs that affect the level of dopamine in the brain can cause the symptoms of stuttering, therefore implicating the neurotransmitter dopamine in the occurrence of stuttering. Clinical trials have

demonstrated that medications affecting dopamine levels can modify stuttering symptoms, highlighting the role of neurotransmitters in stuttering (Alm 2021).

4. *Environmental and Developmental Influences*: Environmental factors also play a role in the onset and development of stuttering. Factors such as stress, family, and school may affect the intensity and duration of the stuttering. Biological factors including anxiety and self-esteem are intricately connected to stuttering which may worsen the situation. Research has indicated that stuttering among children is likely to be aggravated in stressful conditions or in unfavorable educational settings (Iverach et al. 2011).
5. *Emotional and Psychological Factors*: Stuttering is greatly affected by the emotional and psychological aspects of the individual. Due to the child's heightened awareness of their speech problems, they may get frustrated and embarrassed, which in turn worsens the situation. Thus, emotions regarding stuttering may lead to a cycle where the fear of speaking results in stuttering, and stuttering intensifies the fear. Some findings revealed that children who stutter have a heightened level of emotional reactivity and sensitivity, indicating that emotional regulation plays a role in the disorder (National Institute on Deafness and Other Communication Disorders 2010).
6. *Speech Motor Control*: Speech motor control problems may involve the inability to control the muscles and movements of the body responsible for speech production as controlled by the brain's motor system. Some children have motor speech control problems and may have fast language development, which may present more pressure on their developing nervous system. Also, children who stutter may have other developmental issues, including attention deficit hyperactivity disorder (ADHD) or language difficulties that may complicate the child's stuttering in numerous ways (American Speech-Language-Hearing Association 2020).

3.3 Development of Stuttering in Children

Stuttering is not a simple process and is often characterized by specific phases during its development. All phases are different from one another. Let us understand the development of stuttering to provide parents and educators with a comprehensive understanding of how stuttering evolves in children based on current research and clinical observations.

3.3.1 Normal Dysfluency

In the initial years of childhood, it is quite typical for children to have normal dysfluencies while speaking. Such speech disorders are normal and part of the child's developmental stages and do not present a cause for alarm. Some of the normal dysfluencies are whole word repetitions (example: *I-I want that*), interjections (example: *um, uh*), and phrase repetitions (example: *Can I can I go?*). These are seen in fewer than one in every ten words that are spoken and are characterized by fluent and easy flowing repetitions that are not associated with any strain.

At this stage, children may repeat syllables or words several times, but the repetitions are even and do not sound forced. There is no evident attempt, and the child does not appear to be aware of these dysfluencies. For instance, a child may stammer and say, "I-I-I want the ball," with normal, regular, and easily tuned speech. In many cases, such dysfluencies may be seen in children who may be overexcited, may be sleepy, or may be in a state of ideational dysphoria. Ideational dysphoria refers to a state where the child is dissatisfied with spoken messages and wants to speak perfectly. Here, children may repeat words till they get things right, as per their own ideas. Such dysfluencies are mostly harmless and do not require any treatment since they tend to get resolved on their own.

3.3.2 Borderline Stuttering

As children go on to develop their speech and language more, some may display some possible symptoms of stuttering. This stage consists of the speakers producing more than 10% dysfluencies in their speech. The types of dysfluencies at this stage include part-word repetitions (e.g., *b-b-banana*) and single-syllable whole word repetitions (e.g., *I I I want*).

Such children in the borderline stuttering stage may repeat sounds or syllables more than twice, but they do not talk with much tension. For instance, a child may use the word "go" many times as in "Can we go go go to the park?" But it is said without strain or effort. These children may not be conscious of their dysfluencies, and their reactions are typically mild, if they notice them at all. These children need to be followed up to see if the dysfluencies continue and/or if they worsen.

3.3.3 Beginning Stuttering

As stuttering moves to the next level, known as the beginning stuttering stage, even more noticeable changes are seen in the child. This stage is characterized by the heightened tension and pressure visible in the speaker's hurried speech, prolongations, and blocks. It may become fast and uncoordinated, and the child may present physical indicators of stress such as frowning or having problems saying certain words.

For example, a child in this stage might say, "I w-w-w-want to go home," with tension and effort. They usually occur when the child is trying to express a difficult or long word, and the child may increase the rate of speech, the loudness, or use eye blinking or head shaking to attempt to stop stuttering. Stuttering becomes more noticeable, and children may begin to become self-conscious and may even complain about their speech impediment. It is at this stage that the child should be taken for early intervention to avoid worsening and further development of the stuttering.

3.3.4 Intermediate Stuttering

This type of stuttering is the next level of the disorder, in which children demonstrate a great deal of avoidance behaviors and negative feelings. Besides the dysfluencies that are observed in the initial stage of stuttering, children at this level begin to avoid speaking situations or specific words that they expect would lead to stuttering. Strategies that can be used to convey avoidance include using fillers, changing words, or staying silent.

For example, a child may not want to say their name because it makes them stutter, or the child may opt to use simpler words instead of complex words. This stage is also characterized by more fear and anxiety about speaking. The child could begin to feel that they are shameful and that they have failed, which is likely to affect their self-esteem. Physical cues, including the frequency of blocks and observable difficulty, are more noticeable, and the child's total communication is affected.

3.3.5 Advanced Stuttering

Advanced stuttering is mainly noticed in adolescents and adults, but it can occur at any age. This level is characterized by well-entrenched speech patterns as well as other effects that are emotional and psychological. Severely affected children and adolescents with advanced stuttering have severe blocking, prolonged repetitions, and a lot of avoidant behaviors. They struggle physically when they speak and their speaking is filled with tension; thus, communication is not easy and may be painful for them.

By this stage, most people have a well-defined perception of themselves as stutterers, which in turn leads to severe anxiety, isolation, and low levels of involvement in different activities. The effect on self-esteem and social life may be significant, and severe stuttering may be treated by combination methods that include both the classroom and counselling. Interventions may involve speech therapy, cognitive behavioral therapy, and support groups to assist people with management of the condition and enhancement of their quality of life.

3.4 Characteristics of Stuttering

It is important for educators, speech-language therapists, and parents to understand the characteristics of stuttering to be in a position to support children who have this speech difficulty. Stuttering in children, for instance, is accompanied by core behaviors, secondary behaviors, and emotional features which make the disorder more complicated.

3.4.1 Core Behaviors of Stuttering

Stuttering is accompanied by several types of speech dysfluencies, which may alter the process of communication and interaction in the society. Let us review the types of stuttering dysfluencies in detail to improve the understanding of the phenomenon and its effects, especially on children.

3.4.1.1 Types of Stuttering Dysfluencies

1. *Repetitions*

Repetitions are the easiest to recognize as a form of stuttering where sounds, syllables, and/or words are spoken more than once in a natural speech routine. This may involve the repetition of single phones, such as *k-k-kite*; syllables, such as *ba-ba-ba-ball;* or words, such as *and-and-and*. This creates an effect of broken speech, and the speaker may end up feeling frustrated and or even uncomfortable.

Example: A child attempting to say "basketball" might stutter as *ba-ba- basketball.*

2. *Prolongations*

Prolongations are the process of lengthening a sound within a word for a much longer time than would usually be expected. This type of dysfluency is characterized by the fact that the vocal tract is open; however, the sound production is slow, and the speech becomes drawn out and tense.

Example: To attempt to say the word "slide," a child might lengthen the first sound: *ssssslide.*

3. *Blocks*

The blocks are defined by their inability to make sound for a specific amount of time. These are a total arrest of the verbal narrative where the person knows exactly what he or she wishes to say, but the words simply get stuck in the speech muscles.

Example: A child might struggle to start the word "please," resulting in a noticeable pause before the word is spoken.

4. *Interjections*

Interjections are sounds or words that are uttered in the middle of a speech to create a pause or to postpone it in some way. Some of the generally used interjections include filler words like "um," "uh," "like," and "you know."

Example: "I um need to go uh to the store."

5. *Avoidance Behaviors*

Those who stutter often develop ways to avoid situations and words that trigger the stutter. Due to this, they may use other terms that are related to the intended word or use long descriptions to avoid using a particular word that would make them stutter.

Example: A child might use "dad's car" instead of "automobile" if they tend to stutter on the latter word.

6. *Circumlocutions*

Circumlocutions are when one tries to explain or define a word instead of using the actual word. This happens due to the fear of stuttering. This can result in the formation of complex sentences that present the message in a roundabout way.

Example: Instead of saying "refrigerator," a child might say "the thing where we keep our food cold."

3.4.1.2 Physical Characteristics Associated with Stuttering Dysfluencies

- Muscle Tension: Sometimes, alongside block, there is an increased muscle activity or tension in the muscles used in speech production, specifically in the vocal folds.
- Disrupted Breathing Patterns: People who stutter may also have some problems with their breathing, which includes interrupted exhalation or difficulty switching to inhalation during speaking.
- Articulatory Dysfunctions: The areas that assist in controlling the flow of speech involve the correct positioning of certain structures like the lips, jaw, and tongue, but the timing of these structures' movement is faulty in stutterers.
- Low-Frequency Tremors: Some adults who stutter exhibit tremors in the muscles of the neck, jaw, and lips, which are not typically present in younger children who stutter.

3.4.2 Secondary Behaviors of Stuttering

Secondary behaviors, also known as accessory or associated behaviors, are reactions that develop as coping mechanisms to manage the core behaviors of stuttering. These behaviors can be both motor and verbal and occur automatically due to the attempts of speakers to overcome their speech difficulties. Secondary behaviors in stuttering, which at first are meant to help the child cope with the fluency disorder, may become habitual and have adverse effects on the child's communication and psychological state. Knowing these secondary behaviors is important for helping those who stutter, as well as children who have stuttering problems. Other behaviors in stuttering are the extra features that are evident along with the primary speech deviations. These behaviors which are learnt as a way of coping can greatly affect a person's communication and their social and emotional state.

Secondary behaviors are usually adopted by the affected individual as a way of trying to overcome the problem of speech. These behaviors could help to gain some time or to feel that one is in control during the moments of stuttering. At first, they may assist the individual to at least have the confidence to voice out his or her opinions without being interjected. Such strategies can be useful in the short term, which helps to create an impression of competence. However, they do not solve the fundamental problem of stuttering and may even become counterproductive over time.

Overtime, these coping behaviors are learned, and hence, it becomes very difficult to unlearn them even if the core stuttering has been dealt with. Secondary behaviors can become ingrained as habits and are elicited when the subject is speaking without having to be told to do so. Behaviors such as touching the fingers or clenched fists become automatic reactions when the person is likely to stutter. These behaviors do not help to reduce the stuttering but rather perpetuate the dysfluency, and thus, it becomes challenging to attain smooth speaking.

Secondary behaviors may thus bring attention to the existence of stuttering, and this may cause the person to become more self-conscious and nervous in social settings. Conflicts that are evident with these behaviors can therefore affect the child's confidence and their desire to engage in conversation.

Behaviors like eye blinking or facial grimaces make stuttering more noticeable, potentially leading to teasing or negative reactions from peers. So, students may avoid social activities that can cause them embarrassment, which in turn limits their chances of practicing and learning social skills and making friends.

Hence, the management of secondary behaviors is very crucial to tackle the social and emotional aspects of stuttering. This needs support from parents, teachers, and therapists who build the child's confidence and strengthen the child's coping mechanisms, thus reducing the impact of these behaviors.

3.4.2.1 Types of Secondary Behaviors

- Eye Blinking: Blinking of the eyes, either rapid or forceful, is a common secondary behavior associated with stuttering. This is a reflexive action to release tension and get back to normal fluency. For example, a child might blink repeatedly while trying to say a challenging word.
- Head Movements: Nodding or shaking the head while speaking are other secondary responses noticed in stuttering. These movements may occur during an attempt to get past a block or repetition, which suggests the patient's attempt to continue speaking and the struggle to maintain speech flow.
- Facial Grimaces: Generally, there is tension in the facial muscles and grimaces as the child struggles to break the barrier of stuttering. These expressions can represent an internal struggle and physical exertion present while speaking.
- Hand Clenching or Tapping: Frequently, clenching fists or tapping fingers can be observed as physical symptoms of the stress that accompanies stuttering. These actions act as stimuli which usually help to release accumulated tension and, at times, make the speaker feel more self-efficient.
- Foot Tapping: Tapping the foot or moving the legs can be quite helpful as it diverts the traffic from the area of the brain, or the built-up tension associated with stuttering. These behaviors, although helpful at that moment, can build up to be a recurrent practice.

- Other Movements: Other physical activities that may be observed along with stuttering include shifting body weight or fidgeting. These behaviors are the consequences of phonemic speech disruption and are the patient's efforts to restore fluency.
- Irregular Breathing Patterns: During stuttering, the child may display signs of disrupted respiration, which may include taking short breaths or abrupt pauses in the middle of a breath. These disruptions are the results of having to struggle in the process of speaking.
- Holding Breath: Some of the children may hold their breath momentarily before attempting to speak, especially if the word or sound they are about to say is challenging.

3.4.3 Feelings and Attitudes in Stuttering

Stuttering is not only a speech disorder, but it comes with a lot of emotional and psychological complications. Thus, people who stutter may have several negative feelings and attitudes that influence their lives and cause a lot of discomfort. Such feelings and perceptions can worsen the speech disorder, forming a cycle that is hard to interrupt. Thus, it is important to comprehend these factors to be able to help individuals who stutter effectively.

3.4.3.1 Common Emotional Responses

1. *Anxiety*: Anxiety is one of the most widespread feelings that is connected to stuttering. This is usually brought about by the fear of the occurrence of stuttering episodes, especially in social or performance situations. Listeners may make the speaker feel self-conscious, which in turn increases their stress levels and increases the distortions in their speech. For example, a child can be nervous to give a speech in front of the class and be afraid of stammering and being laughed at by the classmates. This creates anxiety and the development of negative emotions about stuttering and about speech tasks in the child's mind.
2. *Shame and Embarrassment*: Shame and embarrassment are quite usual, especially when the stuttering happens in front of other people or when it is crucial to express oneself. This can result in a strong desire to stay away from speaking scenarios as much as possible. For instance, a teenager who is a stutterer could be made to feel very uncomfortable when he or she is unable to order food in a restaurant, leading him/her to avoid such situations in the future.
3. *Frustration*: Due to this, one gets frustrated when he or she is unable to put thoughts into proper words. This can cause the patient to feel frustration, helplessness, and irritation with themselves and the overall situation.

For example, a child can get frustrated when he/she wants to tell a story to his/her friends and knows what to say but cannot say it smoothly.

4. *Low Self-Esteem*: Stuttering is a condition that may persist throughout life and can affect a person's overall confidence. They may view themselves negatively because of their speech impediment, therefore losing their confidence. For example, an adult who

stutters may have low self-esteem as he or she feels that they are unable to communicate well or are not as good as other people in this aspect.

5. *Isolation*: Due to the unpleasant situations connected with speech, people who stutter may avoid communication. Such isolation results in loneliness and further emotional distress. For instance, a student can become a social recluse in order to avoid exposing himself or herself to situations where they may stutter.

3.5 Sheehan's Iceberg Analogy

Joseph Sheehan was one of the first psychologists and researchers in the area of stuttering. His experience in studying and treating stuttering was both clinical and very much a personal one. Sheehan was born in the early part of the twentieth century and was himself a stutterer. This personal experience affected his professional practice and therefore made him one of the leading figures in the analysis of stuttering.

Sheehan's iceberg analogy is one of the best-known referential models of stuttering as a multifaceted phenomenon. Sheehan linked stuttering to an iceberg, where the part that can be seen above water represents visible and observable speech disruptions, and a much larger part under the water symbolizes the emotional and psychological aspect. This analogy is useful as it shows that the surface behaviors are just a very small aspect of the overall experience of stuttering.

The genesis of the iceberg analogy was rooted in Sheehan's practice and interactions with people who stutter, in addition to his own experience as a person who stutters. He realized that there were many aspects to stuttering, and the physical outcomes were just the tip of the iceberg. Sheehan and many other people had unseen psychological problems that were not easily comprehensible to the people around them.

Sheehan noticed in his practice and research that stuttering was not only the disturbed speech fluency, the so-called blocks, repetitions, and prolongations that everyone could see. It was also about the fear, shame, guilt, and anxiety that were concealed and simmering under the veneer. These feelings were usually buried deep and often affected the lives of people who stuttered, including their behaviors, self-worth, and social interactions.

For instance, Priya, an eight-year-old, often experiences repetitions and blocks. When giving a class presentation, she could state, "I-I-I went to the p-park" with fixed face and hand movements. Priya was unable to perform classroom-related speech tasks due to her fear of her classmates, which made her avoid participating in any such activities. This turned her into a shy and isolated student. Priya's teacher often reminded her to raise her hand and read aloud; however, Priya seldom did because she did not want her classmates to laugh at her stuttering.

As depicted by Sheehan's iceberg analogy, the extent of stuttering is well explained, meaning that there is more than what meets the eye and that is the major psychological aspect of the disorder. Sheehan explained that stuttering consists of two major elements:

1. *Visible Part of the Iceberg*: These are observable stuttering behaviors, which are the main/core behaviors of stuttering. These can be easily seen by anyone around the person who stutters. The core behaviors that have been identified include repetitions, prolongations, and blocks.
2. *Hidden Part of the Iceberg*: These are the underlying feelings, attitudes, and perceptions of a stutterer toward his/her stuttering. This encompasses the emotional and psychological dimensions of speech disorder that are not easily observed yet have a profound effect on an individual. These negative emotions could be fear, shame, guilt, anxiety, hopelessness, and isolation. The identification of these factors is important, particularly in helping those who stutter get the best support possible.
   (a) *Fear*: Most commonly, children who stutter have a fear of speaking situations. This fear can be attributed to past experiences, such as being teased or judged for their speech. For instance, a child can fail to answer questions set by the teacher in class due to the fear of stuttering in front of their peers.
   (b) *Shame*: It arises when children incorporate negative attitudes of others toward them because of stuttering. They may be quite self-conscious regarding their speech and will attempt to avoid stuttering. For instance, a child may not want to make new friends because they feel ashamed of how they speak.
   (c) *Guilt*: The feeling of guilt can occur when children believe that they are not living up to the expectations of their parents, teachers, or even themselves. They may blame themselves for their stuttering, supposing that they should be able to speak normally. For example, a child could easily develop guilt for being unable to memorize a poem and recite it in school.
   (d) *Anxiety*: Stuttering can be accompanied by anxiety, which can be both anticipatory and situational. Anticipatory anxiety is when a child is fearful of a speaking event that is to happen in the future, while situational anxiety takes place during the actual speech. For instance, a child might experience palpitations in his or her chest and sweating of the palms before presenting a case in a class.
   (e) *Hopelessness*: It becomes a problem when children lose faith that their stuttering will get any better. This feeling can make the child lose interest in speech therapy or opt not to practice the speech exercises that have been given. For example, the child may refuse to attempt to communicate during a conversation because he or she thinks that it will not make any difference.
   (f) *Isolation*: Isolation is a consequence of avoiding social interactions in order to avoid stuttering. Children may stay away from group work, celebrations, or even playing with their friends. For instance, a child may prefer playing by himself or herself during break time than participating in a group game where he or she will have to speak.

More than the visible part, it is these covert feelings and attitudes that are related to the process of stuttering that make the speech difficulty stand out as an almost untreatable condition with poor prognosis and high relapse rate.

3.6 Understanding Stuttering Through the International Classification of Functioning Model

The International Classification of Functioning (ICF) model is a conceptual model for health and disability developed by the WHO that gives a clear understanding of health and disability. This model incorporates the biopsychosocial approach, which takes into consideration the biomedical aspects of a condition as well as the effects of the condition on the person's ability to engage in different activities. The ICF model has been used to expand the knowledge on many health conditions, and this includes stuttering. The ICF model conceptualizes health and disability using three interconnected domains: The ICF defines the components of body functions and structures, activities and participation, and environmental and personal factors.

1. *Body Functions and Structures*: This domain relates to the actions of body systems and structures of the human body. This entails the neurological and speech motor components of the system that are involved in the normal flow of speech.
2. *Activities and Participation*: This domain deals with the performance aspects and participation in the roles of life. For individuals who stutter, this involves the ability to communicate effectively, which may be in social, educational, or working environments, among other areas of their lives.
3. *Environmental and Personal Factors*: Environmental factors are the physical, social, and attitudinal factors that surround people in their day-to-day lives. This factor deals with an individual's attributes, like age, gender, ways of coping, and other aspects of personal life. These factors have a significant impact on the extent of how the disorder of stuttering can alter one's life.

3.6.1 Dr Yaruss's Application of the ICF Model to Stuttering

Dr J Scott Yaruss, a leading scholar in the domain of stuttering, has extended this model to the study of stuttering to help explain the effect of the disorder on people's lives. His work underlines that stuttering is not only the interruption of speech fluency but also the overall effect on a person. Thus, Dr Yaruss has shown how stuttering impacts an individual's functioning, participation, and quality of life, going beyond the mere description of the symptoms of the disorder through the ICF framework.

3.6.2 Body Functions and Structures in Stuttering

The ICF model's body functions and structures domain relates to the physiological and anatomical factors of stuttering. Dr Yaruss's work supports the idea that stuttering is related to disturbances in the neural mechanisms that are responsible for speech. Studies have also shown that there are differences in the brain activation patterns of people who stutter in certain areas associated with speech motor coordination and time. These physiological differences can affect the dysfluencies that are typically seen in stuttering individuals, including repetitions, prolongations, and blocks.

3.6.3 Activities and Participation in Stuttering

It is in the activities and participation domain that Dr Yaruss's use of the ICF model enhances the knowledge on stuttering. He notes that stuttering affects the subject's capacity to work and engage in various professions and social relations.

- Communication Effectiveness: Stuttering hinders communication since the client is unable to speak fluently. It affects the ability to convey ideas, communicate, and engage in a conversation or a group discussion. Dr Yaruss notes that these communication difficulties cause avoidance behaviors in such a way that people who stutter may choose not to speak in some situations to avoid stuttering.
- Educational and Professional Impact: According to Yaruss, the research shows that stuttering has an impact on scholarly achievement and work. Stuttering children may avoid joining their peers in class activities, which in turn affects their learning and performance. At the workplace, adults who stutter may avoid speaking parts, which may hinder their growth and satisfaction at the workplace.
- Social Participation: Stuttering can cause individuals to avoid speaking and therefore avoid social interactions, hence isolating themselves. Yaruss notes that people who stutter may stay away from social events or speaking in public because of the fear of shame. This avoidance can limit the possibilities for social contact and support and thus adversely impact one's quality of life.

3.6.4 Environmental and Personal Factors in Stuttering

Environmental and personal factors are vital in determining how stuttering impacts an individual's life World Health organisation (1992). Thus, Yaruss's application of the ICF model proves that these factors should be considered in both the assessment and treatment processes.

- *Environmental Factors*: These include the attitudes and reactions of others toward the person who stutters, the availability of support systems, and the physical environment. According to Yaruss, there is a positive effect of the environment on the listener's attitudes, and it helps in minimizing the effects of stuttering by accepting the stutterers. On the other hand, negative attitudes and lack of support will only increase the difficulties experienced by people who stutter.
- *Personal Factors*: These comprise age, gender, personality, and coping styles. Yaruss also noted that some personal factors such as personal resilience, self-esteem, and one's capacity to deal with stress determine how an individual will deal with stuttering. These

personal factors must be known to come up with intervention strategies that can help each person.

To sum up, Dr J Scott Yaruss has used the ICF model to classify various effects of stuttering, and this model gives a comprehensive approach to various impacts of stuttering. Thus, this model is able to come up with an integrated and individualized plan of intervention within the domains of body functions and structures, activities and participation, and environmental and personal factors. The ICF framework not only helps to explain the phenomena of stuttering but also the ways this model can be used to facilitate the process of enrichment of life of people who stutter. By identifying the specific needs of the individual, providing specific intervention, and educating the people in the affected person's life, more can be done to help people who stutter overcome their barriers and help integrate them into society.

3.7 Living as a Stutterer

Maanav, a 14-year-old boy, has been dealing with the complexities of life and a speech impediment in the form of stuttering from a very tender age. In Maanav's world, interactions are a complicated matter that affects his life at school, at home, and in the community. Indeed, at school, Maanav stutters mostly during lessons when he needs to speak. Spelling out, asking questions, or even engaging in any form of group discussion brings a lot of fear to him.

He often recalls a horrifying and embarrassing moment in fifth grade when the teacher asked him to read a passage from a book. The words just would not flow, and he had found it difficult to speak; "I-I-I w-want to t-tell you a st-story," he said. Everyone in the room stopped talking, and he could feel his classmates staring at him, some in what he could only assume was sympathetic, others puzzled or amused. This incident and some similar ones have restrained Maanav from raising his hand or coming forward to participate in any speaking activities, giving him a sense of isolation and frustration.

Back at home, Maanav gets a lot of comfort from his family members, especially from his mother and sister, as they have always stood by him. Still, even in this context, the story has its twists. Manav's social anxiety is also evident in family gatherings, especially when he is required to talk. His cousins may inquire as to which video game he likes, but the words cannot roll off his tongue as he wants them to in order to express his joy. This constant struggle affects his self-esteem as he can't be as open and as spirited as he would wish to be.

Peer interactions are rather difficult for Maanav, and this is where he struggles most. He stays away from social activities such as parties or group activities where he may be forced to speak. He is worried that due to his speech impediment, he will draw attention to himself in a negative way. Most of the time, Maanav does not interject when his friends are having fun or hatching a plan for the next day, for he is always fearful that he will stutter and, as a result, leave everyone in silence or laugh at him. This prevents him from getting close to anyone, and he gradually pushes people away, making it hard for him to develop close friendships.

3.8 Research Insights on Stuttering

Studying the real-life experiences of people who stutter are many researchers and clinicians, including Dr J Scott Yaruss and Dr Barry Guitar. They have shared diverse aspects of stuttering, which are psychological, emotional, as well as social aspects.

1. *Feeling a Loss of Control*

   A critical area of experience in the lives of people who stutter is the problem of power or control over one's speech. This feeling can be quite overpowering. As stated by Yaruss (2001), as he noted that stuttering is not just about the observable verbal dysfluencies but also about the subjective experience of not being able to regulate one's speech. For Maanav, this implies that no matter how much he would like to speak fluently, his speech often does not oblige. It also applies to the periods of time in which the person anticipates that they will stutter, which results in a continuous state of stress.

   In addition, the aforementioned concept of the iceberg model of stuttering developed by Sheehan (1970) can also be considered, which defines the obvious stuttering behaviors as the tip of the iceberg, while a major part of it consists of the emotional and psychological challenges that a person with such a disorder faces. This is one aspect that forms the hidden iceberg that people cannot notice but is a real issue. Such is the case with Maanav, a boy who stutters. Like many others who experience stuttering, he explains the feeling of losing control over one's speech. According to Dr Yaruss (2001), this loss of control causes individuals to be in a state of anxiety because they do not know when they will experience stuttering again. This instability may lead to the students' reluctance to interact with others, share ideas, or even socialize in classroom settings or other group situations.
2. *Anticipation of Stuttering*

   Another major problem is the expectation or anticipation of stuttering. Guitar (2013) pointed out that the anxiety of stuttering is as bad as the actual stuttering. This expectation is a daily occurrence for Maanav. He has a phobia of speaking in front of people, and as such, he envisions himself in such a situation and gets anxious about how he will handle it. This anticipation results in an anxiety and avoidance pattern since the fear of stuttering leads to behaviors that prevent him from engaging in day-to-day activities.

   The mere expectation of stuttering can lead to the process of self-correction, which worsens the situation. This anticipation can lead to a form of cycle of anxiety and avoidance, to the extent that patients are so anxious about what is coming that they avoid it entirely. For instance, Maanav may experience constant anxiety and fear just at the thought of having to speak at some point, which only complicates the process of clear and coherent speaking. This anticipation is not only regarding the fear of stuttering but also the fear of being judged, being embarrassed, and the possible social effects of stuttering.

3. *Emotional Trauma and Stress*

   The psychological impact of stuttering is still quite heavy. Ramig and Dodge (2009) expounds on the way the emotional phase of stuttering may result in long-term psychological issues such as stress, anxiety, and depression. School and social scenario experiences of Maanav have left him feeling isolated and misunderstood. The fear of stuttering and the feelings of his past mistakes also lead to hopelessness. This emotional trauma also has a negative impact on his psychological health, in addition to the quality of his life.

   Ramig and Dodge (2009) estimated that the emotional problems caused by stuttering may contribute to stress and anxiety to a higher extent. This sort of trauma is usually based on prior negative events like failure, mockery, or rejection. Thus, each time Maanav stutters, he feels fear and anxiety, making it a cycle that is quite hard to escape. It is the emotional trauma that reduces self-esteem and confidence and hampers the ability of individuals to take risks and try out new things.

4. *Secondary and Covert Features of Stuttering*

   Covert features of stuttering are the additional strategies that people adopt when they have a stuttering disorder, while secondary behaviors are reactions that are used to cover up the stuttering problem. These behaviors can be a deeply ingrained part of the condition and are usually as problematic as the stuttering itself.

   Covert features and secondary behaviors are not easy and are quite intricate. Van Riper (1982) stated that secondary behaviors are the coping strategies that have been learnt in response to stuttering and can become part of an individual's natural behavior. These behaviors can be motoric, e.g., eye blinking and finger tapping, or verbal, e.g., using fillers or omissions. Covert features, however, are internalized strategies to hide or conceal stuttering. Some of these include avoiding any speaking situations, substituting words, or using mental tricks to try to maintain fluency.

   Maanav's experience with secondary behaviors comprises eye blinking and hand movement, especially when he expects to stutter. These behaviors, which he uses to facilitate fluent speech, turn the focus toward his speech even more and create an additional barrier in the process of communication. His tactics include not participating in some speaking activities such as raising his hand in class or approaching people he does not know, thus reducing his chances of improving his speaking skills. Such strategies, though helpful in the short run, tend to maintain the fear and anxiety that come with stuttering and make it challenging to work through the root cause.

   Intrinsic features of stuttering entail the covert techniques and feelings that cannot be seen by other people. These include vigilance on speech, the utilization of psychological strategies with the aim of preventing stuttering as well as the psychological facet of concealing the stutter. As pointed out by Van Riper (1982), these covert types of characteristics can be even more handicapping than the overt symptoms because they demand constant attention, as well as produce a considerable amount of psychological strain. Maanav also gets tired at the end of the day, not only from the process of speaking but also from the process of hiding his stutter and dealing with social situations.

Secondary behaviors are physical, like rapid eye movement, tapping fingers, or tensing facial muscles. These are efforts to push through or avoid stuttering instances, but they can be overdone, and then stuttering becomes even more of an issue. These are the behaviors that Maanav exhibits as a result of stress felt in the process of attempting to talk. He may clench his fists or tap his foot without even being aware of it, which makes the process of communication even more difficult.

5. *Verbal Starters and Avoidance Behaviors*

   Frequently, the people who stutter tend to use verbal starters, for instance, "um" or "well," at the beginning of the sentence. These fillers allow them to buy time to gather their thoughts and thus speak more fluently. Maanav employs these starters quite often; however, they do not always help to avoid stuttering. Other strategies include circumlocutions, substituting difficult words, and avoidance, or not talking at all in certain situations. Maanav might opt to use a simpler word or a phrase even if it doesn't accurately express what he wishes to convey in a bid to prevent the occurrence of stuttering.

6. *Social Isolation and Loneliness*

   Stuttering often leads to social isolation and loneliness. This is because each time stuttering occurs, individuals withdraw from social interactions and avoid forming close relationships. Individuals with stuttering often fear being mocked or judged by others, and therefore, they isolate themselves and avoid developing friendships. Due to the fear of stuttering when speaking in public, Maanav is an isolated character who rarely participates in group activities and, therefore, does not have friends to cheer him on. It can result in feelings of isolation and depression that affect the mental health of an individual in a negative way.

7. *Academic and Career Implications*

   Stuttering also affects the academic and career aspects of an individual's life. At school, students who stutter generally tend to avoid speaking up during class and may fear presenting their work, which will lead to poor performance. For instance, Maanav, lacking the confidence to speak out in the class and feeling that he is not able to express himself fully, would not participate in class activities, which would adversely affect his participation grades. Over time, these individuals also avoid these activities in their day-to-day life, which may limit their career growth. Adults who stutter may avoid jobs and positions where they are put in the spotlight to speak or may prefer taking positions that do not demand much speaking in public. This may further limit their employment opportunities and career growth.

8. *Impact on Family Dynamics*

   Speech disorders like stuttering also influence the family's functioning and dynamics. The family members might get annoyed or be clueless about how they can assist the person who stutters. Maanav's family sometimes witnesses his struggle with speech, and this is a painful thing for them to see. At the same time, they are supportive and tolerant, though there are moments of irritation due to breakdowns in communication. Concerns about the child's future and the problems that may arise can be a concern for parents; as for the other children, they might feel envy and irritation because they may feel that much attention is paid to their sibling's stutter rather than to them.

9. *Coping Mechanisms and Resilience*

   Nevertheless, owing to these challenges, many people who stutter find ways of coping and dealing with the situation. Some of the recommendations can entail engaging with speech therapists, attending support groups for stutterers, and working on ways to deal with anxiety and to enhance fluency. Maanav, with his parents' help, has now begun going to a local support group for people who stutter. Here, he is with people who understand his struggles. He also learns new techniques to handle his stuttering and gets motivated by others' experiences and success stories.

3.9 Stuttering Oscillates Like a Pendulum

Like the pendulum, the severity of stuttering and the frequency of the occurrences can be quite different for different people and situations. Due to this, there is no clear pattern of the way a student moves from being fluent to stuttering. This is the reason why understanding variability in stuttering becomes vital in the formulation of intervention strategies. The major sources of variability are speaker variability, contextual variability, and variability due to various situations.

Stuttering has been studied by many researchers, including Yaruss, Bloodstein, Guitar, and Riper. Yaruss and Quesal (2006) proposed the Overall Assessment of the Speaker's Experience of Stuttering (OASES), which is used to assess the characteristics of the speech disorder in terms of the frequency, severity, and consequences of the individuals' stuttering. They also found that stuttering was quite diverse in terms of the experiences of the clients, stressing the importance of tailoring interventions. Their research is important because it underlines that stuttering is not only a problem that affects speech but also emotions and social interaction. All aspects of stuttering should be targeted in effective therapies, with treatments that are individualized to the person's circumstances.

Bloodstein and Ratner (2008) described the nature of the disorder, its causes, and possible ways to treat it. They also describe how the speaking situation affects the stuttering rate, for example, when talking to different persons or when placed under stress. They argued that stuttering can be highly inconsistent, even within the same individual. This is in consideration of the view that stuttering is multifaceted, and thus, factors such as context and personality should be taken into consideration when developing therapy plans.

Guitar (2014) focuses on the neurological and psychological aspects of stuttering. He also described the way these factors affect the differences in the patterns of stuttering. Guitar explains the adaptation effect: reading the same passage several times results in fewer stuttering incidences due to reduced anxiety and increased familiarity with the text.

This highlights the potential benefits of practice and exposure in stuttering therapy, stating that if the person practices commonly in a controlled manner, stuttering frequency may decrease over some time.

Van Riper (1982) focused on the behavioral and psychological features of the disorder. He described how people with stuttering can experience different levels of stuttering depending on their feelings and situations. He also documented case studies that describe how some people may stutter at times of stress but stay fluent otherwise. His conclusions pointed to the importance of affect (emotions) and environment in stuttering and argued that therapy should address clients' concerns about overcoming anxiety and speaking confidently in different settings.

Anderson and Wagovich (2010) established the effects of language proficiency on stuttering variability in children. They concluded that children with better language skills had less fluctuation in the severity of their stuttering, thus, language skills may help to regulate severity. This means that improving the language could be a useful element of the stuttering treatment for children, which may reduce the variability and improve communication.

Ingham and Cordes (1999) reviewed different treatment options for the management of adult stuttering, bearing in mind the differences in clients' characteristics that influence the effectiveness of the interventions. This is because they discovered that the pattern of stuttering differs from one person to another, and this calls for the need to develop a unique plan for everyone as there is no standard one that can be used. This underlines the importance of individualized or even idiographic treatment plans and the clinician's ability and willingness to change the course of treatment based on the needs of the individual who stutters.

Smith and Weber (2017a, b) provided the multifactorial dynamic pathways theory, according to which stuttering is a product of multiple factors, including genetic predispositions, neurological variations, and social factors. They found that these are some of the factors that cause the changes in the stuttering patterns over time. Acknowledging the fact that there are many factors that may contribute to stuttering can assist in the identification of a more global treatment process that considers a wide range of factors that influence the complexity of stuttering.

Conture and Walden (2012) also insisted on a dual diathesis-stressor model that describes how and why individual differences in stuttering occur. They proved that there are differences in the kindergarten and school-age stuttering children's stuttering types based on the level of stress they encounter in different kinds of speaking situations. This model shows that to make therapy effective, it is crucial to consider both the individual's inherent tendencies and the stressful factors that surround them. Stress management and the establishment of speaking environments that are conducive for the stutterer are some of the vital aspects of stuttering treatment.

Research on stuttering variability points to the fact that the disorder is multifactorial and that treatment should be tailored to each individual's needs, considering the context. The variability in stuttering can be of different types. These include:

3.10 Speaker Variability

Speaker variability refers to the differences observed in the patterns and frequency of stuttering between individuals. No two people who stutter are the same, which means the signs and symptoms that are present in one person may not be present in another. This variability is affected by various factors such as the genetic makeup of the individual, the neurological factors, and the personal experiences that one has had.

1. *Genetic Factors*: Stuttering can be inherited, as it is commonly observed that it affects members of the same family. It could be due to genes, since if one of the parents stutters, the child is also likely to stutter. Research has also established that there are certain genes that are linked with stuttering, and this is why some people are more vulnerable to the condition as compared to others.
2. *Neurological Factors*: Studies have revealed that there are variations in the neural networks, especially regarding speech regions in the brains of people who stutter as compared to non-stutterers. For instance, they may use one lobe of the brain for speaking while the other lobe is used for comprehension. Research has also shown that there is a difference in the neural connections of people who stutter as compared to those who do not. These differences can impact the way speech is perceived and generated. Stutterers have been found to exhibit over-activation of the right hemisphere of the brain, which does not usually have an involvement in speech and under-activation of the left hemisphere regions that are generally involved in language.
3. *Personal Experiences*: Everyone who stutters is different and has a different past and experiences with stuttering. For instance, a child who developed stuttering at a tender age and received early intervention might not have the same way of stuttering compared to someone who started later and didn't get help. Hence, the history of the individuals who stutter also contributes to speaker variability. It means that aspects like the age of onset, the level of stuttering, and the previous treatment can together influence the nature and pattern of stuttering.

3.11 Contextual Variability

The term "contextual variability" describes variations in the frequency and intensity of stuttering due to various speaking contexts and settings. Stuttering can be caused by a variety of contextual factors, such as the presence of an audience, the listener's familiarity, the difficulty of the speaking task, and emotional states.

1. *Audience Presence*: A lot of stutterers claim that speaking in front of a group causes them to be less fluent than speaking to one person at a time. This is often related to an increase in social anxiety and the level of self-awareness.
2. *Acquaintance with the Audience*: It is important to note that every individual will stutter in the same manner before a stranger or his/her family member or friend. Knowing

the person helps reduce anxiety and thus creates a comfortable atmosphere for speaking, which in turn might reduce the rate of stuttering.

3. *Complexity of the Speaking Task*: The speaking task's inherent characteristics can affect stuttering. For instance, there are differences between the fluency of speaking in the presence of a script and speaking without one. Stuttering can be aggravated when carrying out tasks that depend on fast and delicate language analysis.
4. *Emotional States*: Emotions also play a huge role in this; stress, excitement, and even exhaustion can severely worsen the stuttering. Stuttering, for example, is a communication disorder that affects a child's fluency; the child may have more dysfluency when discussing an interest but may be more facile when answering questions in a classroom or other pressure situations.

3.12 Environmental and Situational Aspects

Stuttering variations can also be affected by various situations and environmental aspects that are not directly connected to speaking situations. Some of the factors that can be used to explain variability in the rate and severity of stuttering include education systems, support systems, and cultural beliefs.

1. *Cultural Perceptions*: People's attitudes toward their speech and the ways they approach their dysfluency might depend on cultural attitudes towards stuttering and its connotations. It is likely that people will stutter more and will be more anxious in societies that have a negative perception toward stuttering.
2. *Educational Settings*: Stuttering is part of an individual's communication and can be affected by the rules and format of educational contexts (Yaruss & Reardon-Reeves (2013)). For example, anxiety can be reduced, and fluency can be enhanced in a classroom that has a positive environment with regard to stuttering by teachers who know how to manage students who stutter. On the other hand, there is a possibility of exacerbation of stuttering, especially in academic settings where there is a lot of speaking in front of the class.
3. *Support Systems*: An important factor of stuttering management is having support from the community, friends, and professionals like speech therapists and support groups. Therefore, it is evident that strong networks provide people with more adaptive methods of coping, leading to less fluctuation in the degree of their stuttering.

3.13 The Consistency Effect in Stuttering

The consistency effect in stuttering deals with the situation where a person stutters on the same words or sounds in different contexts. It has been well-documented in research on stuttering and is quite helpful in the general framework of the mechanisms of dysfluency. The consistency effect is determined by factors like anticipatory anxiety, conditioning, and the cognitive processes of language.

1. *Preventive Anxiety*: This is when those people who stutter are certain that they will face difficulties when it comes to pronouncing some words or sounds, then become anxious, and this worsens the condition of stuttering. Thus, the premonitory anxiety sets off a chain reaction in which the expectation of stuttering on specific words leads to the actual stuttering when these words are encountered.
2. *Conditioning*: Since certain words elicit stuttering, the body forms conditioned responses, which means that the individual will stutter on the particular words. This conditioning process entails the creation of a relationship between certain words or sounds and the occurrence of stuttering, thus raising the chances of having the person stutter on those words or sounds in the future. For instance, if a child stutters whenever he or she tries to say words that begin with the letter 'b,' the child may get a conditioned response and consequently stutter whenever he or she attempts to say terms such as "ball" or "book."
3. *Cognitive Processing*: The factors that are related to the mental faculties in producing speech can also be responsible for the consistency effect. Stuttering is more frequent when one is speaking difficult or new words because they require more brain power to articulate. This leads to cognitive or other kinds of blocks or even hesitations, leading to the consistency effect.

3.13.1 Instances of the Consistency Effect Include

1. *Utilization of Specific Word Repetition*: An example of this is the scenario where a person stutters on certain words in different circumstances. For instance, a student may have a speech difficulty on the word "presentation" both in class and in conversation.
2. *Sound Patterns*: In the consistency effect, the same phenomenon can also be witnessed in the patterns of sound. For instance, a child can end up stuttering, particularly when trying to say words that begin with the letter S, like school, summer, and sandwich, among others.
3. *Stressful Situations*: The consistency effect usually has a greater effect in situations where there is pressure or stress. For instance, an individual may find it very hard to speak fluently when introducing themselves by their name, as this raises the level of tension that may lead to stuttering.

3.14 The Adaptation Effect in Stuttering

The adaptation effect in stuttering means that when the same paragraph is read or the same passage is to be repeated, there would be a marked decrease in stuttering. This phenomenon stresses the dynamic nature of stuttering and provides some insight into the potential treatment options.

The adaptation effect leads to reduced stuttering due to reduced fear, increased familiarity, and better motor planning.

1. *Alleviated Anxiety*: Repetition of the same speaking task reduces the level of anxiety that one has when performing the task. Over time, the more they become acquainted with the passage, the more confident they become, and therefore, they stutter less. This reduction in anxiety helps in breaking the cycle of expectancy, which is often a major factor that makes the stuttering worse (Yaruss & Quesel (2010)).
2. *Enhanced Acquaintance*: This is when a statement is made with more fluency due to prior understanding of the subject in question. Repetition of a passage improves peoples' understanding of the words and the phrases used in the passage, meaning that less cognitive effort is required to produce speech. It helps in overcoming the initial hitches or the stigma that is usually associated with stuttering.
3. *Enhanced Motor Planning*: Repeating the same passage enhances motor skills such as planning and coordination. It has been noted that through repeated practice, the neural pathways that are involved in speech production become more efficient, thus enhancing the fluency of a person's speech.

3.14.1 Examples of the Adaptation Effect

1. *Iterative perusal*: A good example of the adaptation effect can be seen when people read the same text repeatedly. Initially, it can be observed that stuttering happens more frequently, but as the text is read again, cases of stuttering are reduced.
2. *Delivering Oral Presentations*: It is also possible to note the phenomenon of adaptability when people rehearse speeches or presentations. For instance, a student who has a speech impediment may realize that his/her speech will be smooth if he/she rehearses the speech before delivering it to an audience.
3. *Therapeutic Exercises*: Speech therapists often use the adaptation effect in therapy by telling clients to practice the difficult words or phrases repeatedly. Over time, the clients' speaking skills become more natural because they become accustomed to the specific speaking tasks.

3.15 Comparing Children: Fluent Versus Stutterers

To comprehend the impact of stuttering on a child, it is crucial to examine the differences between children who stutter (CWS) and those who do not stutter (CWNS). It is crucial to analyze multiple facets, including linguistic features, emotional and psychological components, social relationships, academic performance, neurological factors, and hereditary factors.

3.15.1 Characteristics of Speech

The primary distinction between CWS and CWNS is evident in their level of speech fluency. Stuttering is defined by interruptions in the typical progression of speech, such as repeating sounds, syllables, or words, prolonging sounds, and experiencing blocks where the mouth is prepared to speak a word, but no sound is produced. The frequency and severity of these speech disruptions are usually higher in CWS compared to the occasional normal speech disruptions in CWNS. Additionally, these children exhibit variations in their speech rate and rhythm in the following manners (Wagovich & Hall (2010)):

- Children who stammer frequently exhibit an inconsistent speech tempo and impaired rhythm. Their speech can be described as having many pauses, irregular tempo, and sudden beginnings and endings. This inconsistency can cause their speech to sound less smooth and more laborious. Additionally, the speech of children who stutter may exhibit evident exertion, tension, and variations in tone or volume during instances of dysfluency. The following attributes can make it seem like the speaker is straining the voice and hence sounding artificial.
- Normal speaking rate and fluency of speech are characteristic of children who do not stutter. The overall speech of people with greater fluency is more fluid, even in cases when they have typical speech dysfluencies. Normally, CWNS has some dysfluency, which is not severe enough to affect the overall quality of speech. The speech they use is usually casual, and there are no signs of stress or effort in their speech.

3.15.2 Analysis of the Occurrence and Nature of Speech Disruptions

In research done by Ambrose and Yairi (1999), it is seen that CWS experience more dysfluencies than CWNS. CWS usually displays speech dysfluencies, which are part-word repetitions, monosyllabic whole-word repetitions, and prolongations. On the other hand, children with typical speech production will exhibit normal dysfluencies (NDs), which include repeating polysyllabic words, repeating phrases, as well as the use of interjections.

Stuttering is described as a disorder that affects the fluency of speech and is characterized by disruptions in the voluntary control of speech and the timing of speech segments, and these disruptions are more frequent and have specific characteristics in CWS, and this is why it is crucial to have speech therapy that is designed for children with stuttering to target these disruptions. It is ideal to have early treatment because this can lessen the severity of the stuttering and increase speech fluency. The major differences between CWS and CWNS are as follows:

1. *Rate and Type of Dysfluencies*
    - CWS usually have more dysfluencies than CWNS. Research shows that CWS has dysfluency of more than 10 per 100 spoken words. This high frequency is one of the most important and often used parameters by speech language pathologists when differentiating between stuttering and disfluency.
    - CWNS are likely to have less dysfluencies than CWS. CWNS, on average, display fewer than 10 dysfluencies every 100 spoken words. Occasional repetitions, interjections, and revisions may be present in their speech, but these happen less frequently and are generally regarded as normal in the process of speech development.

- The dysfluencies exhibited by CWS and CWNS differ greatly, and this distinction is essential for making a diagnosis.
- *CWS*: The speech disruptions of CWS are frequently more noticeable and encompass:
  - Part-word repetitions: The act of repeating segments of words, for example, saying "ba-ba-ba-ball."
  - Single-syllable whole-word repetitions: The act of repeating complete words with only one syllable, for example, saying "I-I-I want."
  - Prolongations: The act of lengthening sounds within words, as exemplified by the word "sssssnake."
  - Blocks refer to moments when a youngster is unable to create sounds and is typically accompanied by evident stress. These dysfluencies are typically accompanied by physical tension, struggling behaviors (such as eye blinking and head nodding), and an increase in pitch or loudness when repeating or prolonging sounds.
- *CWNS*: The speech disruptions of children who do not stutter are usually milder and consist of:
  - Whole-word repetitions: The act of repeating complete words, for example, saying "Can I can I go?"
  - Phrase repetitions: The act of repeating phrases, such as saying "I want to I want to."
  - Interjections: Including filler words such as "um" and "uh."
  - Revisions: Altering the wording of a sentence, for example, transforming "I want—I need that."
  - Typically, these dysfluencies are characterized by a smooth and calm manner, without any observable indications of physical effort or strain.

2. *The Length and Continuity of Dysfluencies*

CWS: Stuttering dysfluencies tend to be more enduring and can linger for months or even years. If a youngster displays stuttering behaviors persistently for a period beyond 6 months, it is more probable that the diagnosis will be stuttering.

CWNS: Common speech problems are usually transitory and may improve on their own within a few weeks or a few months. They are temporary and do not increase over time.

3. *Emotional and Psychological Factors*

Many of the children who are affected by stuttering face numerous emotional and psychological problems that are likely to influence their well-being in a poor manner. Some of the barriers include heightened levels of stress, lowered confidence, and higher rates of negative emotions when it comes to speaking. The perception and response to speech disruptions vary among different children.

- Children who have an understanding that they have a speech impediment often feel frustrated and shameful, and hence, they avoid speaking. They can get afraid when in speaking situations and resort to some secondary behaviors like averting their eyes or using simpler words.

- CWNS do not have a conspicuous perception of their normal dysfluencies and will not have negative feelings or avoid speaking. Their speech abnormalities are considered within the norm in the process of language development.

4. *Anxiety and Stress*

The present research has documented higher rates of anxiety in CWS in several investigations. Blood et al. (2001a) found in their research that children who stutter often experience a significant amount of concern regarding their speech; this concern may also manifest itself in other social situations as generalized anxiety. Stuttering is thus a source of anxiety, and the child may, therefore, avoid speaking in situations where he or she is likely to stutter.

Stuttering children are usually threatened by speaking situations, and as such, they communicate with difficulty. This nervousness can be evident as "avoidance behaviors," for instance, not raising their hand in class, avoiding certain words or sounds, or not talking at all at some point. The given actions stem from the wish to avoid stuttering and the possible reactions it may elicit from other people. CWNS are not likely to avoid speech or show symptoms of anxiety concerning speech. They may sometimes display typical speech interruptions, but these interruptions are not a cause for major worry or avoidance. The manifestation of physical tension and struggle observed in these youngsters during episodes of worry and stress varies in the following manners:

- CWS sometimes exhibit noticeable indications of physical strain and effort in their speech. These symptoms can appear as facial grimacing, eye blinking, or other bodily motions that occur alongside attempts to speak.
- CWNS usually experience normal dysfluencies without any bodily stress or struggle. Their discourse exhibits a more easy-going demeanor, devoid of any accompanying bodily gestures.

5. *Self-Esteem and Self-Perception*

According to Yaruss and Reardon-Reeves (2007), CWS frequently has lower self-esteem and less favorable self-perception in comparison to their peers who do not stutter. The development of a poor self-image sometimes arises from recurrent instances of unfavorable verbal encounters and societal responses to their speech impediment. Interventions focused on enhancing self-esteem and fostering a positive self-perception are crucial. The combination of speech therapy and counselling can assist individuals with communication disorders in enhancing their self-assurance and cultivating a more positive perception of themselves.

6. *Interpersonal Relationships*

Stuttering can have a substantial impact on a child's social relationships, affecting their ability to communicate with classmates, engage in group activities, and establish friendships. Thus, the variety of stuttering is instrumental in the process of defining the child's capacity to interact with the outside world. It is vital to comprehend the distinctions between the two categories of youngsters.

7. *Consistency and Adaptation*

- CWS: Stuttering can occur consistently in various speech contexts. The consistency effect pertains to the inclination to experience stuttering on the same phrases or sounds. Moreover, CWS may exhibit an adaptation effect, whereby the repetition of reading the same material leads to a gradual reduction in the frequency of stuttering over a period.

- Dysfluencies in CWNS typically exhibit less uniformity and lack the same regular patterns of adaptation observed in CWS.

8. *Interpersonal Connections*

Research has indicated that CWS are more susceptible to social isolation and bullying in comparison to CWNS. In their study, Davis et al. (2002) discovered that children who stutter are frequently subject to distinct perceptions from their classmates, resulting in unfavorable social interactions and exclusion from group activities. Establishing a comprehensive and encouraging social atmosphere is of utmost importance. Disseminating knowledge about stuttering among peers and fostering empathy can effectively mitigate instances of bullying and alleviate social isolation experienced by CWS.

9. *Secondary Behaviors and Physical Concomitants*

Secondary behaviors, or physical concomitants, are frequently observed in children who stammer. These can encompass eye blinks, facial grimaces, head movements, or other physical motions that coincide with instances of stuttering. These acts are frequently efforts to overcome or end a stuttering block.

CWS do not display any secondary behaviors that are linked to their typical dysfluencies. Their speech is devoid of any visible signs of exertion or hardship.

10. *Group Communication*

During social interactions, individuals with CWS may encounter difficulties in keeping pace with the fast tempo of discourse. This challenge might result in feelings of annoyance and a lack of willingness to engage in group conversations. According to Conture and Walden (2012), individuals who stutter may choose to avoid social engagements in order to prevent the humiliation associated with their speech impediment.

CWS: Stuttering can greatly affect a child's willingness and capacity to engage in communication. Children with stutter may exhibit a reduced inclination to partake in conversations, respond to queries in class, or involve themselves in group activities. This effect on communication and engagement is a crucial diagnostic sign.

Typically, CWNS are not affected in their desire or ability to communicate. Typical speech interruptions do not impede their engagement in discussions or educational tasks.

11. *Scholastic Achievement*

It is crucial to emphasize that stuttering can also have an impact on a child's academic achievement, specifically in subjects that involve verbal communication.

In terms of IQ, memory, and overall performance, it is important to note that CWS are not inferior to CWNS. However, though cognitive abilities are usually intact, communication issues may complicate the learning process in an academic setting with the presence of stuttering. It is not unusual for CWS to avoid engaging in school activities, answering questions, or contributing to discussions for fear of stuttering. This might affect their academic performance and become a barrier to their oral communication as well as the acquisition of knowledge. According to Riley and Riley (2000), teachers reported that CWS exhibits less participation in their class than CWNS. Therefore, teachers have the potential to greatly enhance the development of children with communication disorders by creating a favorable learning environment. This can be done by allowing students to participate in the discussion via writing or speaking one-on-one with the instructor. This can help CWS prove its expertise without the pressure of public speaking.

12. *Speaking in Front of an Audience and Reading Aloud*

Oral speaking and reading are common educational tasks that are rather challenging for children with childhood-onset fluency disorder. This means that when the client is in front of an audience, the frequency of stuttering may increase, which is associated with increased anxiety and possible avoidance of such situations in the future. Certain activities can be performed more effectively by people with communication disorders if certain accommodations are provided to them, for instance, more time to prepare for the task or allowing usage of certain devices such as speech-generating devices. Since mistakes are a part of the learning process, creating a positive classroom environment where students are allowed to make mistakes could thus go a long way in easing them from the fear of speaking in public.

3.16 Professionals to Seek for a Child with Stuttering

It is quite a concern for parents and teachers to notice that a child is stuttering in some manner. Thus, in most cases, the management of stuttering requires the intervention of several specialists. Many professionals are involved in determining and assisting young people with stuttering. Understanding the roles of the professionals who perform these tasks will help parents and caregivers to recognize their child's needs and secure the appropriate treatment and intervention. The main focus of this guide is thus on the various professionals involved, their roles, and their parts in the holistic management of children who stutter. The primary provider of care for a child with stuttering is the speech-language pathologist, along with psychologists and other therapists.

Speech-language pathologists (SLP) are essential in stuttering intervention because they provide specialized therapy to improve the individual's speech. Psychologists are involved in the treatment of the emotional and psychological aspects that are usually linked to stuttering. Moreover, other personnel, like the occupational therapist and the special education teachers, may provide additional input. It is allowable for the employed staff to give drugs if considered necessary and monitor the drug's administration. All these professionals have different skills and perspectives about the child, thus providing complete care for the child.

3.17 Interdisciplinary Approaches to Treating Stuttering

Stuttering is known to affect several aspects of a child's development, including speaking fluency, social interaction, and emotional health.

Therefore, it is crucial to integrate a multifaceted management approach in this regard. This approach involves the participation of numerous clinicians, every one of whom is concerned with different elements of the affliction. The integration of several specialists may lead to the development of a more extensive and individualized approach in the management of the child, which will lead to better results. Stuttering is best controlled when it is addressed early, meaning that early intervention is crucial in the management of the condition. The effects of stuttering on a child's communication skills and overall development can be lessened greatly if therapy is introduced at an early age. It also looks at the emotional and social aspect of the child, and this is the reason early intervention is very effective.

SLPs, psychologists, and other relevant specialists help the child in building self-esteem and healthy communication skills while in the company of other children, teachers, and parents.

Speech-language therapists: Therapists who are most useful in the intervention process of children experiencing stuttering are the SLP. They use research procedures that aim at the improvement of the free and efficient use of speech and communication skills. Because speech-language pathologists are qualified professionals who assess the child's speech, they establish specific aspects of stuttering and develop individual treatment plans. The two techniques generally used in helping a child to go through phases of stuttering are fluency shaping and stuttering modification. SLPs also provide important teaching and guidance to parents and other carers, where they help teach them how to set up an environment that is beneficial for the child's development of communication.

Psychological Support: Emotional and psychological problems are usually associated with CWS. This is because CWS have great difficulty in expressing themselves and often experience anxiety, frustration, and low self-esteem. Concerning these issues, psychologists are essential in solving them through counselling and other special therapies with the aim of improving the mental health of the child and building up their emotional strength. Another technique used to help young people develop proper positive thinking patterns and reduce the amount of concern related to the fluency of speech is called cognitive behavioral therapy. Cognitive behavioral therapists complement the extensiveness of the treatment plan by dealing with the affective aspects of stuttering.

It may be noted that parents are often majorly concerned about the rehabilitation of the child. It is very useful to inform the parents about the stuttering and involve them in the therapy process since it enhances the efficacy of the interventions. It is common for professionals to provide parents with training on how to encourage their child's communication development at home, create a positive and encouraging environment and support the methods introduced during treatment sessions. Having a parent participate, enhances the kid's compliance with the processes of therapy and gives the kid stability and a sense of consistency.

The results of the treatment for stuttering are long-lasting and improve the means of producing groups of speech sounds and also other factors. When conducted effectively, therapy will enhance the child's level of confidence, social relations, and performance in school. Stuttering therapy encompasses the child's verbal and emotional self; it empowers young people and helps them develop excellent communication skills that could prove advantageous in the foreseeable future. The use of a multifaceted approach ensures that records of all the aspects of a particular disease are given enhanced consideration so as to produce a durable improvement in the quality of life of the child in question.

3.18 Emphasizing the Importance of Speech-Language Pathologists

SLPs are the key personnel who conduct the assessment and diagnosis of children with stuttering Yaruss (2021). Their job begins with the examination that involves the analysis of the child's magnitude of fluency, the frequency and type of stuttering behaviors, and other accompanying phenotypes that might be physical or emotional. For this data, SLPs use assessment procedures and tools, written tests, and observations with the child and the child's parents, if possible. Such an evaluation is very important in the development of an individual treatment plan that addresses the child's needs in detail.

There are specific measures adapted by SLPs for each client depending on the test outcomes. These are aimed at meeting the requirements of each child individually with the help of plans that are developed for him/her alone. It contains clear goals, methods of intervention, and outcome measurements that may be expressed quantitatively. Specialists like speech-language pathologists employ approaches including fluency shaping, which revolves around training the child in new techniques that help in the fluency of speech, as well as stuttering modification, which works to change the kind of stuttering habit that interferes with communication. It is flexible in a way that the devised plan changes based on the progress and needs of the child as he or she grows.

The direct therapeutic approaches that SLPs use involve the following therapeutic approaches that ensure that CWS can manage the condition well. Several frequently employed strategies include:

- *Fluency Shaping*: Some of the elements of this technique include teaching the child to speak in more refined ways and at a slower rate. Exercises may involve the deliberate and unhurried articulation of words, the gradual and soft initiation of vocalization, and the uninterrupted production of sounds.
- *Stuttering Modification*: This strategy seeks to decrease the intensity and occurrence of stuttering by altering the manner in which the kid stutters. Methods encompass deliberate stuttering, whereby the child purposefully stutters to exert authority over the

behavior, and pullouts, whereby the child acquires the skill to transition out of a stutter gracefully.

SLPs frequently utilize cognitive and behavioral interventions to assist children in effectively coping with the anxiety and frustration that accompany stuttering. These strategies may encompass relaxation techniques, positive self-talk, and desensitization exercises.

Parent and caregiver training is crucial, as SLPs understand the need to include parents and caregivers in the therapy process. They offer instruction and direction to assist parents in establishing a nurturing domestic setting that fosters the child's growth in their communication. These instructions may involve instructing parents on how to demonstrate deliberate and calm speech, offer encouragement, and facilitate occasions for the kid to apply their speech abilities in everyday scenarios. It is crucial to involve the parents in the treatment plans to enhance the goals put in place and ensure consistent support to the child.

Additionally, SLPs work in partnership with staff members of a school to guarantee that the child's communication needs are met within the academic setting. Thus, there is a need for constant assessment and subsequent adjustment of the therapy procedures when managing stuttering. This includes monitoring the child's learning progress as well as evaluating the kind of changes that need to be made to the therapy plan. SLPs regularly evaluate the child's speech and language development over time in relation to therapy goals and modify strategies used to help the child progress. This guarantees that the treatment persists to be effective and flexible to accommodate the kid's changing needs.

The key tasks of SLPs include helping children develop confidence in their communication skills, among others. SLPs practice several procedures, and in each of the processes, they encourage the child to encourage the children to speak better and with confidence. The raised self-esteem is beneficial for influencing the child's social interactions, academic performance, and other aspects of life.

3.19 Role of Psychologists in Managing Stuttering

1. Addressing the emotional and psychological aspects: Stuttering can significantly affect a child's emotional and psychological well-being. Children afflicted with stutter may encounter emotions of anger, shame, and unease, which can have an impact on their self-worth and interactions with others. Psychologists have a vital role in addressing emotional and psychological issues related to stuttering. They equip the kid with the necessary tools and methods to effectively deal with the obstacles associated with stuttering.
2. Cognitive behavioral therapy (CBT) is one of the most common techniques applied to treat stuttering in therapy. CBT seeks to change the negative thought patterns and behavioral patterns associated with fluency disorder. Psychotherapists involve children in the change of thought patterns that negatively affect the ways of communication, which helps develop appropriate strategies for handling challenges and reduce anxiety and fear related to speaking. Face-to-face with real-life situations, CBT is used in

increasing children's ability to persevere and build confidence so as to improve their communication.

3. Therapeutic guidance and assistance: The use of counselling is helpful in providing psychological help to the children who have this problem of stuttering. Specialists in this field offer children a safe environment where they can share emotional and speaking concerns connected with stuttering. Individual or small group counselling may be used to discuss feelings, understand the child's experience, and learn ways to reduce their anxiety and anger concerning their stuttering. Besides, counselling gives young people the opportunity to get acquainted with others who have gone through the same experience, helping them to create a common purpose and support each other.
4. Family therapy and education: Consequently, stuttering has an influence on the child as well as on all members of their immediate family. Speaking with the parents of a child who stutters is a common task for psychologists, as they use family therapy and education to help the parents understand the impact of this disorder on the child's emotions and teach them how to be supportive in the right manner. Group therapy sessions can be useful in treating family aspects, if there are any, that are causing the child's worry or tension. Such sessions should help to develop constructive speaking between relatives and provide feasible strategies for creating a progressive home atmosphere.
5. Social skills training: Every child who is affected by this speech disorder may face some form of social dysfunction and may tend to avoid situations that require verbal interaction. Teachers and educational psychologists can play a crucial role in the process of providing the children with adequate lessons in social skills as they can help form adequate communication processes and boost the children's social self-esteem. This training may entail participation in role play, presentation on how to communicate, and the articulation of verbal skills in different social settings. Thus, enhancing children's social skills can lead to more confidence in social settings and situations.
6. Another revolutionary component that is usually incorporated in the stuttering therapy lessons is stress management and exercises, since stress is known to be a key factor in enhancing stuttering. Teachers inform kids in many ways and techniques to relieve stress and relax, such as deep breathing, being mindful, and progressive muscle relaxation. It is noted that such strategies can help to relieve children from the physical and psychological burden of stuttering, leading to the elimination of all the resulting negative changes and improvement of the general state and the quality of the spoken language.
7. Another goal of the work carried out in the subject area of psychological support is to help children become more resilient and have high self-esteem. Psychologists collaborate with children to cultivate a constructive perception of themselves, identify their aptitudes, and establish attainable objectives for their communication. Psychologists enhance children's self-esteem and fortitude, enabling them to confront the difficulties of stuttering with assurance and resolve.

3.20 Treatments for Stuttering

Behavioral therapies are the main treatment for stuttering, but drugs may be included in a comprehensive treatment strategy. Medications are typically used for severe cases of stuttering that have a major negative impact on a child's quality of life, and when other therapies have not produced satisfactory outcomes. It is noteworthy that the utilization of drugs for stuttering is relatively seldom and generally regarded as a final option. Several drugs have been investigated for the treatment of stuttering, including:

- Antianxiety drugs: These drugs can alleviate the anxiety and tension commonly associated with stuttering. Reducing anxiety levels in children may lead to a decrease in the frequency and intensity of their stuttering episodes. Frequently employed anxiolytic drugs comprise selective serotonin reuptake inhibitors (SSRIs) and benzodiazepines. Some antidepressants have been prescribed off-label to treat stuttering, especially when it is accompanied by notable anxiety or sadness. These drugs have the potential to enhance mood and alleviate anxiety, which may result in improved speech fluency.
- Antipsychotic drugs: In exceptional circumstances, antipsychotic drugs may be recommended for the treatment of severe stuttering. Since such drugs affect the neurological aspects of the illness, they may help to manage the neurological aspects of stuttering, which arise from the imbalance of dopamine in the brain. However, the administration of antipsychotics is usually limited because of the potential side effects of the intervention.

Taking drugs for stuttering opens the door to options like a decrease in anxiety, improvement of mood, and less severe stuttering attacks. However, these are some of the benefits that the human body gets to enjoy while using the drugs to enhance their performance and productivity. However, they come with probable risks and side effects. These side effects range from drowsiness, changes in body weight, to changes in behavior. The overdose of some drugs might cause dependency or other negative impacts when the usage of the medicine is continued for an extended period. In terms of the prescription of medication for a child who has a case of stuttering, consultation with a healthcare practitioner with a focus on pediatric neurology or psychiatry should be made. A thorough evaluation should be conducted with regard to medication provision and identification of the apt choice. Supervision is important when medicine is given to assess its effectiveness and monitor for unwanted effects. Adjustment in the dose or the type of drug used may be needed based on the reaction of the child to the drugs.

Thus, medication for stuttering should not be regarded as the single panacea for the problem. It should be used with behavioral therapy given by SLPs and psychologists in cases of disability. The combination of pharmacotherapy and psychotherapy approach might be more beneficial because it is capable of addressing both the neurobiological and behavioral aspects of stuttering. This proves that the formulation and integration of this extensive strategy can help enhance the efficacy of the treatment plan.

Parents and caregivers should therefore be involved in the decision-making process, especially in the administration of any medication for stuttering in their child. Discussing openly and honestly the likable features of the potential change, undesirable things that could occur, and other options, while talking to healthcare providers is very important. Getting consent on the therapy intervention is very crucial because it helps provide parents a detailed understanding of everything regarding the therapy as well as make them comfortable with the chosen therapy type.

3.20.1 Alternative Treatments

1. Support groups: Group and peer interactions are particularly helpful for young people with stuttering. Such groups ensure that young people have platforms where they can share their experiences, practice their speaking skills, as well as get support from people who understand them. It can be provided by an SLP, a psychologist, or any other trained person. On interaction with peers, children's self-esteem develops, leading to a reduction in feelings of seclusion, enabling the child to feel they are part of society.
2. Music and art therapy: Music and art therapy offer young people who stutter unique ways of self-communication and, as a result, improve their skills. Some elements of music therapy include singing, playing musical instruments, or rhythmic speech aimed at improving fluency and coordination. Art therapy helps the child to be able to express themselves emotionally/psychologically by mainly involving them in artwork like drawings, painting, and similar forms of artwork. Both forms of therapy possess the potential to reduce anxieties, enhance the ways of expressing one's feelings, and provide various ways of interaction.
3. Establishing good relaxation practices, like yoga, meditation, deep breathing, etc., can help the children manage the stress and anxiety that comes with stuttering. Such techniques help to have a break and sharpen senses, which can be helpful when endeavoring to pay more attention to breathing and speaking patterns in youngsters. Indeed, training one's mind to be mindful and/or practicing relaxation exercises can be beneficial as it may lead to better flowing speech and overall well-being.
4. Aids and technologies can help young people who stammer. By using speech generating devices (SGDs), children with severe stuttering can have a chance to be communicative and interact with others in some way. Also noteworthy is the fact that there are many applications as well as software tools designed to aid children in the task of improving their speaking skills and even their fluency. Thus, these technologies can be used in combination with traditional therapies to enhance the child's communicative skills.

Some families apply some integrated and supplementary therapies, including acupuncture, homeopathy, or even herbal treatment, as a technique for handling the stuttering. While these therapies have not been scientifically proven to be effective, the following families have found these therapies to be useful adjunct therapies. It is important to discuss with the doctors the impact of any of the nontraditional approaches being taken on any of the diseases, to determine whether it is safe and will not impede other forms of treatment. A comprehensive approach to managing stuttering in children requires the involvement of several therapists, where each therapist focuses and brings their expertise on specific dimensions of the disorder. SLP, a psychologist, and other related team members work together to establish an effective treatment program that addresses the child's speech disorder, social-emotional development, and other domains. The parents and caregivers can help a kid manage the challenges of stuttering, as well as the objectives connected with it, by seeking appropriate therapy and getting the necessary help.

3.21 Status of Stuttering in India

As common as stuttering is, its manifestations, perceptions, and management differ across cultures and economic status. Due to the diversity of languages, people's awareness about speech difficulties in India varies. Hence, it is necessary to understand all the particularities of stuttering to offer appropriate intervention.

3.21.1 Prevalence and Demographics

Stuttering currently affects more than 1% of the global population, with vast differences across regions and cultures (Sharma & Kumar (2016)). In India, a country of over 1.45 billion with 122 major languages exceeding 1500 with the inclusion of dialects, the aspects of stuttering occurrence and embodiment can be rather diverse. Praveen et al. (2011), in their study estimated the frequency of stuttering to be about 1%. This work recognizes that stuttering is more common in boys than in females, with the male-to-female ratio being approximately 4:1. The occurrence of stuttering differs significantly in different states and regions of India. Varghese et al. (2024) carried out a cross-sectional prevalence study on the urban districts of Karnataka. They revealed that the prevalence of stuttering in school-going children was 1.68% with a ratio of 2.4:1 among males and females, respectively. They found no significant association between socioeconomic status and linguistic structure on the prevalence of stuttering. Such differences can be attributed to differences in consciousness, healthcare facilities, and beliefs regarding speech disorders.

3.21.2 Age and Onset

Stuttering is normally seen from the age of two and may extend to 5 years. It had long been a conventional opinion in India that those who stammer should be allowed to recover from it without professional help. This cultural approach often leads to a late presentation of the child to seek help from a professional, owing to the cultural belief that the stuttering would reduce over time as the child grows older. However, by adopting the wait-and-see approach, the stuttering condition may be aggravated and may even get harder to manage. Over time, as it is recognized that stuttering may not improve naturally, the important time and opportunity for early intervention is lost, which might make treating the stuttering more difficult.

3.21.3 Cultural and Societal Perceptions

According to Indian Stammering Association, stuttering in India significantly reflects the cultural and societal beliefs and how individuals who stutter will be treated or how they will perceive themselves. Some of the consequences of stuttering include rejection, discrimination, and emotional challenges. There seems to be a lack of knowledge and awareness about stuttering in different parts of the country. Preconceptions about the causes of stuttering that can be subversive are rampant. For example, the assumption that stuttering occurs because of supernatural phenomenon or bad karma contributes to the formation of negative attitudes towards stuttering. The ways society perceives mental health and the support such patients can expect to receive from their culture or family have a significant impact on those who are more/less likely to ask for help and how much help they will receive. Stuttering has several untoward effects on an individual's psychological state, including reduced self-esteem, social anxiety, and depression. It is also common to find many Indian children who stutter, encounter severe bullying and harassment by fellow pupils in school, which augments their speech disorders and poor performance in academic activities. Adults who stutter may face discrimination in the workplace and may find it hard to remain employed. Pronunciation is a critical area of concern, and stammering is significantly affected by gender in the context of the Indian population. Self-focused attention and gender expectations have it that females who stutter may face more hurdles due to cultural norms and prejudices. Here, self-focused attention refers to a heightened awareness of oneself, specifically one's thoughts, feelings, behaviors, or physical sensations, often in social or performance-related contexts. In the context of stuttering, self-focused attention can lead individuals to become overly conscious of their speech patterns, which may increase anxiety and exacerbate dysfluencies. Cultural expectations and biases may impact women who stutter more strongly. Societal norms around female communication styles and expectations for smooth, fluent speech can intensify self-consciousness and social anxiety in women who stutter. This heightened self-awareness may lead to increased negative self-evaluation, further compounding difficulties in communication and social interactions.

3.21.4 Speech Therapy and Intervention Accessibility

As a rule, the availability of speech therapy is significantly higher in urban areas than in rural ones. Many big cities like Mumbai, Delhi, and Bangalore have clinics for speech and language therapy, which are conducted by a number of professionals. On the other hand, such clinics are often scarce in rural settings, thus making it difficult for people to get early and efficient assistance. The cost of getting speech therapy might well stand in the way of seeking help for many families in India. The civil facilities and the non-profit organization do their services free or at a concessional price, but self-paid and personal therapy sessions may be highly expensive. It has become possible in recent years to provide teletherapy and digital solutions to improve the supply of speech therapy.

However, even though the obtained results and the levels of knowledge in India are increasing, speech therapy remains a topic that is either considered socially unacceptable or taboo. Parents are highly hesitant to take their child for speech treatment; many of them do not bother to do so because of the social stigma and misconceptions surrounding it. Such cautiousness often persists until the challenges intensify. However, by then, early opportunities for intervention and action may have been lost. Resolving cultural issues and increasing awareness of the benefits derived from childhood intervention are critical for improving results for children who stammer.

3.21.5 Obstacles in Education and Employment

Stuttering presents certain challenges in learning and working processes that can be potentially disabling. The need to communicate in those situations might exacerbate the stuttering and, hence, affect the learning capability and career productivity. In a school environment, children who have been diagnosed with stuttering will find it hard to participate in any activity that involves the use of oral words, such as making presentations, reading aloud, and joining class discussions. Due to the rudimentary understanding and perception that educators have about the disorder, a child's academic performance can suffer. Studies (Erickson and Block 2013; Mulcahy et al. 2008) have shown that stuttering negatively impacts an adolescent or young adult attending a tertiary institution. Essays, oral exams, group debates or discussions, and even presentations are often rather difficult. It has emerged with time that students who stutter avoid taking classes and careers that require much speaking in a bid to avoid such challenges. A person with a speech disorder may suffer from discrimination in the employment sector, especially in promotions.

In general, students who stutter may experience challenges with reading, writing, and auditory processing of sounds and syllables, although their foundational skills in reading and writing, especially in the early stages, are often comparable to those of their peers. Teachers have observed that students who stutter tend to struggle more with words or syllables beginning with strong consonants. This difficulty does not typically stem from an academic learning issue but rather from the elevated anxiety associated with stuttering, which can impact their comfort and confidence during reading activities. This anxiety, often due to concern over classmates' reactions, can further affect fluency. Studies by Sami et al. (2025) found no significant difference between verbal IQ and performance IQ in children who stutter, suggesting that intellectual abilities remain within normal limits, similar to other children without speech impairments. While academic performance as a whole may not be significantly impacted, students with stuttering often face greater challenges in verbal subjects and activities, as noted by Pınarcık and Sarı (2013).

Advanced learners with stuttering in India have said that they suffered discrimination at workplaces, including being passed over for a promotion and unfavorable attitudes from employers and coworkers.

Counselling and support are crucial to improving the standard of living of those with a stammer. Some of the Indian groups and projects are involved with promoting awareness, helping those who have fluency disorder, and fighting for their rights. One such Indian organization is *The Indian Stammering Association (TISA)*, which is an organization dedicated to addressing and supporting individuals who experience speech impediments, especially associated with major or minor stuttering. TISA provides support groups, meetings, and information for those who stutter and their relatives. It also advocates for the rights of stammerers and tries to play a role in reducing prejudice to stammering. Social groups enable individuals who stutter to share with others, educate themselves and their peers, as well as practice their speech in a friendly environment.

Research has indicated that people with stuttering who participate in support groups derive a lot of benefits, including increased self-confidence and reduction of the psychological impact of stuttering (Manning 2010). Public awareness of stuttering is also very low, which indicates that there is a need to alter cultural perspectives and remove the stigma attached to this condition. Apart from this, TISA, along with other speech therapy centers, raises awareness through workshops, social media, and public events. According to Mehta et al. (2019), awareness programs play a big role in heightening the level of understanding and attitude toward stuttering in the public.

Government policies and activities play an important role in the provision of support and services to individuals affected by stuttering. India has brought out several regulations and distinctive initiatives for the benefit of people with speech difficulties, including people who stutter. The Rights of Persons with Disabilities Act (2016) provides general rights and safeguards for people with disability in India, including those having speech and language processing impairments. The legislation promotes equal opportunity in education and employment and permits the development and establishment of mainstream educational facilities for students and workplaces for persons with disability. The National Institute for Empowerment of Persons with Multiple Disabilities (NIEPMD), located in Chennai, offers different programs and services to individuals with disabilities, including speech therapy and rehabilitation services for individuals who stutter. Besides, it also undertakes research and training activities to improve the quality of the care and support offered to disabled persons. Lastly, the Integrated Child Development Services (ICDS) is a government-sponsored program that provides health, nutritional, and educational support to children and mothers. The program provides intense services to children who have demonstrated language and speech impairments with a primary focus on early identification and subsequent appropriate management of these conditions.

In conclusion, it is possible to say that cultural, sociological, and economical factors influence stuttering in India. While progress has been made in terms of raising awareness and opportunities for help, priorities and barriers exist in the attempts to change for the better and eliminate prejudice in access to these services. There remains a need to create a culture of inclusion by paying attention to the needs and challenges related to stuttering in India, in particular.

References

Alm PA. Stuttering: a disorder of energy supply to neurons? Front Hum Neurosci. 2021;15:662204. https://doi.org/10.3389/fnhum.2021.662204.

Ambrose NG, Yairi E. Normative disfluency data for early childhood stuttering. J Speech Lang Hear Res. 1999;42(4):895–909. https://doi.org/10.1044/jslhr.4204.895.

American Speech-Language-Hearing Association. Practice portal: fluency disorders. 2020. Retrieved from https://www.asha.org/Practice-Portal/Clinical-Topics/Fluency-Disorders/

Anderson JD, Wagovich SA. Relationships among linguistic processing speed, phonological working memory, and attention in children who stutter. J Fluency Disord. 2010;35(3):216–34. https://doi.org/10.1016/j.jfludis.2010.04.003. Epub 2010 May 6. PMID: 20831969; PMCID: PMC2939037.

Blood GW, Blood IM, Maloney K, Meyer C, Qualls CD. Anxiety levels in adolescents who stutter. J Commun Disord. 2001a;34(5):417–31.

Blood GW, Blood IM, Tellis GM, Gabel RM. Communication apprehension and self-perceived communication competence in adolescents who stutter. J Fluen Disord. 2001b;26(3):161–78. https://doi.org/10.1016/S0094-730X(01)00094-3.

Bloodstein O, Ratner NB. A handbook on stuttering. 6th ed. Clifton Park: Delmar Cengage Learning; 2008.

Carlson EB. Stuttering therapy: an integrated approach to fluency disorders. Pro-Ed; 2013 Boston, MA.

Chang S-E, Erickson KI, Ambrose NG, Hasegawa-Johnson MA, Ludlow CL. Brain anatomy differences in childhood stuttering. NeuroImage. 2008;39(3):1333–44.

Conture EG, Walden TA. Dual diathesis-stressor model of stuttering. In: Guitar SF, McCauley RJ, editors. Treatment of stuttering: established and emerging approaches. Philadelphia: Lippincott Williams & Wilkins; 2012. p. 49–72.

Davis S, Howell P, Cooke F. Sociodynamic relationships between children who stutter and their non-stuttering classmates. J Child Psychol Psychiatry. 2002;43(7):939–47. https://doi.org/10.1111/1469-7610.00093.

Erickson S, Block S. Peer relationships and stuttering in school-aged children. J Fluen Disord. 2013;38(1):45–59.

Guitar B. Stuttering: an integrated approach to its nature and treatment. 4th ed. Philadelphia: Lippincott Williams & Wilkins; 2013.

Guitar B. Stuttering: an integrated approach to its nature and treatment. 4th ed. Philadelphia: Lippincott Williams & Wilkins; 2014.

Ingham RJ, Cordes AK. On watching a discipline shoot itself in the foot. J Speech Lang Hear Res. 1999;42(4):879–82. https://doi.org/10.1044/jslhr.4204.879.

Iverach L, Menzies RG, O'Brian S, Packman A, Onslow M. Anxiety and stuttering: continuing to explore a complex relationship. Am J Speech Lang Pathol. 2011;20(3):221–32. https://doi.org/10.1044/1058-0360(2011/10-0091).

Manning WH. Clinical decision making in fluency disorders. Clifton Park: Delmar Cengage Learning; 2010.

Mehta K, Suresh R, Chandrasekhar M. Prevalence of stuttering among primary school children in Mysuru district: a cross-sectional study. J Indian Speech Lang Hear Assoc. 2019;33(1):5–9. https://doi.org/10.4103/jisha.JISHA_8_19.

Mulcahy K, Hennessey N, Beilby J, Byrnes M. Social anxiety and the severity and typography of stuttering in adolescents. J Fluen Disord. 2008;33(4):306–319. https://doi.org/10.1016/j.jfludis.2008.12.002.

National Institute on Deafness and Other Communication Disorders. Stuttering. 2010. Retrieved from https://www.nidcd.nih.gov/health/stuttering

Pınarcık Ö, Sarı H. Evaluation of newest facts on stammering according to the definitions. Karaelmas J Edu Sci. 2013;1:33–42. https://dergipark.org.tr/en/download/article-file/2160847.

Praveen BR, Deepthi R, Kumar K. Effect of speech rate on stuttering frequency. J Indian Speech Lang Hear Assoc. 2011;25(1):14–8.

Ramig PR, Dodge DM. The child and adolescent stuttering treatment and activity resource guide. Clifton Park: Cengage Learning; 2009.

Riley GD, Riley J. A revised component model for diagnosing and treating children who stutter. Contemp Issues in Commun Sci Disord. 2000;27:188–99. https://doi.org/10.1044/cicsd_27_S_188.

Sami R, Ramzy S, Tarek Orabi G. Assessment of verbal and nonverbal cognitive abilities in children with stuttering using 5th edition Stanford Binet. Appl Neuropsychol Child. 2025; 1–8. https://doi.org/10.1080/21622965.2024.2448009

Sharma R, Kumar A. Anxiety and avoidance behaviors in school children who stutter: an Indian perspective. J Child Adolesc Behav. 2016;4(3):213–9.

Sheehan JG. Stuttering: research and therapy. New York: Harper & Row; 1970.

Smith A, Weber C. How does a stuttering event come to pass? Evidence from neuroimaging studies. J Speech Lang Hear Res. 2017a;60(3):327–41. https://doi.org/10.1044/2017_JSLHR-S-16-0211.

Smith A, Weber C. How stuttering develops: the multifactorial dynamic pathways theory. J Speech Lang Hear Res. 2017b;60(9):2483–505. https://doi.org/10.1044/2017_JSLHR-S-16-0343.

The Indian Stammering Association. Resources. n.d. Retrieved from https://stammer.in/resources/

Tichenor SE, Yaruss JS. Stuttering as defined by adults who stutter. J Speech Lang Hear Res. 2019;62(12):4356–69. https://doi.org/10.1044/2019_JSLHR-19-00137.

Van Riper C. The nature of stuttering. Englewood Cliffs: Prentice-Hall; 1982.

Varghese AL, Devania P, Kunnath L, Balasubramanium RK, Bajaj G, Karuppali S, Bhaskaran U. Prevalence of stuttering among school-age children in Dakshina Kannada district of Karnataka, India. Clinical Epidemiology and Global Health. 2024;22:101327. https://doi.org/10.1016/j.cegh.2024.101327

Wagovich SA, Hall NE. Language ability and verbal diversity in children who stutter: changes over time. J Fluen Disord. 2010;35(3):222–31. https://doi.org/10.1016/j.jfludis.2010.04.003.

Wingate M. The structure of stuttering: a psycholinguistic analysis. New York: Springer; 1964.

World Health Organization. International statistical classification of diseases and related health problems. 10th ed; 1992. Retrieved from https://icd.who.int/browse10/2019/en

Yairi E, Seery CH. Stuttering: foundations and clinical applications. 2nd ed. Boston: Pearson; 2015.

Yaruss JS. Evaluating treatment outcomes for adults who stutter. J Commun Disord. 2001;34(1–2):163–82. https://doi.org/10.1016/S0021-9924(00)00049-6.

Yaruss JS. It's (almost) NEVER breathing in stuttering therapy! McKinney: Stuttering Therapy Resources; 2021.
Yaruss JS, Quesal RW. Overall assessment of the speaker's experience of stuttering (OASES): documenting multiple outcomes in stuttering treatment. J Fluen Disord. 2006;31(2):90–115.
Yaruss JS, Quesal RW. Overall assessment of the speaker's experience of stuttering (OASES): documenting multiple outcomes in stuttering treatment. J Fluen Disord. 2010;35(2):140–51. https://doi.org/10.1016/j.jfludis.2010.04.002.
Yaruss JS, Reardon-Reeves NA. Stuttering and the school-age child: practical ideas for treating children in schools. McKinney: Stuttering Therapy Resources; 2013.
Yaruss JS, Reardon-Reeves NA. Early childhood stuttering therapy: A practical guide. Stuttering Therapy Resources, Inc.;2007.

Understanding Stuttering in School

4

Abstract

The chapter discusses recognizing and managing stuttering in educational settings. It highlights the crucial role of teachers in the early identification and support of students who stutter. The chapter covers various age levels—preschoolers, school-aged children, and teenagers—and explains the signs and symptoms specific to each stage. Emphasis is placed on identifying red flags that warrant referral to a speech pathologist or psychologist. The chapter also elaborates on the psychosocial features of stuttering for school-age children and teenagers.

Keywords

Stuttering in school · Preschool children · School-age children · Teenagers Psychosocial impact

Stuttering is characterized by its variability, which means that the rate and severity of stuttering may be high at some times and low at other times. It is quite apparent when the child stutters at home and how he/she engages while stuttering at school. An understanding of these differences is critical for parents, teachers, and speech-language pathologists to work with the child who has a speech disorder involving repeated or prolonged production of certain sounds, syllables, or words.

Children who stutter often stutter relatively less at home, as it is more natural to them. Satisfaction with the comments that are supportive and empathetic from the adjacent persons of family will reduce the anxiety of the speaking member to speak fluently, which in turn will lead to lesser episodes of speech disruptions. A child may feel comfortable and have less interruptions, encouraging them to speak when around parents or siblings that do not criticize or scold the child. While speaking in front of an audience is challenging, there are other

R. Kaur, *Navigating Childhood Stuttering*,
https://doi.org/10.1007/978-981-96-6206-7_4

different challenges that are created by a school environment that can aggravate stuttering. The non-optimal conditions designating the protesting type of attitude are the fear of negative evaluation of the stutter, increased anxiety due to the expectations for greater verbal involvement, and presence of peers which may lead to more frequent and severe episodes of stuttering.

Children who stammer at the *school setting* may be more conscious and comparatively shy when speaking due to the embarrassment of their speech condition. The need to read aloud or answer questions, or participate in discussions that might arise, could be very demanding. This often results in increased levels of stress and development of struggling behaviors, which may include making faces, blinking of the eyes rapidly, or miming to clear a stuttering chord. However, interactions with peers as well as teachers in school, along with hindered or facilitated situations, can cause fluctuations in stuttering. Also, peer-related anxiety may lead to avoidance behaviors, instances where kids avoid speaking or participating in classroom activities with a hope of avoiding a stutter. These disparities explain the importance of understanding the specific characteristics of stuttering in a learning context to be able to provide proper support and intervention.

4.1 The Role of Teachers

Teachers are particularly in a core position of identifying which child is having a stuttering problem and supporting the child appropriately. A teacher's understanding and awareness of the condition can significantly impact the child's learning process and development. Several studies indicate that teachers often notice signs of stuttering in children in the number of repetitions, prolongations, or blocks in the class activities. By swiftly identifying these indicators, educators can accelerate appropriate referrals to speech-language pathologists for precise and detailed evaluation and intervention.

Additionally, the educators can enthuse a positive school environment that can minimize the anxiety and pressure associated with verbal communication. Measures like increasing the duration of reaction time, providing an option other than oral presentation to children who stutter, and promoting turn-taking can increase the comfort and confidence of children with stuttering issues in their overall experience of school. Teachers can also educate other peer groups of the child about stuttering. This further aids in changing people's attitudes toward the issue and reduce the chances of mockery. This aids in raising a culture of respect and inclusivity. By understanding and implementing these strategies, educators can positively influence the quality of life for children suffering from the effects of stuttering.

4.2 Societal Implications

Teachers play a critical role of influencing other cultural themes and policies concerning stuttering on behalf of their students. Professionals in the teaching fraternity, especially those who understand about children with stuttering, can help these children by advocating for them and by enlightening the school administrators, management, and other important persons regarding the special needs experienced by CWS. Such lobbying may lead to formulation of supporting policies or programs that will provide for accommodations for CWS. This includes speech therapy resources and services, teacher training, and education about stuttering and other.

Moreover, instructors can help expand the knowledge of people suffering from stuttering, by eradicating myths surrounding this condition and reducing discriminatory attitudes toward those who stutter. One of the ways teachers can influence parents, students, and the community about the people who stutter is by providing an inclusive environment for them in school. Such measures can lead to a more accepting society where children who stutter get equitable opportunities to grow to the best of their ability.

Moving deeper into the aspects of the identified attributes of stuttering in learning institutions, it is imperative to note that teachers play a highly significant role in the lives of children who stutter. Thus, it is vital for teachers to isolate the barriers which are inherent to stuttering and to work toward the positive outcomes of the students with the help of early identification of the students who stutter, creating the mentally conducive environment for these children and lobbying for conducive policies.

4.3 Stuttering Seen at Preschool Level

Preschool children are typically those who are between the ages of three and five. They are in the most important stage of speech and language development. Typically, children at this stage can communicate using whole sentences and retain a lexicon of around 1000–2000 words. They can express their thoughts and emotions, inquire about things, and participate in basic conversations. Preschoolers can acquire fundamental academic skills, such as letter and number recognition, understanding of time-based ideas (such as yesterday, now, and tomorrow), and learn to develop early reading abilities through storytelling and other interactive engagements.

In terms of speech requirements, preschool needs include active involvement in group conversations, rapid responses to inquiries, obedience to directions, and engagement with peers during both play and organized activities. Teachers anticipate that students will effectively convey their requirements, articulate their thoughts, and participate in social communication actively. Efficient communication is fundamental to acquiring knowledge, participating in social interactions, and promoting self-confidence. Hence, it is crucial for educators to acknowledge good speech and language development in this age group so as to detect any variations that could indicate the presence of stuttering.

4.4 Stuttering Severity in Preschool-Aged Children

While understanding the traits of stuttering among preschoolers, it is essential to identify the predominant degrees of stuttering at this developmental period. As mentioned earlier, stuttering can be classified as borderline, beginning, intermediate, and advanced. Each level corresponds to variable levels of severity and complexity.

At this preschool stage, children may largely experience *normal nonfluency*. Thus, at this level, it is common to display typical nonfluencies, and this majorly is a natural part of speech and language development. These normal dysfluencies are prevalent among children between 2 and 5 years and incorporate the repetition of complete words or phrases, interjections, or fillers and other blocks. These dysfluencies are less frequent and are marked by smooth, relaxed repetitions, and the children exhibit no evident physical strain or exertion.

Undoubtedly, teachers can distinguish between normal nonfluencies and stuttering-like dysfluencies by keenly observing the dysfluencies for their frequency, nature, and characteristics.

Normal nonfluencies are not very frequent and are found less than ten times per hundred words; they are usually fluent and non-tense. Stuttering is a disorder in which the frequency of disruptions that occur in spoken words is higher, including repetitions of parts of words, for example, "b-b-b-ball," prolongation of sounds, for example, "sssnake," and blocking which is often combined with tension and effort, as well as secondary movements, such as blinking or head movements. In addition, children who stutter may have signs of frustration or shame regarding their speech, a feature absent in children without speech disorders. By paying much attention to these attributes, the educators can quickly take note of the young people who may need further evaluation and help.

Borderline Stuttering: Children who stutter at the preschool age are usually in the borderline stuttering group. In this phase, stuttering is sometimes characterized by many repetitions and prolongations but without evident tension or struggle. Preschoolers with borderline stuttering exhibit the following characteristics:

1. Excessive Repetitions: Children may have a tendency of reproducing the sound, syllable, or word more than twice in one go. For instance, a child may say "b-b-b-ball" or "I-I-I want" when in a conversation.
2. Loose and Relaxed Dysfluencies: At this stage, the dysfluencies are characterized by the absence of muscular contractions or effort. The child may not show signs of discontent or even shame.
3. Limited Awareness: Most preschool children with borderline stuttering have little or no insight into their speech problems. A person who stutters need not exhibit signs of discomfort in the usual sense owing to their speech difficulty.
4. Incoherent Fluency: Stuttering could be inconsistent; that means that there will be periods of normal speaking and then there will be periods of stuttering. The variability might be due to differences in the child's level of arousal, fatigue, or stress.

5. Parental Concern: Parents may notice that the child is repeating things and prolonging them, but they may not notice much effect on their child's desire to speak or engage in activities.

Borderline stuttering is commonly the initial phase during which parents and teachers become aware of a child's speech difficulties. Identifying this at an early stage can be quite useful in preventing the advancement to more severe stages of stuttering.

4.4.1 Beginning Stuttering

Some preschool children may present some early signs of stuttering, in a way that they are in a borderline category of stuttering. The onset of stuttering is marked by increased muscular rigidity and increased awareness of speaking tasks. The features of initial stuttering encompass:

1. Accelerated and Irregular Repetitions: Repetitions accelerate and can be irregular. They may also involve changes in the speed of repetition. The child may say "b-b-ball" with increased speed and with more force when saying the word.
2. Prolongations and Blocks: Apart from the reduplication of phonemes, the child may also produce phonetic processes such as syllable prolongations, for instance, "ssss-nake," and phonemic omissions, where the child fails to produce sounds.
3. Physical Struggle: Some physical signs of effort, like facial grimacing, frequent blinking, or head movements, become more apparent. These acts imply that there is a lot of effort being made to use words to make a point.
4. Emotional Reactions: Children can have feelings of anger, shame, or anxiety toward their speech. They can have adverse reactions to their own speech interruptions.
5. Heightened Consciousness: As opposed to borderline stuttering, the kids with first stuttering are more conscious of their speech difficulties. This consciousness might lead to the development of secondary behaviors and the process of evasion of situations that include talking. Preschool stuttering is a sensitive period when it is most likely to address the speech problems and the feelings that go with the disorder. At this stage, speech therapy aims at decreasing physical strain and improving the way of communication.

4.4.2 Intermediate and Advanced Stuttering

Intermediate and advanced stuttering is rarely observed in preschool children, but it is possible when the stuttering becomes worse and there is no intervention or help. The severity of stuttering in these levels is higher, and there are severe emotional and social effects. It is defined by a higher frequency of the so-called avoidance behaviors, with the speaker actively trying to avoid certain words or speaking situations. Children can be under more physical stress and may have problems that are often characterized by the frequency of blockages and prolongations. Emotional reactions—fear and shame, for instance—become more significant. Normally, this level requires a lot of speech therapy and support to help manage the verbal behaviors and their related feelings.

Advanced stuttering is a rare condition that is not seen in preschool children to a great extent. It is more frequent in the elder children and teenagers. It includes very ingrained speech patterns, substantial impediments, and widespread avoidance tactics. The child at this stage may be very much aware of the fact that they are stutterers, a situation that leads to anxiety and may avoid interacting with other people. Moderate and severe stuttering calls for an extensive therapy that encompasses speech therapy alongside counselling. Children in the preschool toddlers' category who stutter are likely to stutter at the borderline or emerging stage. The aim of this article is to identify the signs and symptoms at these stages and the importance of early intervention to prevent the worsening of the condition and to improve a child's fluency.

4.4.3 Signs and Symptoms of Stuttering in Preschool

Knowing the signs and symptoms of stuttering in preschool-age children helps prepare the teachers and caregivers be in a better position to help the affected child. The following are the symptoms that should be noted by teachers so as to help the children:

1. Frequent Phonological Repetitions: The use of the initial sounds or syllables of words in a phrase, as in "b-b-b-ball."
2. Prolongations: The process of phonetic lengthening in which the time taken to articulate the sounds in syllables is increased as in the case of the word "sssssnake."
3. Interruptions are the absolute stoppages of speech, or temporary silences, which are known as blocks when a child cannot make a sound.
4. Physical Struggle: Visibly suppressing physical effort while presenting, for instance, squinting, blinking, or shaking the head.
5. Avoidance: A level of discomfort in engaging in speaking activities, for instance, not responding to questions or not contributing to group discussions.
6. Variations in Pitch or Volume: Swelling and thriving of pitch or volume when stuttering.
7. Negative Reactions: Shame, frustration, or discomfort through rejection in being able to express oneself when faced with struggles.
8. Inconsistent Fluency: The investigations of the fluency of speech, namely, the increase of the frequency of pause or hesitation, especially when the communication takes place in a stressful context or when there is a high level of pressure.
9. Utilization of Fillers: The use of the verbal time fillers including "um," "uh," or "er" to delay the start of speaking.

10. Self-correction is a process of trying to correct or restart a conversation because one feels that there is an error or have phrased it the wrong way.

4.4.4 Red Flags for Referral to a Speech Pathologist

If a preschool child displays any of the following warning signs, it is crucial to obtain an assessment from a speech-language pathologist:

1. Prolonged Stuttering: Otherwise defined as stuttering that lasts for more than 6 months without showing any signs of alleviation.
2. One can develop long-term stuttering if there is a family history of stuttering or other speech issues.
3. The child shows signs of anxiety, agitation, or discomfort in connection with speaking.
4. Excessive and Intense Dysfluencies: Many intense attacks of stuttering.
5. Manifestation of Bodily Strain and Struggle: Apparent physical signs of stress and effort in the course of speaking.
6. The child has avoidance behaviors and does not talk or avoids talking in certain situations for fear of stuttering.
7. Secondary Behaviors: Use of other strategies including eye blinking or head nodding as a way of coping with the stuttering.
8. Stuttering is having a negative impact on the child's social relations as the child is unable to communicate and join in group activities.
9. Stuttering is always there, irrespective of the context or situation.
10. Continual concern displayed by parents or teachers about the child's speech and developmental milestones.

The general teachers and caregivers can also help in the early identification of the preschool children who stammer, and support them, if they are well informed and conscious of the signs and symptoms. If early intervention is made, then it will greatly help in the child's development in terms of communication and in the overall quality of life.

4.5 Stuttering Seen at School Level

Difficulties that are related to stuttering in school-aged children are different from difficulties seen in preschool children. During their primary education and even in other subsequent classes, the demands for the children's communication skills are high. They are expected to engage in more elaborate and formalistic speaking tasks, such as group discussions and debates, and to express themselves eloquently. To help children through this, teachers should gain more insight into the characteristics of stuttering in children of this age in order to identify the children who stutter and to help them in the right way.

Children between 6 and 12 years of age, referred to as school-going children, are expected to have enhanced speech and language development as compared to the toddlers. At this level, children's vocabulary is generally larger, the structures of their sentences are more complex, and they are more articulate and expressive. It is for this reason that they can convey complex ideas, understand different grammatical structures, and be a part of deeper conversation.

Children of school-going age are required to do many speech-related activities as part of their schoolwork. These skills include reading aloud, participating in class discussions, answering questions, making presentations, and working in groups. Effective oral communication is important to excel academically and fit in socially. Teachers expect these children to be able to state their ideas in a specific manner, give proper reactions to prompts and questions in a logical and assertive manner, and interact with their peers and other people in general.

The speech needs in school are higher than in preschool. The current understanding of the young preschoolers' language development is that they learn through playing and simple verbal communication, but school-age children must deal with more structured and complex speech situations. Moving from one environment to another, particularly to the classroom, may be quite a challenge for children with stuttering because the demands and social interactions are much higher in this setting and thus may experience deterioration in their speech fluency.

4.5.1 Developmental Levels of Stuttering in School-Aged Children

While in childhood and attending preschool, natural speech disruptions occur very often, and it is usually difficult to distinguish stuttering from natural fluency. However, as the child grows older and starts attending school, the natural disruptions of speech are rare as compared to chronic stuttering. At this period, children who stutter can be classified into early childhood development or borderline stuttering type, less frequent, beginning, moderate, and advanced stuttering type, which is more significant.

1. Children in the initial phase of stutter are more noticeable in their stuttering as opposed to preschool children. These stutters are the short and unsystematic ones, the sustained ones, and those of blocks. Children also display signs of physical aggression, brain stress, and feelings like irritation or shame.
2. In the intermediate level of stuttering, children are more excessively likely to avoid certain phrases or speaking situations on purpose. The impact of psychological barriers of stuttering is seen basically in the form of increased fear and embarrassment. Muscle tension and the appearance of other reactions that occur simultaneously with the main tic are usually present.
3. More advanced stuttering that requires professional help is not as frequent in younger children but can be present in older youngsters. At this level, the degrees of difficulty

are very high, the patterns are very frequent, and the attitudes toward speaking are predominantly negative. Self-consciousness in children may manifest in complex evaluation of the stuttering condition and subsequent constant worry or withdrawal from social life.

4.5.2 Key Signs and Symptoms of Stuttering in School-Aged Children

The stutters that are manifested and the concomitant symptoms documented in preschool children are also exhibited by school-going children. However, the demand for verbal or spoken language alongside social expectations, especially inside a school, may add other challenges or even display other behaviors. Teachers should be cognizant of these symptoms, particularly in situations such as reading aloud, delivering oral presentations, taking oral exams, engaging in elocution, performing on stage, and responding to questions in class:

1. At this level, children who do stammer tend to present with more frequent repetitions, prolongations, and pauses while reading aloud in class. People may have problems when trying to start reading or have issues when coming across some terms, which can be reflected in the body as signs of tiredness.
2. They are likely to stumble or stutter more during oral presentation because of the self-induced pressure to speak fluently in the presence of their classmates. Repetitions can be rapid, and sounds can be sustained or appear as blocks, which are normally associated with signs of children's distress and their attempt to produce sounds with observable muscular strain.
3. With reference to the oral exam model, the child who stammers may find it difficult to answer questions on time. People may use onomatopoeic features such as hesitating and stammering, or they may use a lot of filler words like "um" or "uh," which are employed to gain much time.
4. It may be further worsened by elocution contests or stage performances, as a lot of these activities involve high levels of pressure and exposure. Very often, children may decide to exclude themselves from such opportunities altogether or, if they do participate, experience severe dysfluencies.
5. If children with fluency disorder are questioned in a classroom, they tend to delay, pause a lot, and stammer when answering. They will avoid putting up their hand or participating in talks so that they cannot be forced to speak in a way that stutters.
6. Apparently, in a group setting, children may show a tendency toward shyness or an increase in the stammering frequency, more so when it is their turn to speak. A concern of how other students will respond may even make their anxiety worsen and cause more stuttering.
7. Dyadic communication with peers and teachers in regular daily interactions can also become a way of paying attention to or drawing focus to stutters. For instance, children

may use strategies such as choosing to speak in simple words or even avoiding talking at all, to contain their speech difficulties.

4.5.3 Red Flags for Referral to a Speech Pathologist

There are specific red flags that teachers ought to be alert to when referring a student to an SLP. All the red flags described here resemble those of preschool kids and can also be used for kids attending school.

1. Continuous Stuttering: Subtle stuttering that occurs for a period that is over 6 months, and which shows no signs of easing requires professional attention.
2. Family History: The presence of family history of stuttering or some other speech disorder increases the likelihood of long-term stuttering.
3. The child has moderate to high level of anxiety or stress whenever he/she is to speak. This can be evidenced in actions like avoiding talking to others, not volunteering to speak in class, or physically reacting like sweating or shaking when it is their turn to speak.
4. Severe Dysfluencies: This is a term used to describe a massive instance of stutters where the instances of stutters and the intensity of the experience are rather high. These episodes include the two types of dysfluencies: the sound and syllable dysfluencies, which include the repetitions of sounds and syllables in word, and lexical dysfluencies, which include the repetition of words and the use of the filled pauses and long silent pauses. The severity is worse especially for events that involve pressurized speaking such as speaking in public or responding to questions in class.
5. Physical Struggle: Articulatory concomitants of physical tension and effort in speaking, namely, wincing facial expressions or other facial movements, frequent blinking, head motions, or any other continual movements supplementary to movement in the vocal tract that indicate considerable effort in speaking.
6. The child self-protects, avoiding talking and specifically avoiding certain speaking situations or words by regularly being inattentive or using many "umms" or not speaking at all. This includes not raising their hand to answer a question, not engaging in debate, guessing, or not engaging in activities that require the use of the mouth.
7. Secondary Behaviors: The use of passing movements of eyelids, inclination of the head or finger drumming, and other similar mannerisms in place of stuttering. These actions are attempts to get unstuck from a speech block or to reduce the stress that stuttering causes.
8. Stuttering causes a poor performance by the child in class and interferes with the child's participation in school activities. This includes the barriers that one may face while doing oral tests, doing group reading match activities, or presenting on finished books, mercy chores, etc., which lead to low academic accomplishment and less participation.

9. Dysfluencies are present constantly in different contexts and settings, or in other words, both in natural and seminatural communication. Thus, the results indicate that stuttering is not situational anxiety but a prevalent issue.
10. Parental Concern: Continuous self-uncertainty on the part of parents as to the child's use of language and development milestones. This may include the child's demonstration of disapproval or reluctance to speak or avoid social contact due to concern over stammering.

4.5.4 Red Flags for Referral to a Psychologist

1. Chronic Worry and Tension: Daily and chronic concerns and apprehension that are associated with speaking or interaction with other persons that do not resolve even after having gone through initial Speech therapy practices.
2. Depression or mood swings may present as a shift in one's mood, usually swinging from one extreme to another. The child may experience feelings of sadness, irritability, or loss of feelings and interest in what they previously enjoyed.
3. Behavioral Issues: Emergence of new behavioral challenges or any signs of escalation of existing issues linked to frustration caused by speech may signal deeper emotional or psychological struggles.
4. Social Anxiety: Social anxiety disorder is a more severe and chronic form of fear in social situations, leading to a high amount of avoidance behaviors.
5. Chronic Low Self-Esteem and Poor Self-Image: The youngster persistently remains vulnerable to feelings of helplessness or low self-esteem and so develops a negative self-image.
6. Academic Decline: Outward decline of performance in academic work that may not be solely due to stuttering, which may be triggered by some form of stress or an emotional or psychological ailment.
7. Bullying and Teasing: Persistent cases of bullying or teasing in areas, such as stuttering that cause emotional pain, require psychiatric help to build the child's ability to cope with such experiences.
8. Severe Social Anxiety or Isolation: Mental health disorder that significantly impairs functioning in the educational environment and makes it impossible for students to interact with their classmates, who then avoid any form of social interaction both in and outside the classroom.
9. Excessive Preoccupation with Stuttering: Preoccupations and obsessions with stuttering that are recurrent and distressing, which interfere with social, occupational, or other important areas of life and functioning.
10. If the child experiences a worsening of the stuttering as a result of family factors, there may be a need for a family counsellor or therapist to address problems that may affect all the members of the family.

4.6 Stuttering Seen Among Teenagers

Adolescence is a unique stage in the life of an individual where he or she experiences a series of changes in physical, psychological, and interpersonal development. These years are very important for the definition of personal identity and for setting up the bases of long-term communication. Teenage stammerers are often in a worse position than children because the demands made on their speech are higher in various learning and interaction environments. It is paramount for parents, teachers, and friends of the affected adolescents to learn more about the specific nature of stuttering as a way of helping the affected adolescents.

Youth are expected to engage in such forms of communication and interaction that are somewhat more complex than those of young children. They undertake discussions, group tasks, oral reporting, and class activities requiring effective and confident expressions. These activities are intended to develop the students' analytical skills, voice their opinions, and simplify complex concepts effectively.

Aside from the academic requirements, the adolescents also participate in cocurricular activities including drama clubs, debate societies, and sports, which often involve use of oral language. The social processes at high school are more subtle. The emphasis is made on forming deep relationships and navigating through social networks. It is important that efficient communication is had in such cases, and stuttering can hinder a teenager's ability to fully participate and express themselves confidently. Students are expected to take on more academic challenges as they go through middle and high school. Students are expected to deal with more complex material, complete a vast amount of work assignments, as well as prepare for various examinations. Stress and anxiety induced by the academic pressures can be quite intense and therefore increase the intensity of the stuttering condition. Oral assessment, such as tests, class attendance, and group work, are areas that require verbal communication, which adds to the stress prevailing among adolescents with a stuttering disability.

Adolescence is a period of the most significant changes in the body in connection with the beginning of sexual development. Hormonal changes may affect one's personality, the amount of energy one has, and one's temperament, which in turn determines the manner in which one communicates. Adolescents may develop increased levels of affective reactions, including increased anxiety or stress, which can complicate the state of stuttering. Physiological changes like the development of secondary sexual characteristics can also lead to self-consciousness and worries about one's looks, which, in turn, can worsen a teenager's confidence in verbal communication.

Adolescents are continuously engaged in the process of constructing their sense of self, actively investigating their personal identity, and seeking their place within society. This phase includes more interaction with peers, the pressure from peers, and the desire to be accepted by the peers. Stuttering can be detrimental to a teenager's interpersonal relationships, thereby affecting their social interactions, social development, overall social experience, and applying themselves in social situations as well as expressing themselves without ease. Auditory vagary and loneliness may be induced by the fear of being judged or being laughed at for the way one speaks.

The need for independence and autonomy is also another factor that affects personality development during adolescence. Stuttering is a speech disorder that affects adolescents and in turn they may lack the confidence to express themselves or even stand up for themselves, thus affecting their ability to deal with social and academic problems. The negative perception about stuttering may lead to feelings of shame and embarrassment, which lead to low self-esteem in young people thus affecting their mental health and well-being in the future.

4.6.1 Levels of Stuttering in Teenagers

In adolescent development, clients normally incur an intermediate or advance state of stammering. Adolescent stuttering can range from mild to severe where it causes various levels of interference with the activities of the adolescents. Although reaching an understanding of the different extents of stuttering may be helpful in identifying correct therapies and modes of support.

1. *Mild Stuttering*: Children with slight stammering may occasionally prolong phonemes or use a word, but such cases do not interfere with the communication ability of the child. Speaking situations might cause slight nervousness in some cases, and while a person might stutter, he/she does it efficiently without being much bothered by the stutter as it does not intrude with their tasks.
2. *Moderate Stuttering* is a type of stuttering that exhibits more often and more observable types of dysfluencies, including repetition, prolongation, and blocking. Young people at this stage can become anxious and overcritical, particularly in terms of how they are viewed by others and in academic situations. They might use coping strategies like the regularization of language use or failure to talk in certain conditions.
3. *Severe Stuttering*: In definitions of stuttering, severe stuttering is used to describe a situation where people stutter often and with great impact. Frequently experiencing pauses or displaying some level of physical endeavor in their speech that can include blinking or head movement. Those teenagers, who suffer from a severe stammer, can experience significant degrees of concern, loneliness, and difficulties in performing academic and social activities. As to the impact on their self-esteem and mental health, it might be rather profound.

4.6.2 Context-Specific Signs and Symptoms

As it is with school children who stutter, the signs and symptoms in teenagers are recognizable too. However, adolescents might face supplementary difficulties and take actions due to the increased verbal expectations and societal pressure.

Some of them include:

- Debates and Public Speaking: Stuttering often worsens when the person has to speak to an audience, because of the stress this causes. It can lead to one not going for discussions in debate or public speaking occasions.
- Oral Presentations: These are characterized by particularly distinct and long repetitions, prolongations, and blocks in the speeches. It is also seen that during interaction, adolescents are likely to use several blocks, fillers, as well as introductory phrases.
- Oral Exams: Multiple delays in the response, many stops during the performance, and corrections of the speaker.
- Timidness to take part in elocution contentions and theatrical displays. In case they decide to take part, then the extent of the condition known as stuttering will be aggravated.
- Classroom Questioning: Shyness or even refusal to go ahead and raise their hand or participate in a discussion.
- Group Discussions: Demonstrate a low level of contribution to discussions, often avoiding any speaking opportunities.
- Daily Encounters: They avoid informal conversations and interactions and become socially awkward or agitated and thus socially isolated.
- Bullying and Social Conflicts: Hence, teenagers who stammer are amongst the most vulnerable groups of children to bullying and other kinds of social difficulties. They may also get teased or scorned by their peers, hence developing more fear and isolation. The teenagers did establish that the existence of bullying makes stuttering become worse and leads to behaviors of avoidance and isolation. Thus, unpleasant experiences must be minimized by teachers and peers, making the environment more inclusive.

4.6.3 Intensification of Stuttering in Teenagers

Fluency disorder or stuttering, which may be observed during early childhood, can reoccur or become worse during the puberty stage. This occurrence can be confusing and distressing to adolescents as well as to parents of adolescents. It is essential to note that adolescence is a period of considerable changes, and, depending on the particular factors, this phase might be accompanied by the reemergence or aggravation of stuttering. These are the following risks of worsening of stuttering during adolescence:

1. It is possible that the onset of puberty will lead to changes in the brain and therefore decrements in aspects such as speech. These physiological changes might at times cause a *reemergence of a previous stutter* or indeed make a preexisting stutter become worse or manifest after a period of fluency has been achieved.
2. Academic stress is deemed to be high since adolescents' experience more significant social and academic pressure as social creatures. Stuttering might thus be worsened by the pressure to conform and the fear of being assessed. Stuttering may be elicited by

factors such as stress, for instance, while presenting an idea, during a social meeting, or while writing an exam.
3. Neurological Development: The brain of an adolescent is still in the developmental stage, particularly the part of the brain that regulates self-control and cognitive function. These transitional changes may cause changes in speech and the flow of words.
4. As people become adolescents, they become conscious of themselves and, therefore, sensitive to their own speech. This consciousness can in fact create a feedback negativity loop that leads to stuttering and further apprehension of stuttering.
5. The increase of speech frequency and complexity, in the course of adolescence, potentially increases the visibility of stuttering. For instance, during intricate social interactions, an adolescent is under a lot of pressure to produce clear language free from stutters.
6. Stuttering may develop, possibly due to the changes in the social dynamics of a particular culture. Subsequently, in later stages of childhood and subsequently, as social interactions grow and people become more concerned with what their peers think, they may experience greater stress to speak "perfectly." Ironically, this pressure results in an even higher amount of stuttering than when they are relaxed and there are a number of reasons for this.
7. Identity Formation: Teenagers are currently in a developmental phase where they are establishing their individual personalities. There is a conflict during this period because people who stammer may come to accept stammering as one of the characteristics of their personality or may view it as a disability. This could affect the rate at which stuttering occurs within the affected individual, although it is possible that this internal battle might merely manifest in psychological effects such as anxiety and/or depression.
8. Occasionally, stuttering may be limited by medical disorders, which appear as the side effects of drugs consumed during adolescence.

4.6.4 Red Flags for Referral to a Speech Pathologist

1. Prolonged Stuttering: Eventually, the adolescent is characterized to present a stammering of certain words that lasts for a period of not less than six consecutive months with no signs of recovery. This covers episodes of repeating, extending and/or interrupting speech patterns which in various contexts hinder the flow of the communication process.
2. Severe Dysfluencies: Severe and severe/paroxysmal stuttering, especially when the speaker is to speak before an audience, make oral presentation, or attend a social event. This includes strong somatic expressions of fight, including facial tension and movements that go along with it (e.g., eyelid flutters, head nods).
3. The teenager exhibits intentional de inhibitory behaviors, for instance, the teen consciously avoids speaking situations so that they do not stutter or even avoids certain terms that the teen knows they stutter on. This may mean not participating in class

discussions and arguments, not submitting oral assignments, or using nonspecific words such as "um" and "er" to prolong discussions.

4. The academic record of individuals who stutter exposes the significance of the impact that this disorder has on the academic performance of the teenager. Stuttering results in an inability to take part in oral exams, read aloud, actively contribute to group discussions, or presentations resulting in a drop in the person's performance, and they will not be as involved in class activities as they used to be.
5. Continuous concern formulated by the parents, teachers, or caregivers focusing on the teenager's speech activity and developmental achievements: This includes the awareness of the variety of signs of the teenager's current mood as being annoyed, not willing to communicate, or changes in the conduct which are known to be linked with the speaking ability.

4.6.5 Red Flags for Referral to a Psychologist

1. A child develops persistent fear and agitation, and these are related to the task of speaking or social scenarios. In addition, these symptoms do not seem to get better even after the first attempt at speech therapy. Such symptoms may entail panic episodes, the shunning of social activities, or great amounts of anxiety when speaking is required.
2. Melancholy or Mood Swings: Signals of depression or recurrent changes in mood, for example, constant outbreak of feeling sad, becoming easily irritated, loss of interest in performing activities, and changes in eating and sleeping patterns, all of which may be attributed to the emotional impact of stuttering.
3. Behavioral Issues: The manifestation of aggressive behaviors, oppositional, or defiant behaviors; withdrawal from students' usual activities; and overall mood changes may be attributed to the feelings of frustration that often accompanies stuttering. Examples are misbehavior at school or at home or having some difficulties in interacting with peers and family members.
4. Vulnerable poor self-regard and negative self-image are evidenced by the teenager who often complains of feelings of hopelessness, worthlessness, and guilty feelings for stammering. This can be observed, for instance, in the form of self-seclusion or unwillingness to engage in activities that are new to them.
5. Adolescent who experiences bullying or teasing because of their stammering are often left with a problematic state of emotions and generally need a psychologist. This ranges from school phobia, refusal to attend social functions, and significant change in behavior or mood due to negative peer relations.

Therefore, it is important to identify the need to refer teenagers who stammer to speech pathologists and or psychologists so that they can be helped as soon as possible. Proper and detailed help can hence respond to both the speech and the emotional problems, helping teenagers to develop efficient speaking abilities and to improve their well-being. Thus, it is crucial to name these signs, so parents and educators would be able to provide teenagers with the required amount of care and attention they need.

4.7 Psychosocial Features of Stuttering for School-Age Children

Stuttering is more than a disorder of fluency; it has severe psychological and social implications for children who stammer. Understanding of these psychosocial factors is vital to parents and teachers to help children in regard to their education and environment. This section provides comprehensive review of the psychosocial factors associated with stuttering among school-going children.

4.7.1 Emotional Impact of Stuttering

Stuttering in school-aged children might result in many emotional problems. Several researchers have highlighted the high prevalence rate of negative effects including anxiety, irritation, and embarrassment, among students who stammer. These styles of thought and such unpleasant feelings normally intensify during puberty. Craig et al. (2003) have investigated children who stutter and found out that they show high levels of social anxiety compared to their peers who do not stutter. It often stems from one's fear of getting low grades and the anticipation of having a stutter in social settings. The study found that this worry may lead to avoidance behaviors and children may stop speaking in class or engaging in activities where they fear they may start stuttering

Blood et al. (2001) also examined the pattern of emotions in children who stutter and noted that such children fully experience increased frustration and humiliation. They can develop negative emotions about themselves and their self-worth, which harm their self-image and self-perception. The study done on the characteristics of stuttering, therefore, indicated that the chronic nature of this diagnosis could lead to a cyclical pattern of negative feelings where the anxiety about stuttering has the impact of making the speech dysfluency even worse, leading to an increase in unpleasant feelings.

4.7.2 Social Impact of Stuttering

Difficulty in speaking has severe implications for social life, since a child may have difficulties in making friends and being understood by other children. A child who stammers is socially handicapped, and there are long-term consequences for the social status of the child. Research conducted by Langevin et al. (2009) shows that kids who stutter receive more bullying and teasing than their peers, who do not experience stuttering. This study showed how bullying affects social relationships, since CWS may tend to avoid interacting with other pupils to avoid being bullied. The researchers also emphasized the importance of a supportive school environment that could prevent such cases of exclusion and bullying. Erickson and Block (2013) paid much attention to the impact of stuttering on peer relationship. By own experience as well as through findings of other researchers, Davis et al. (2002) noted that young people with speech disorders often face difficulties in initiating and maintaining friendships because of stuttering. This may lead to feelings of loneliness and social exclusion. The study also found that fostering positive attitudes and understanding from fellow students improved the social interactions of students who stutter.

4.7.3 Academic Impact of Stuttering

Stuttering also comes with effects touching on a child's academic performance as well as participation in other school related activities. Stuttering fear may lead to negative attitudes toward speaking assignments, this in turn limits a child ability to demonstrate what he/she has learnt and his/her engagement in the class. Guitar (2013) studied the impact of stuttering on the performance of a child and discovered that children who stutter were more likely to avoid certain tasks and therefore could not read out in class, answer a question in front of the class and/or present before the class. Exempting or avoiding particular activities results in poor academic performance and poor contribution to the class discourse. In their study, Guitar (2014) outlined that teachers should provide suggestions and aim for equity in class to help CWS.

In their research, Yaruss and Reardon-Reeves (2002) looked at the academic performance of children who stutter and found that these children tend to perform worse in areas that call for speaking aloud. Hence, the study prioritized early identification and interventions, such as Individualized Education Plans (IEP), in enhancing the learning of children who had stuttering difficulties. The researchers suggested that speech treatment in association with classroom accommodations can significantly promote youngsters' academic outcomes.

4.7.4 Psychological Impact of Stuttering

The psychological effects of stammering do not stop with the dramatic emotional and social effects that are associated with the condition. Long-term psychological outcomes include constant fear, low mood, and feelings of low self-worth. Both Craig and Tran (2005) conducted longitudinal assessments of children with the aim of monitoring factors of psychological health of people who stammer from childhood to adulthood. The study established that there is a significant possibility that people who stutter experience anxiety and instances of sadness than people who do not stutter. According to the study, there is a necessity for early, more focused and consistent psychological support to help kids with stuttering develop appropriate coping mechanisms and improve their psychological health in the future.

Smith et al. (2014b) studied the self-esteem of children and stuttering. During the study, it was established that the child with speech disorder, particularly those who stutter, lose self-esteem because of their disorder and the challenges that they encounter in their social interactions. The study stressed the need to develop a "circle of care" for children who stammer, which included their family, teachers, peers, and such individuals to ensure that their self-esteem and confidence was boosted.

4.7.5 The Role of Family and Teachers

The major support and care offered by family and teachers play an important role in offering the children who stammer solutions for managing the psychosocial challenges arising from the disorder. Several socioeconomic studies have postulated that a *tender embrace* has a role to play in reducing the nasty impacts of stuttering. Manning and DiLollo (2017) discussed the role of family support in the processes, which concern children with speech disorders. In a number of studies that have been conducted, it has been illustrated that when families provide emotional support and encouragement to their children, this helps the children to be more capable of coping with the challenges that come with stuttering. According to the study, the education that parents should be given is regarding stuttering and the necessary tools that they should have to effectively help their children.

In the same study, the authors stressed the role of teachers in supporting students' learning among children with a stammer. This study revealed that the organization of classroom environment by teachers with special knowledge in stuttering can greatly improve the educational interactions of these children. The researchers noted that teachers should be trained in how best to support children who stutter and the right methods that can be employed to ensure that such children participate in classroom activities.

4.7.6 Peer Support and Social Inclusion

Peer support and friends are essential in the social integration of children with stuttering disorder and should be encouraged. According to research, the enjoyment of pleasant interaction with peers has been found useful in reducing the damaging impact of stuttering and enhancing social acceptance. Murphy et al. (2007a) explored the efficacy of the peer support programs for children with stuttering difficulties. From the research, they established that peer support groups provided a safe haven for youths to share experiences and thus build on their confidence in their interpersonal communication skills. Furthermore, they help in the dissemination of knowledge and understanding of stuttering among classmates, hence creating a friendly learning environment.

Conture and Walden (2012) examined the relationship between social inclusion and children diagnosed with a speech disorder that involved stuttering. The findings showed evidence that youths who feel accepted by their peers have low levels of social anxiety (SA) and high levels of social acceptance and relationship participation (SARP), thus encouraging them to participate more in school functions. The study also brought to light the importance of giving policy and program support in schools to support and encourage the kids to embrace diversity.

Consequently, the psychosocial dimensions of stuttering in children and adolescents of school-going age are complex and multifaceted. Stuttering can impact the child in terms of personal, social, and academic performance, as well as the mental and emotional aspects of the child. In this case, it is pertinent for parents and teachers as they assist children who stutter to have a full understanding of these effects at an individual level.

4.8 Psychosocial Features of Stuttering Among Teenagers

Stuttering, as mentioned earlier, may progress or become worse during the period of adolescence, resulting in observable psychological distress. Adulthood is marked by gender-specific physical, sexual, and psychological transformations that may exacerbate the difficulties seen in young people who stammer. Thus, the knowledge of the psychosocial impact of stuttering for teenagers would be beneficial for parents, teachers, and peers to provide adequate support to such children.

4.8.1 Emotional Impact of Stuttering

Stuttering is manifested in increased emotional problems among adolescents who already have such tendencies. Such ones include higher levels of anxiety, frustration, shame, and lower levels of self-esteem.

- Anxiety and stress: Young people suffering from stuttering often have higher degrees of social phobia. The kind of anxiety exhibited here is mainly due to the anticipation of negative evaluations and adjustment of expectations to include shyness in social encounters that results in speech difficulties, hence the use of avoidance strategies. Studies revealed that people with stuttering in their teenage years have a high risk of suffering from social anxiety disorder (SAD) and generalized anxiety disorder (GAD) (Craig et al. 2003; Smith et al. 2014a, b). Adolescent anxiety disorders can reduce the quality of life and impede simple social contacts and school performance.
- Experiencing frustration and shame: The struggle to speak fluently goes on, and it is accompanied by feelings of frustration and embarrassment. Often, adolescents tend to internalize the negative responses of their peers, and it may lead to the deterioration of their self-esteem and confidence levels (Blood et al. 2001; Stamurai 2020). This may result in the students, especially the disabled, avoiding the act of speaking in class or mingling with other students, thus the feeling of exclusion increases.

4.8.2 Social Impact of Stuttering

The social impact of stuttering is described as severe since the ability of teenagers with this speech disorder to form and maintain relationships is impaired; hence, they experience loneliness.

- Bullying and taunting: Children and youth who stammer are more vulnerable to acts of retaliation such as teasing and being bullied. Negative social experiences may lead to individuals avoiding social interactions and hence avoiding going to school or social events. Research has shown that the adolescent stuttering individuals experience increased levels of social rejection and negative peer perceptions that critically affect the child's social functioning in the future (Langevin et al. 2009; Ghai and Mueller 2021).
- Maintaining friendships: Peer relationships are cited to be challenging to youth who stutter, more so when it comes to forming friendships. Stuttering problem ensures that an individual does not organize themselves to speak during events or fail to attend some events because of fear that they will stutter. Such a concern can lead to feelings of loneliness and social isolation (Erickson and Block 2013; Stamurai 2020). Intentional relations with other people are crucial for developing competency in interpersonal relations, and the deficiency of such interactions may impede the development of proper relatedness.

4.8.3 Academic Impact of Stuttering

Stuttering can considerably impact the learning ability of an adolescent in school, especially when used in carrying out tasks that require speech.

- Avoidance of speech tasks: Students who stutter tend to avoid speaking tasks often or perform those tasks less frequently than their peers because of stuttering. Failure to attend class may lead to lower quality in class work and poor involvement in class work. Teachers have a central role in identifying such patterns of avoidance and providing necessary support to foster their participation (Guitar 2014; Stamurai 2020).
- Decreased scholastic achievement: It has been reported that fear of stuttering may cause developmental and academic difficulties in adolescents. Studies have shown that those youths who stutter may have lower grades in areas of learning that require some level of verbal interaction. This emphasizes the importance of early focused intervention and special education approaches that may help these students (Yaruss and Reardon-Reeves 2002; Stamurai 2020).

4.8.4 Psychological Impact of Stuttering

The consequences that stuttering has on the psychological aspect are numerous and include chronic anxiety, sadness, and low self-esteem. Therefore, it would be possible to feel hopelessness due to the constant struggle with stuttering and other challenges faced in interactions. The signs of this state can include disinterest in social activities, shift of the sleeping schedule, irritation, and frustration. These symptoms of depression can significantly harm the overall quality of life in an adolescent in the long run (Craig and Tran 2005; Stamurai 2020).

It is a common characteristic of adolescents who stutter to develop a negative perception of themselves due to their speech difficulty, causing poor self-esteem and negative self-perception. A negative self-perception may also develop with a decline of self-esteem that, in turn, can be reinforced by negative reactions of others. It can persist through childhood, adolescence, and effectively to adulthood, significantly affecting the individual at a personal level as well as in professional life (Smith and Weber 2017; Stamurai 2020).

4.8.5 The Role of Family and Teachers

Family and teacher support is highly relevant if teenagers who stammer have to cope with the psychosocial challenges of their difficulty.

- Emotional support is required from family members as they are the close ones who are mostly involved in the support of the patient. Parents may assist through the creation of a supportive and understanding environment within the home, encouraging open communication, and seeking professional help if needed. They give parents information and resources that will enable them to meet the needs of the child with regard to stuttering (Manning and DiLollo 2017; Stamurai 2020).
- Support for teachers: Specifically, the position of teachers is significant since they are the main pillars of support for teenagers who stutter at school. To a certain extent, teachers can reduce the stress linked with speaking responsibilities: establishing a classroom environment that is friendly to students who stutter, as well as adopting specific strategies such as providing extra time for speaking or offering other methods of speaking in their classes. There is a need to give training to the instructors in the identification of requirements of students with a stammer with a view of how to handle them appropriately. This training is essential for the academic as well as social development of these kids (Healey et al. 2007; Stamurai 2020).

4.8.6 Peer Support and Social Inclusion

Ensuring the children's social incorporation and providing support to one another are vital for the adolescents' social and emotional growth when they stutter.

- Self and mutual support allows the teenager to willingly share one's experience and, at the same time, improve their communication, thus increasing their confidence. These groups also play a role in helping spread knowledge and understanding among fellow students and in the process create a more welcoming environment for all students around them (Murphy et al. 2007a, b; Stamurai 2020).
- Promoting social inclusion: It is important to advocate for courtesy and understanding in school settings as the negative consequences can be more pronounced when teenagers with a stutter are involved in social engagement. Early intervention measures and programs that pursue and promote social inclusion help reduce instances of bullying and social exclusion and thus enable these children to fully participate in a number of school activities (Conture and Walden 2012; Stamurai 2020).

References

Blood GW, Blood IM, Maloney K, Meyer C, Qualls CD. Anxiety levels in adolescents who stutter. J Commun Disord. 2001;34(5):417–31.

Conture EG, Walden TA. Dual diathesis-stressor model of stuttering. In: Guitar SF, McCauley RJ, editors. Treatment of stuttering: established and emerging approaches. Lippincott Williams & Wilkins; 2012. p. 49–72.

Craig A, Hancock K, Tran Y, Craig M. Anxiety levels in people who stutter: a randomized population study. J Speech Lang Hear Res. 2003;46(5):1197–206. https://doi.org/10.1044/1092-4388(2003/093).

Craig A, Tran Y. Chronic and social anxiety in people who stutter. Adv Psychiatr Treat. 2005;12:63–8. https://doi.org/10.1192/apt.12.1.63

Davis S, Howell P, Cooke F. Sociodynamic relationships between children who stutter and their non-stuttering classmates. J Child Psychol Psychiatry. 2002;43(7):939–47. https://doi.org/10.1111/1469-7610.00093

Erickson S, Block S. Peer relationships and stuttering in school-aged children. J Fluen Disord. 2013;38(1):45–59.

Ghai B, Mueller K. Fluent: an AI augmented writing tool for people who stutter. In: Proceedings of the 23rd International ACM SIGACCESS Conference on Computers and Accessibility (ASSETS '21) ACM. 2021. p. 1–8. https://doi.org/10.1145/3441852.3471211

Guitar B. Stuttering: an integrated approach to its nature and treatment. 4th ed. Lippincott Williams & Wilkins; 2013.

Guitar B. Stuttering: an integrated approach to its nature and treatment. 4th ed. Lippincott Williams & Wilkins; 2014.

Healey EC, Gabel RM, Daniels DE, Kawai N. The effects of self-disclosure and non-self-disclosure of stuttering on listeners' perceptions of a person who stutters. J Fluen Disord. 2007;32(1):51–69.

Langevin M, Bortnick K, Hammer T, Wiebe E. Teasing and bullying experienced by children who stutter: toward development of a questionnaire. J Speech Lang Hear Res. 2009;42(2):154–71.

Manning WH, DiLollo A. Clinical decision making in fluency disorders. 4th ed. Plural Publishing; 2017.

Murphy WP, Yaruss JS, Quesal RW. Enhancing treatment for school-age children who stutter I: reducing negative reactions through desensitization and cognitive restructuring. J Fluen Disord. 2007a;32(2):121–38. https://doi.org/10.1016/j.jfludis.2007.02.002.

Murphy WP, Yaruss JS, Quesal RW. Enhancing treatment for school-age children who stutter II: reducing bullying through role-playing and self-disclosure. J Fluen Disord. 2007b;32(2):139–62.
Smith A, Weber C. How stuttering develops: the multifactorial dynamic pathways theory. J Speech Lang Hear Res. 2017;60(9):2483–505. https://doi.org/10.1044/2017_JSLHR-S-16-0343.
Smith A, Goffman L, Sasisekaran J, Weber-Fox C. Language and motor abilities of preschool children who stutter: evidence from behavioral and kinematic indices of nonword repetition performance. J Fluen Disord. 2014a;41:22–40. https://doi.org/10.1016/j.jfludis.2014.05.003.
Smith KA, Iverach L, O'Brian S, Kefalianos E, Reilly S. Anxiety of children and adolescents who stutter: a review. J Fluen Disord. 2014b;40:22–34. https://doi.org/10.1016/j.jfludis.2014.01.003.
Stamurai. Stuttering therapy app. 2020. Retrieved from https://stamurai.com/.
Yaruss JS, Reardon-Reeves NA. Stuttering and the school-age child: practical ideas for treating children in schools. J Fluen Disord. 2002;27(2):203–15.

Understanding Stuttering at Home

5

Abstract

The section *Understanding Stuttering at Home* explores the impact of the home environment in significantly influencing the onset, persistence, and management of stuttering. Similar to the previous chapter, this section recognizes and emphasizes stuttering but focuses specifically on the home environment. It highlights the crucial role of parents and family members in identifying stuttering and improving the quality of life of children who stutter. The section also provides research insights on understanding the impact of the home environment on stuttering.

Keywords

Stuttering at home · Variety of environments · Family composition · Situational triggers Role of parents

It is often mentioned that stuttering occurs in schools and other public and academic environments but the role of home environment for the emergence, manifestation, and therefore, regulation of stuttering is crucial. In the household, interactions with other family members, the presence of persons who have an authoritative position, and the emotional climate can influence the frequency and the severity of stutters. Foreigners, close ones, friends, and teachers should clearly understand what characteristics of stuttering are shown in a domestic environment. This knowledge assists them in the process of providing proper help and setting a proper attitude toward children who stutter.

The nature of the change in the stuttering process is such that it is extremely changeable as a regular feature and even more so within the framework of one's own home. The degree and frequency of stuttering might depend on several circumstances, such as the existence of members of relatives, the kind of conversation, and the emotional state of the person.

R. Kaur, *Navigating Childhood Stuttering*,
https://doi.org/10.1007/978-981-96-6206-7_5

5.1 Variety of Environments

Stuttering is less severe when the child or the adult is in familiar environments. Kids may realize they stutter less at home than at school because they are less stressed or maybe more familiar with the environment they are in. In contrast, individuals may experience a higher rate of stammering in parental or sibling company, or when referring to relatives, owing to social pressures.

5.2 Family Composition

Stuttering can be influenced by the structure of one's family. Children might experience different stuttering frequencies, depending on their interlocutors' attitudes. For instance, a calm and encouraging demeanor from family, for example, from mothers or siblings, may lessen stuttering. However, authoritarian or critical remarks from family members, such as from a strict father or a critical grandma, can increase the stuttering.

5.3 Conversation Type

There is a great variation in stuttering, depending on the kind of discussion taking place. Small talk, casual conversations, and conversation on topics other than those that are anxiety-evoking will cause the individual to stutter less. On the other hand, topics that involve argumentation, performance assessment, problem-solving, or discussing issues that the child may regard as sensitive or that invoke high energy states will result in increased stuttering.

Stuttering also depends on the emotional aspect. Both children and adults make higher frequency of stutters whenever they find themselves in a stressing situation. Discourse related to a problematic area or when the speakers are disputing something increases emotional pressure and thus the level of speech dysfluency.

Stuttering may be a hindrance when it comes to speaking at public events such as parties or any related social events. Stuttering becomes more probable in situations where the listeners' number is higher. The attitude of the listeners to the speaker is also important. When one is speaking in front of a large congregation or when they are in a position where they have to engage in conversations in public, there is always that pressure, which pushes the person to enunciate every word, and that is when the stuttering becomes worse.

The perception of people in the family can determine the extent, frequency, and how severe the child's stuttering is. It is commonly known that children are influenced by their parents, and thus authority and pressuring style of child-rearing often contribute to the high number of children who stutter. A strict father or any dominating role model at home can set up an environment of high pressure and stress. Some children feel anxious or dreadful about their fluency of speech since stuttering results from fear of making mistakes. Persistent pressure to attune to the expectations of fluent speech without making any errors will increase the rate of speech dysfluency. In the same way, if parents set higher standards for the child or make unsavory remarks regarding the kid's performance, the child's stress level may rise. The above anxiety stems from the pressures of having to meet these expectations as the child experiences the fear of failing and therefore disapproval. Essentially, children living in communication-restrained families or, more specifically, families where communication is dominated by authoritative people who demonstrate poor empathetic or supportive behavior may have more problems regarding stuttering.

Studies show that a child's speaking ability is often hindered by a nonempathetic or supportive environment. Secondly, the attitudes of the authoritative members of the families where the child is from might also influence the child's emotional reactions that characterize the disorder. When a youngster comes to understand that their stuttering is eliciting either disappointment or annoyance from their parents, this can heighten their stress levels and make for an even worser speech difficulty. To overcome the impact of authoritarian parents or other authoritative figures in the familial environment, one has to create an environment that will make the child feel safe and understood. Promoting open conversations, being encouraging in the right way, and helping to remove pressure from the stuttering can help in easing the child and managing the dysfluency.

5.4 Situational Triggers for Stuttering

There are situations that can trigger stuttering and make it worse. These triggers often occur during stressful, emotionally charged, or major life events.

1. All the stress and pressure resulting from tests and academic performance can greatly worsen the symptoms of stuttering. The existence of phobia toward failure and the use of strict rules and high standards for the learners may lead to the creation of an environment that is full of stress, leading to increased dysfluency. Trigger topics can include grades, performance, or future academic endeavors.
2. Delicate Conversations: Some of the matters that are sensitive may include relationship issues, peer pressure, or personal issues, and it is especially challenging for teenagers. These conversations may become quite charged and therefore may increase the speakers' anxiety levels and, thus, stuttering frequency. For instance, issues to do with relationships, friends, or even problems with fellow students may be compelling without resulting in more off-task talk.
3. Family quarrels or even simple discussions might cause stress for all the members included. However, it is even worse for people who stutter. Thus, the emotional state of an individual during an argument may lead to increased severity of stuttering, due to difficulties in speaking during stressful situations.

4. Oral presentations, as well as social functions, can be nerve-wracking for individuals who have a stutter. The fear of social evaluation, or simply the possibility of committing mistakes in public, increases anxiety and, therefore, the severity of stuttering. Public speaking may be quite challenging in any case, but interactions that incorporate oral presentations within the family or at school or other community gatherings might be particularly challenging.

5.5 Research Focusing on Understanding the Impact of Home Environment on Stuttering

Research carried out to establish the effects of the home environment on stuttering is quite informative. All these works stress the importance of support and understanding in the management of stuttering.

In a study by Craig and colleagues (2003), a clear relationship was identified between the structure of the family and the degree of stuttering in children. The analysis indicated that the children who were exposed to higher levels of parental pressures and criticism had a higher tendency of manifesting severe stuttering.

Unfortunately, the children who received positive reinforcement and help from their parents had fewer speech disruptions. Yairi and Ambrose (2005), in their research, sought to examine the effects of parental attitudes on the emergence of stuttering. It was therefore observed that children whose parents displayed affirmative and tolerant behavior had improved skills to deal with their stuttering. This was because research found that parental support plays an important role in the creation of a supportive environment for children with a speech disorder that is characterized by stuttering and pausing.

In their rejoinder, Manning and DiLollo (2017) established that family communication patterns are useful in the understanding of the development of stuttering. According to their research, families that were more open and encouraging had children with less incidents of stuttering. Thus, the research hypothesis suggested that with a reduction in communication pressure and the creation of a friendly environment, fluency could be significantly improved. Conture et al. (2006) examined the linkage between stress and childhood stuttering. The present research indicated that higher stress in the home environment tends to be associated with higher rates of stuttering among children. The researchers noted that stress management techniques should be used, and the home environment should be made comfortable to reduce the cases of stuttering.

Jones et al. (2008) focused on the impact of family therapy on children who have a stuttering disorder. Their research showed that family therapy, focusing on communication and stress management, significantly reduced stuttering in children. The researchers concluded that it is necessary for all the family members to be involved in the process of the therapeutic intervention in order to achieve good management of the stuttering.

5.6 Early Detection

Parents have to pay attention to the language development of the child and report any signs of stuttering to a professional as early as possible: Failing to recognize and act early can be disastrous.

1. Establishing a conducive environment: This means that there is a need to ensure that the environment at home is one that is supportive without ridicule. Parents should encourage communication, should provide feedback to the child, and should not put too much pressure on the child to speak flawlessly.
2. Acquiring knowledge: The parents should ensure that they get information on the aspects of stuttering. Understanding the nature of stuttering and the factors that go with it may help parents be of more help to their child.
3. Promoting positive communication: Parents should also model good communication skills and help the child to feel that he or she is safe to share his or her thoughts and feelings without the fear of being judged. This entails practicing tolerance, paying keen attention, while listening and giving positive feedback.
4. It is crucial to help the child in dealing with their stress and anxiety. Parents can teach their child how to reduce stress, create a calm atmosphere at home, and make sure that the child has an opportunity to do some activities that can help reduce stress.
5. One needs to seek the services of SLPs and other professionals who have a focus on stuttering with a view to get help. These professionals can give the patient a tailor-made treatment and support to help in controlling the stuttering.
6. Family involvement: In this case, it is recommended that the entire family be involved in the therapeutic process, which could be more effective. It can improve the family's communication, reduce stress, and create an environment that is beneficial for the child.
7. Enhancing self-esteem: Parents should ensure that their young children build up their confidence and self-esteem. Encouraging a child, playing with them, praising them for the things they do, and helping them when they are sad or upset will help build their self-esteem.
8. There is a need for parents to fight for their child at school and in other places. This entails engaging the educators in a bid to put into place the required changes, as well as ensuring that the child gets the support they require.
9. Parents should celebrate small victories and keep the hope that their child can handle the condition of stuttering. They should always encourage their child and patiently nurture the improvement of the child.

Stuttering at home is influenced by several factors, such as the environment, the presence of parents, situational factors, and family relations. This means that when parents understand these elements, they can improve their child's coping mechanisms when they stumble. Several measures may help to prevent the occurrence of stuttering, such as developing a supportive environment and seeking the services of SLPs and psychologists when stuttering occurs in the home.

References

Craig A, Hancock K, Tran Y, Craig M. Anxiety levels in children and adolescents who stutter. J Speech Lang Hear Res. 2003;46(5):1197–1206.

Conture EG, Kelly EM, Walden TA. Temperament, speech, and language: an overview. J Commun Disord. 2006;39(5):279–95.

Jones M, Onslow M, Packman A, O'Brian S, Hearne A, Williams S, Ormond T, Schwarz I. Extended follow-up of a randomized controlled trial of the Lidcombe program of early stuttering intervention. Int J Lang Commun Disord. 2008;43(6):649–61.

Manning WH, DiLollo A. Clinical decision making in fluency disorders. 4th ed. Plural Publishing; 2017.

Yairi E, Ambrose N. Early childhood stuttering. 2nd ed. Austin: Pro-Ed; 2005.

Management of Stuttering in School and Home

6

Abstract

This chapter focuses on a comprehensive approach to stuttering management through collaboration with professionals, generalization of learned skills, and emotional and social support. It highlights the essential roles of speech-language pathologists (SLPs), psychologists, and counsellors in providing holistic care for individuals who stutter. Emphasizing the importance of teamwork, the chapter explores how parents, teachers, and other professionals can work together to ensure the consistent application of therapeutic strategies across different environments.

As the most detailed section, the chapter is divided into speech therapy techniques, followed by management strategies for school and home. It highlights specific strategies tailored to these environments, offering general therapy approaches that can be implemented to support fluency and help prevent the occurrence of stuttering. Key sections include the generalization of skills in everyday contexts, fostering emotional well-being and social participation, and understanding the underlying speech mechanism. Practical techniques for managing stuttering are discussed in detail.

Keywords

Stuttering management · Speech therapy techniques · Stuttering management in classrooms · Stuttering management at home · Emotional and social support

R. Kaur, *Navigating Childhood Stuttering*,
https://doi.org/10.1007/978-981-96-6206-7_6

6.1 A Tale of Inspiration

The story starts in Halifax, West Yorkshire, with a boy who had to face his teenage years with the drawback of stuttering. This speech disorder affected his ways of interacting with other people and expressing himself. These interactions were often characterized by distinctiveness, as well as isolation from friends. He recalls being an odd child, with a large birthmark and prescription glasses that were too large for his face, and as such, he always felt different from his peers.

Notwithstanding these initial difficulties, a pivotal moment arose from an unforeseen medium, music. His father was not aware of this; he bought him Eminem's "The Marshall Mathers LP" record at the age of nine without knowing the contents of the album were explicit. The child became fully involved in the record, trying to remember every single word and mirrored Eminem's vocal flow. This was very effective for him since it helped him to create a pattern in his speaking and in due course, he overcame the stammer. The person is the famous singer/songwriter Ed Sheeran who found solace and healing in music.

Although Ed was a child with a speech impediment, he transformed into a confident performer which was not easy. He faced oppression and discrimination, but he persevered due to his strong commitment and passion to share his music with others. He struggled through small and almost unheard-of pubs and even took to the streets to beg for his audience and hone his skills until he got an opportunity.

At present, Ed Sheeran is considered to be one of the most popular singers in the world, thanks to his beautiful voice and heartfelt lyrics. However, he is not ashamed of the background from which he came or reluctant to share about the challenges he had to overcome. Many a time, he uses his page to inspire and empower others, especially the children going through similar situations. During the 9th Annual American Institute for Stuttering Benefit Gala, Ed recounted his personal experience and offered the following advice: "Accept and embrace your idiosyncratic behavior. Stop trying to be fashionable. Self-acceptance is the act of accepting the parts of yourself that you try to cover."

In reflection, Ed promoted the values of self-acceptance and determination. "Just be yourself and let out your peculiarities, for being out of the norm is a wonderful trait," he remarked explaining how his nontypical traits have helped him become innovative and achieve his goals. He routinely encourages people with stuttering to seek treatment but without the mentality of being limited by it. He opines that one should treat stuttering as something which one has to struggle to change and get the right treatment for and not as a burden in life.

Ed Sheeran's story is a perfect testimony to the power of perseverance and music's ability to create change. From being a child with speech disorder to being a world-renowned artist, he is an inspiration to people with speech impediments. Thus, one can see that despite the significant adversities, with the right guidance, it is feasible to accomplish great goals and achieve great results.

6.2 The Greek God of Bollywood

Another striking story is of a person of fame who overcame many of the barriers during life and accomplished more than most of us. This is the real-life story of courage, perseverance, and the power of honest folks, from a boy with a speech impediment. This narrative is not just of one person's success but an enthralling account that has inspired many people in the world.

Ever since this person was a child, he had faced the challenges of stuttering, a speech disability that has always been considered as a limitation to a person's dreams. He shared his problems, explaining what frustration and isolation meant for him as a person who is not a fluent speaker. However, instead of considering these issues as a part of who he is, he chose to confront them. He had a dream of becoming an actor which he held on to at his best and worst times.

He was not a man to sit back and accept the situation as is. Thus, he sought help from speech therapy classes. This signified the beginning of a very deep journey of discovery and transformation in him. He spent a lot of time working on the clarity of his speech, which is a clear indication that change is a process that requires commitment.

"Strength Through Struggle"

The journey to fluency was long and arduous and every step he had to take was a new kind of challenge. However, he did not give up, and with each problem, he persevered with the spirit of a fighter. He devoted himself to reading aloud and to reading every book, magazine, and novel he could lay his hands on. Through constant practice, he developed communication skills, turning every stumbling block into a stepping stone.

He challenged the world with great confidence and did not allow the doubt and judgment of society to hold him back. As he embraced his true self, he stood up without any fear, and instead of focusing on his stutter, he became the focus of everyone's attention as a symbol of power. He changed the lives of many people, and his story showed that if one is honest and patient, the barrier to success is possible to overcome.

Hrithik Roshan is one of the most gifted and acclaimed actors of the Bollywood film industry, and this handsome man is the exceptional individual described above. Hrithik is very much aware of the fact that every word that he utters holds a lot of weight. He used it to spread awareness of stuttering and took the mantle of a spokesperson for people with the same issue. Hrithik's message conveyed a distinct idea: All words have power, and every speaker is meant to be heard.

"United in Empowerment"

Besides his success in the movie industry, Hrithik also claimed leadership roles in raising awareness of people with speech problems. He became a role model of hope, who inspired people, especially the youth who face speech difficulties, through his money and fame. Hrithik made many families see him as a hero after he financially supported and helped in setting up a speech therapy center for young people.

The change of Hrithik Roshan from a youth with a speech problem to a famous actor worldwide is a clear indication that people cannot be limited if they are willing to overcome such barriers as depicted here. What he was able to accomplish is an exemplary example of how much therapy and help from professionals can help. Hrithik's story shows that being true to oneself and accepting one's identity is the final victory.

A Beacon of Hope

Hrithik's dedication to championing the cause of individuals with speech impediments goes well beyond the glamour of the Bollywood industry. He has emerged as an emblem of optimism and empowerment, employing his vocal prowess to motivate and elevate others. His unwavering commitment to this cause has firmly established his reputation in the hearts of millions, not only as an actor but also as an advocate and a source of inspiration for future generations.

"I Embraced My Journey, So Can You!"

Hrithik Roshan's message to the world is uncomplicated yet profound. He says, "Thank you for accepting my personal journey and you can also accept yours!" It encourages the readers to embrace their real self and every word of it. Together, those who are empowered can gather and support each other, share the sorrow and joy of the journey.

Lessons from the Journey

Hrithik Roshan's story is an inspiring case of what can be accomplished when a person decides not to be defined by their limitations. His life and his work represent the spirit of man and the possibilities of the future that are available to anyone willing to work for it. Hrithik has well established that anyone has the ability to bear any challenge and achieve their goal as long as they work hard, get help, and believe in themselves. It is also worth pointing out the positive effect of professional treatment that can be seen in Hrithik Roshan's case. He had a lot of speech therapy which was quite important in his development. It endowed him with the techniques and strategies that could help to improve his speech and boost his confidence in his speaking skills. The case of Hrithik exemplifies the importance of seeking help from other people as well as the difference that treatment can make. Self-reflection helps to remember that professional help can greatly contribute to the solution of the issues and achievement of personal objectives.

It is, therefore, hard to miss the lesson that Hrithik's story offers on the importance of resilience and persistence. Hrithik was willing to strive for better speech despite numerous challenges, which is another aspect of endurance. Hrithik's case is a great example of the fact that real strength is not in avoiding challenges but in tackling them head-on and not giving up, even if the road is steep and treacherous. His determination and the effort that he put in to achieve his goal is a motivation to us to pursue our dreams and goals with a lot of determination.

Thus, I think there is one big lesson that everybody can learn from Hrithik's experience—the lesson of self-acceptance and self-appreciation. This made it possible for Hrithik to transform what can be perceived as a disability, that is, the stammer, into a strength. He showed that one has to be real and accept oneself to be well developed and successful in life. From Hrithik's story, one gets the notion that one should embrace the various attributes that one has and use them as a foundation to build a rewarding and meaningful life. Hrithik Roshan's commitment to the cause of people with speech disorders and his efforts to create awareness about the condition underline that it is important to use one's star power for the betterment of others. His devotion to helping speech treatment centers and supporting the fight for the rights of the speech-impaired is the best evidence of the importance of being involved in the community. His case, therefore, shows that success is not only personal but also has a trickle-down effect on other people's lives.

Hrithik Roshan's journey from being a child with a speech disability to one of the most successful actors in Bollywood is a clear example of the power of determination, stubbornness, and seeking professional help. The reader is also shown the importance of treatment, hard work, and acceptance of who one truly is. His constant efforts to promote the welfare of speech impaired and to create awareness among the masses about speech disorders make him a role model and a source of inspiration for many. The essence of his message to the world is straightforward yet very meaningful: "I have fully embraced my personal journey, and you can do the same!" Hrithik Roshan celebrates the fact that anyone can change, achieve their goals and dreams if only they have the courage, the determination, and the right help.

6.3 Management of Stuttering

The treatment of stuttering aims at improving the communication skills of people who stutter and reducing the impact of stuttering on their day-to-day activities. It is necessary to pay attention not only to the treatment of speech disorder but also to the emotional, social, and educational development of people who stutter. Effective management of the child requires the participation of parents, teachers, SLPs, and sometimes other professionals. The goal is to create an environment that supports the learners' confidence and effectiveness in expressing themselves.

6.3.1 The Role of Early Identification and Intervention

Therefore, early diagnosis and treatment are significant factors in controlling the stuttering problem. It is for this reason that early identification of stuttering is usually favorable to the child's odds of recovery. This stage is where parents and teachers come in. They are usually the first to identify that there is a problem, for instance, repeated whole sounds, syllables, or words; prolonged sounds; or blocks in which a child seems to have difficulty coming up with a word. These are the early warning signs that if identified and referred to an SLP can result in timely and appropriate intervention. It usually starts with an assessment done by the SLP, in which the severity and the type of disorder will be determined. This assessment aids in identifying the child's needs and thus come up with a suitable treatment plan for the child. The SLP will liaise with the child, the child's parents, and teachers or caregivers to ensure that the strategies that may help the child to improve his or her fluency and overall communication are put in place. It is important to note that early intervention emphasizes not only enhancing speech development but also on the child's self-esteem as well as managing any adverse side effects that are related to stammering.

6.3.2 Creating a Supportive Environment

The creation of an appropriate environment is crucial for the success of the stuttering management. Such an environment, both at home and in school, is one where CWS feel secure, welcomed, and free to be able to explain their speech impediment. This fosters positive self-image which makes them free to express themselves without any fear of stigma or ridicule. Thus, parents and teachers can contribute to the formation of such environments by demonstrating polite and tolerant interaction.

For example, at home, parents can facilitate open communication by permitting the children to say what they need to say without frequent judgments or corrections. They should try to understand *what* their children are saying and not *how* they are saying it. Parents need to listen to their children carefully and not criticize them for the wrong use of grammar. Modelling calm and slow speech can also assist the children to remain relaxed and feel less pressurized in speech tasks. Positive reinforcement and celebrating small successes can help raise the child's morale and make the child want to practice more on his or her communication skills.

At the school level, there are ways through which teachers can help students who stutter, which includes establishing an inclusive, empathetic, and understanding environment. It is crucial for teachers to be informed of the problems that students who stutter experience and help them. This includes letting these children have more time to present or find another way to contribute to the class. Teachers can also raise awareness among other students about children who stutter to minimize persecutions and social exclusion that CWS often face.

6.3.3 Collaborating with Professionals

Management of stuttering is usually not a one-man show and may need the assistance of other professionals, mainly speech language pathologists. SLPs are professionals who diagnose and manage cases of speech disorders such as stuttering. They employ the best practices to enhance the client's speaking and language skills and, therefore, enhance communication. As a rule, the SLP works with the child on a set schedule, and during the sessions, the child practices certain methods that help them manage the stuttering. Thus, parents and teachers should communicate with the SLP to ensure the continuity of the strategies in different contexts. It can include reporting on what was observed and reporting on the progress made, and even on how the strategies that are being used need to be modified. At times, other professionals like psychologists or the counsellors may be called in if there are any emotional or psychological complications with regard to the stuttering. These professionals can also give more support to the child and teach them how to manage stress and other issues.

Self-help groups and other social networks could also be of immense help in dealing with stuttering. Socializing with people who have gone through the same ordeal is therapeutic as the individuals can share their experience. It is understood that these groups can provide children and their families with a sense of belonging and also help in alleviating the feelings of loneliness.

6.3.4 Promoting Generalization of Skills

One of the major difficulties in treating stuttering is to teach the client to apply the learned techniques in everyday life. Generalization is the ability to apply the strategies learned in therapy to new situations and with new communication partners. This is important to guarantee that the effects of therapy are long-lasting and that the individual is able to communicate in all facets of their life.

Both parents and teachers are of great importance for generalization. They can help the child to use the speech strategies in different situations, which are at home, at school, and in the community. For instance, in the family setting, parents can involve children in discussions during dinner time, while educators can encourage students to participate in group discussions that are held in class. It is also useful to identify relatively low-stakes situations for practice, which the child is likely to find less threatening.

Regular feedback and positive reinforcement are important to improve the use of speech strategies. Encouraging the child for their efforts and progress, instead of the final outcome, helps in motivating them to keep practicing further. Giving the child positive criticism and constructive feedback enables a child to develop right skills without feeling discouraged.

Besides structured practice, there is spontaneous practice which is equally important. This entails using speech strategies in most aspects of life, for instance, when conversing with peers, when in a restaurant, or when responding to questions in class. The aim of these strategies is to ensure that they become a natural part of the child's communication repertoire.

6.3.5 Supporting Emotional and Social Development

Treating stuttering is not only the enhancement of the fluency of speech but is the enhancement of the emotional and social aspects of the person as well. Stuttering is a speech disorder that affects a person's confidence, causing the affected individual to experience frustration, shame, and isolation. These are some of the issues that lead to considering emotional and social aspects that are important in management of stuttering.

The members of society, especially parents and teachers, also play their part by building up the children's confidence and ensuring that the children accept themselves. Children who stutter should be made to know that stuttering is only one part of them and in no way affects their value or potential. Positive reinforcement of children's hobbies and abilities can make them more confident in themselves.

Another factor that should not be overlooked is the opportunities for social interactions. Promoting children's involvement in group activities, clubs, and teams as well as other social activities can assist them to enhance their social skills. It also helps children to learn from each other and support one another as peers.

Therefore, the most important factor in assisting children who stutter in overcoming social difficulties is to create a comfortable atmosphere. Teachers can support the diversity of students in the classroom by enhancing the students' awareness of other people's feelings, as well as the rights of each individual to be respected by others, while parents can support this by demonstrating appropriate interpersonal relations. This also enables the child to have a say in decision-making regarding his or her communication and thereby boosts the child's confidence.

6.4 Understanding Speech Therapy Techniques to Manage Stuttering

The role of speech therapy techniques in the management of stuttering cannot be overlooked as it helps to enhance the fluency of an individual's speech. However, it is imperative to stress that these strategies should be used only by a qualified SLP. Even though parents and teachers can help and encourage the use of strategies implemented in therapy, trying to apply them on your own without a professional's help may cause more harm and worsen speech difficulties.

SLPs are skilled personnel who deal with the identification, evaluation, and management of speech and language disorders such as stuttering. SLPs have the knowledge to design therapy plans which are specific to clients who stutter. Attempting to use speech therapy techniques without the supervision of an SLP can lead to several adverse effects as follows:

1. *Exacerbation of Stuttering*: Abuse of techniques may make the situation even worse than before as far as stuttering is concerned. For instance, the erroneous application of fluency-shaping strategies may enhance the level of tension and thus increase the number of dysfluencies.
2. *Development of Maladaptive Habits*: Maladaptive habits such as avoiding certain words, using excessive filler words, tensing facial muscles, irregular breathing patterns, and avoiding speaking situations may cause CWS to acquire improper speech patterns which are hard to eradicate. Some of these may hinder the communication process and the long-term improvement of speech.
3. *Increased Anxiety and Frustration*: Using the techniques wrongly can cause the person to become more anxious and frustrated and this in turn worsens the situation of stuttering. Some people may become frustrated and begin to doubt their own speaking skills and further lose confidence in their ability to speak fluently.
4. *Lack of Progress*: People should not expect to immediately see the changes they want when it comes to their speech with the guidance of an SLP. Such expectations can result in the patient giving up on the hope of feeling any better and losing the motivation to engage in the therapy.

6.4.1 Understanding Stuttering and the Speech Mechanism

Before understanding the therapy techniques, it is essential to first describe the general functioning of the speech mechanism in the child. This foundational knowledge can be useful in debunking the whole process of speech and help in eliminating the fear and anxiety linked to stuttering. This helps in expressing the main ideas of speech production using simple images and examples. Through the understanding of speech mechanisms and speech machines, children can easily comprehend the idea of speech control. It is also important to note that an understanding of how speech is being produced can enhance the effectiveness (or rather the efficiency) of the given techniques in treatment and consequently minimize the probability of relapse (reoccurrence of stuttering).

6.4.2 The Speech Machine

The speech mechanism, also commonly known as the "speech machine," is made up of several components that are integrated in the way that they coordinate in the production of speech. These parts are the brain, lungs, vocal cords, and articulators which are the tongue, lips, and palate.

- Brain: The brain is the part of the body that regulates speech. It executes the ideas we wish to convey and sends commands to the muscles that are involved in speech. In this case, when a person has a desire to speak, the brain initiates the specific regions to plan and utter the words.
- Lungs: The lungs are used in providing the airflow which is crucial for speech. As we speak, we blow out air from our lungs and this air goes through the vocal folds and into the vocal tract. This airflow is very important since it forms the basis of sound production.
- Vocal folds: The vocal cords which are situated in the larynx or voice box vibrate to produce sound when an airflow is passed through it. The tension and the position of the folds in between the vocal cords can alter to bring about different pitches and loudness.
- Articulators: There are various structures that are involved in the production of speech, and they are the tongue, lips, teeth, and palate. These structures modify the sound produced by the vocal folds into specific speech sounds or what we call phonemes. The movement of articulators is rather critical in defining the speech's clarity and comprehensibility.

Hence, speech is a well-coordinated activity of all these parts. If one component of the speech machine does not work in harmony, then there is stuttering. This further helps in the demystification of the problem in children which will lessen their fear of having speech difficulties.

6.4.3 Speech Analogies

Analogies are the comparisons of two things where one is explained in terms of the other. They assist in breaking down concepts in a way that is easier to understand by comparing them to other things. Analogies have been employed extensively in education since it helps in the breaking down of complex ideas into models that are easier to comprehend and memorize. Since children are more likely to learn faster and better when concepts are compared to something they can easily understand, analogies can be of great use in speech therapy.

Speech analogies in stuttering are specific kinds of comparison which are used to explain some aspects of speech. They help the child in understanding the procedures that are involved in speaking and the methods that could be used to boost the child's speaking. Thus, these processes can be made easier and more entertaining for the children who stutter using the analogy.

Here Are a Few Effective Analogies

1. *The Lily Pad Analogy*

Considering that every word or sound, which needs to be produced, is a lily pad and the child is a frog who has to jump from one lily pad to another. Just like a frog who should be ready to jump from one lily pad to another, the child should get prepared to smoothly move from one sound to another while speaking. Sometimes, the frog may take its time to jump, or it may jump too fast which may increase the probability of falling into the water. Likewise, in case of stuttering, if the child rushes or hesitates too much, then the likelihood of stammering increases.

For instance, when saying the sentence, "I am going to eat an apple," imagine every word in the sentence as a lily pad. The child must try to achieve fluidity in the movement of words from one to the other, just like a frog that leaps nimbly from one lily pad to another. When the frog or, in this case, a child's speech stumbles or leaps out too fast, it will fall into the water which is a symbol for a stutter. This is the case when the transition from one word or sound to another is not seamless. The frog may take time to jump, and in the process, it may wobble, overbalance, or jump hastily and fail to catch the lily pad and end up falling into the water.

Thus, if every word is visualized as a lily pad, children can work on proper and fluid movement from one word to another, like a frog planning and performing a jump. This visualization assists the students to appreciate the role of preparation as well as control in speech, to minimize on pauses, or hurriedness that culminates in stuttering.

2. *The Thumb and Finger Opposing Analogy*

Imagine a gesture in which the thumb and the index finger are pinched together. If an individual combines them in a very delicate and fluent way, then they do not cause any conflict. However, if you push them together or try to make them meet at a certain time, they may well fail or collide. Stuttering works in a similar way to the thumb and finger.

Smooth speech is produced by soft and gentle pressure: When the thumb and the finger, that is, vocal folds, make gentle contact with each other, then it embodies fluent speech. This slow and coordinated movement enables the vocal folds to vibrate in a manner that enables them to produce sound without straining.

For instance, when saying the word hello, one should try to place the thumb and the index finger together, gently at the initiation of the word hello toward the "h" sound. This is useful in starting the sound in a smooth and tension-free manner.

Getting stuck is visualized as overlapping or inaccurate contact: If the thumb and finger (your vocal folds) touch or seize violently and then either miss or hit each other, this will cause tension and pauses in the speech. This is a type of disruption where the vocal folds fail to initiate the sound properly, as in the case of stuttering.

For instance, speaking fast, to articulate the word hello, will sound more like "h-h-hello" because the articulators are not coordinated well, thus leading to stuttering. In such situations, decreasing stress and practicing gentle contact can work wonders.

3. *The Blown-Up Balloon Analogy*

Just like a balloon, lungs are like an air sac. When the air is pumped into a balloon and then released slowly, the balloon is deflated in a rather gentle and relaxed manner. However, if too much or too little pressure is applied, it results in producing a hissing sound and the balloon deflates in a manner that is not smooth. The speech process is very similar to this.

Smooth speech can be compared to controlled airflow: When the air from the balloon (human lungs) is let out in a slow and steady manner, this is equivalent to speaking fluently. This gradual release allows the speaker to have a constant supply of air, which is important for the continuity of speaking. For instance, before saying the sentence "I like to play," the child can take a deep breath and, while saying the sentence, release the air slowly. This assists in ensuring that there is continuity of the speech.

Getting stuck is equivalent to rapid air release: In this case, when the air is let out of the balloon (lungs), it may cause irregular and loud popping sounds, which stand for stammering. The airflow control issue can be defined as the rate and consistency of air release affecting the fluency of speech. For instance, when saying "I like to play," if the child forces their breath, then it comes out as "I l-l-like to p-p-play," due to the inconsistency in the airflow that causes stammering. Hence, exercising control over breathing is useful in ensuring that there is fluency.

4. *The Traffic Light Analogy*

Picture a traffic light where green means one is allowed to proceed, yellow means one should slow down, and red means one should stop. The speech that is described as smooth is like obeying the traffic lights to minimize the occurrences of accidents.

Smooth speech: Adhering to the traffic light signals means that one is speaking fluently. Green is when one is speaking without any difficulties, yellow is when one feels some stress, and red is when one should stop and take a breath if necessary. For instance, while speaking, sometimes one may feel tense, and in such a case, imagining a yellow light will help to calm down. If one is at some point where they feel unable to proceed, imagining a red light will help and, in such cases, it is important to break a few minutes before going further.

Getting stuck: If one does not obey the traffic signals that are the speech cues, then one may end up causing speech accidents, stammering included. Disregarding information on slowing down or pausing, when necessary, may cause disturbances in speech. For instance, if you do not pay attention to the signals and speak the sentence "I am going to school" without pausing, it may sound like "I a-a-am g-g-going to s-s-school." Thereby, the traffic light signals ensure fluent speech.

6.4.4 Implementing These Analogies

These analogies are usually employed by SLPs in the first few therapy sessions to describe the speech mechanism to the child prior to introducing the stuttering therapy techniques. Using such analogies, parents and teachers can also describe the mechanisms and processes of speech to children. These analogies, undoubtedly, give a better picture of speech concepts and thus make them easier to understand and handle. Due to the frequent use of these analogies during exercises and real-life speaking, children can gain better control over their speech and decrease stuttering occurrences.

Comparison and imagery are backed up by research in cognitive behavioral methods of speech therapy. Various research has indicated that children achieve better success when they know the mechanics of their speech and have pictures of speech production in their mind as they try to practice the techniques used for the management of stuttering. For instance, Guitar (2014), in his work, stresses the use of cognitive restructuring in the treatment of stuttering, wherein the role of thinking and constructing images of the speech processes is pivotal in the therapy.

With these analogies, parents and educators can help the children to understand their speech mechanism and empower them to better manage their stuttering using simple and relatable examples. This approach not only helps to explain the way speech is being processed but also provides children with enough knowledge and techniques to regulate their speech.

6.5 Fluency-Shaping Techniques

Fluency-shaping techniques are ways and methods used in the speech therapy of a person who stutters with the aim of achieving fluency. These techniques follow a rationale of focusing on modification of the entire speech production process to achieve fluent and well-controlled speech.

While the other set of techniques, called stuttering modification techniques, focus on correcting stuttering during the moments when it occurs, fluency shaping is an approach that is aimed at preventing stuttering before it occurs, through the creation of fluent speech patterns. Fluency-shaping techniques are intended to change the general speech mechanism to support fluent speech. This approach is concerned with changing the speech aspects that lead to stuttering and thus help individuals to speak more fluently and with fewer breaks. These techniques include the use of certain speech functions and strategies include easy onset, gentle voicing, prolonged speech, and breathing exercises. Using these techniques leads to gaining greater control over speech, thereby significantly reducing the instances of stuttering.

6.5.1 Techniques Following Principles of Fluency Shaping Are

I. *Easy Onset*

Easy onset is when the speaker begins to produce sound gradually and without a harsh break. This aids in preventing tension that can accompany the initiation of speech. This technique tries to avoid the situation where the vocal folds close suddenly in a tense manner, which is associated with stuttering. Research has indicated that easy onset can be useful in decreasing the occurrences of stuttering (Onslow and Packman 1999).

When employing easy onset, the individual starts to speak with a whisper and builds up the intensity of their voice. This gradual onset minimizes the chances of getting stuck in the first word of a sentence and therefore prevents a block or stutter. The main goal is to initiate the speaking process in a slow and calm way, which can gradually progress faster speaking.

For instance, if a child is about to mention the word "apple," the child should begin with "aa-a" sound which is very soft before connecting it to the correct pronunciation of the word. This approach prevents sudden onsets, which can trigger stuttering.

II. *Gentle Phonatory Contacts*

The gentle contact of articulators is another vital practice applied in speech therapy to aid people who stutter to pronounce words with fewer stutters and less strain. This method is centered around the way various structures (like lips, tongue, and palate) are involved in the production of speech as they meet each other. This technique targets at helping individuals to relax by using tender, delicate touches on the face and neck, when forming speech sounds, in a bid to prevent the physical strain that may cause stuttering.

The rationale behind applying gentle articulatory contacts is to avoid the physical tension and pressure that are usually associated with the articulation of speech sounds in individuals who stutter. Stress and forceful contact can worsen the stuttering as the articulators have a harder time sliding from one sound to another. Gentle articulatory contacts help to:

1. Reduce physical tension: With the help of light and gentle contacts between the articulators, the whole tension of speech muscles can be reduced. This reduction in tension assists in making the passage from one sound to the other and from one word to the other easier.
2. Enhance speech fluency: Light contact helps with more polite and light communication which does not cause interferences and makes speech smoother. This technique is useful in minimizing the instances where the articulators collide in a rather harsh manner.
3. Improve coordination: The gentle contact of the articulators assists in the development of more precise control and coordination of the motor mechanisms of speech. This is because the control is enhanced, thereby enabling the production of accurate speech.
   - Lips: For bilabial sounds like /p/ and /b/, the lips are advised to just touch without firm pressure between them. Example: Miming the word "pat" and saying the /p/ sound with the lips.

- Tongue: For the sounds that require the tongue to touch some part of the mouth like /t/ and /d/, individuals are taught to place the tongue gently on the alveolar ridge which is the region between the upper teeth and the hard palate. Example: Saying the word tap with the light contact of the tongue with the alveolar ridge for the /t/.
- Palate: In the case of velar sounds like /k/ and /g/, individuals must pay attention to the fact that the back part of the tongue is slightly touching the soft palate. Example: The instruction to say the word "cat" while slightly raising the back of the tongue for the /k/ sound.

III. *Prolonged Speech*

Prolonged speech is a technique that allows the speaker to speak more slowly; this gives the speaker more time to form words and coordinate their speech muscles efficiently. This technique increases control and flow by enabling the speaker to speak slowly and deliberately. Prolonged speech has been one of the most investigated techniques for the improvement of fluency and is probably the most widely used.

Ingham et al. (2001) conducted a study that depicted how participants' stuttering frequency reduced when they practiced prolonged speech, which shows the benefits of the method in encouraging fluent speech. As for the speech muscles and cognitive processes, fast speech is tiring and may lead to stuttering. Slowing down speech helps the speaker to control the rate of speech, thereby synchronizing the breathing and phonation hence improving on the fluency of speech.

IV. *Controlled Breathing Exercises*

Diaphragmatic breathing, also known as abdominal or belly breathing, is the control of breath support for speech using the diaphragm. Breath control helps in regulating the flow of air and this is quite important in speaking fluently.

Breath control is one of the most significant elements of speech production. Thus, there are factors such as irregular or shallow breathing which affect the smooth flow of speech leading to stuttering. Diaphragmatic breathing ensures the availability of constant supply of air in the lungs, hence enabling the smooth and continuous flow of speech. For example, to practice diaphragmatic breathing, place one hand on your stomach, inhale, and exhale slowly so that your stomach goes up and down with the breathing. These consistencies are helpful in ensuring that there is a constant flow of air which prevents blockages.

A popular method to incorporate airflow control and the coordination of the other muscles involved in speech is the *airflow technique* and the *modified airflow technique*. The modified airflow technique is an airflow control strategy in stuttering therapy to control the airflow during speech production to increase fluency. This technique is helpful in the case of stuttering because it tends to ease the physical strain linked with speech to start up and enhance the fluency of speech.

The modified airflow technique involves the control of breathing and the control of speech, wherein the two have to be in synchronization. The central concept is that one should try to speak on a breath of airflow to avoid sudden strain on the vocal cords that usually leads to stammering. This way, the child is encouraged to initiate speech with less stress, and thus there is less chance of stuttering.

V. *Rate Control*

Rate control is one of the strategies that entail reducing the rate of speaking with the aim of achieving more fluency, less pressure, and ess rush, which may worsen stuttering. This technique helps in ensuring that the speaker takes a reasonable tone in his or her communication.

A rapid speech rate enhances the cognitive and physical load of speech production, which results in speech errors. Through reducing the rate of speaking, one can pay much attention to each sound or word to be spoken without stumbling.

6.6 Stuttering Modification Techniques

Stuttering modification involves improving fluency by treating stuttering episodes directly. Unlike fluency shaping, stuttering modification techniques help teach the individuals to adjust better to their speech and to deal with their stuttering as the stuttering episodes occur. These methods assist in changing the person's perception about their speech and managing the fear and nervousness that is commonly linked to stuttering.

Stuttering modification therapy is the most acknowledged approach to the disorder; the Van Riper approach is the most popular. Created by one of the most famous speech therapists, Dr. Charles Van Riper, this approach focuses on stuttering modification and changing one's attitude toward the fluency issue (Van Riper 1982):

1. *Identification*: The first stage is the identification of the individual's specific stuttering episodes and awareness of the same. This includes learning of the different types of dysfluencies which include blocks, repetitions, and prolongations, along with knowledge on the situations that aggravate the stuttering and the awareness of the physical and emotional responses to stuttering.
2. *Desensitization*: This stage focuses on reducing the many fears and anxieties that are related to stammering. These are voluntary stuttering where one intentionally stutters in a certain area while talking it out. Here, the person with the stuttering problem discusses the issue and confronts places or situations that the individuals tend to avoid due to fear of stuttering.
3. *Modification*: The stuttering episodes are directly discussed in the following manners in this context:
   (i) *Voluntary stuttering:* This is the deliberate vocalizing of stuttering by intentionally repeating or extending certain sounds or words. This technique enables individuals with stuttering disorders to at least manage the stuttering and minimize the occurrence of anxiety when they experience unexpected stuttering. Hence, people can try to

stutter deliberately to reduce their anxiety toward stuttering. This helps them feel the stuttering in a safe environment, which weakens the effect of involuntary stuttering in their lives. It also assists in controlling their response to stuttering, and therefore, this becomes less of a factor that hinders their communication. Sheehan (1970) has shown that voluntary stuttering can be used to reduce clients' sensitivity to stuttering incidents. Thus, purposeful stuttering in a low-anxiety situation may help decrease the general anxiety related to stuttering and consequently enhance one's coping skills.

(ii) *Cancellations:* This means repeating and rehearsing a word that is likely to be stuttered before speaking the word. The stutterer retraces it in his mind and then speaks it aloud. This technique is corrective in nature and enables the individuals to speak fluently, thereby reducing the future likelihood of stuttering. If the person stutters on a word, they cease speaking (stop the stutter), wait for a few seconds saying or thinking the word (silently or softly), and then say the word without a stutter. This helps to accentuate fluent speech patterns and minimize the chances of the stutter being repeated in future speech. Van Riper (1982) pointed out that cancellations were instrumental in altering stuttering behaviors. The results indicated that individuals who were engaged in cancellations avoided stuttering more often while they had more control over their speech.

(iii) *Pull-outs:* Better known as "slide-outs," these focus on the transformation of a stuttered word in progress while the child is speaking it. The individual progressively departs from the stuttered word through the smooth transition into non-stuttered speaking. This technique enables control of stammering as it occurs without having to stop and start over. During episodes of stuttering, the client does not stop making sounds but smoothly transitions from the stuttered sound or syllable into the rest of the word. This technique decreases physical exertion and serves to help the person retain the rate of speech.

Both fluency-shaping and stuttering modification approaches have their unique advantages and can be applied in concert as components of a stuttering management system. The combination of these techniques makes it possible to meet the specific needs of each person who stutters and the difficulties he/she has. A blended approach of fluency shaping and stuttering modification provides the client with a balanced method for managing stuttering. For example, a person may apply fluency-building strategies such as easy onset and pause for breathing to build up a fluency strategy. In cases of dysfluencies, they can use stuttering modification methods like pull-outs, cancellations to reduce stuttering in real-life situations.

6.7 Other Approaches to Stuttering Therapy

A. *Psychological Therapy*

Stuttering can also have psychological impacts that include anxiety, low self-esteem, and social isolation. These psychological problems require the services of a psychologist:

(i) *Cognitive behavioral techniques (CBT)*: Such techniques are sometimes used in stuttering to help treat the other effects that come with the condition. CBT assists the clients in changing the cognitive and behavioral processes that are linked to fluency disorders. It helps in identifying ways of combating stress, changing negative thinking patterns, building coping mechanism for anxiety, and improving confidence. These methods entail cognitive restructuring, where people are taught to recognize and fight negative thoughts, beliefs, and behaviors concerning stuttering. Thus, by changing negative beliefs into positive and more accurate ones about one's communication competence, a person's overall self-perception can be boosted. Further, CBT employs behavioral strategies like exposure therapy that expose patients to progressive real-life speaking situations that trigger anxiety to help them regain confidence and stop avoiding public speaking.

(ii) *Supportive counselling*: Besides therapy, counselling is another significant aspect of stuttering treatment as it helps clients to vent their feelings, tell their stories, and get comfort from other people, including counsellors. The counselling sessions are aimed at treating psychological issues, increasing self-acceptance, and coping with the difficulties of stuttering. Support groups also help in this by providing a place for peers to talk to and learn from those who have been through the same ordeal.

(iii) *Support groups and clubs*: Peer support groups help clients to find and share their experiences, as well as to get the necessary information. These platforms provide support and hope and often make people feel understood and less alone.

(iv) *Acceptance and commitment therapy (ACT)*: The self-help approach that ACT offers is to let go of the desire to change the stammer and instead learn to live well in accordance with one's values. It fosters tolerance, consciousness, and understanding of one's flaws and shortcomings, which in turn decreases the negative feelings that are associated with stammering.

B. *Complementary Therapeutic Approaches*

In addition to traditional speech therapy and psychological interventions, several other therapeutic approaches can enhance stuttering treatment and improve communication skills:

1. Electronic devices: Devices such as delayed auditory feedback (DAF) and frequency-altered feedback (FAF) give real-time feedback and alter the auditory feedback in a way that helps the person to speak fluently.
2. Medication: There is no pill to completely cure stuttering. Some medications that help manage the dysfluencies are:
   - Dopaminergic medications: These modulate dopamine circuits and have previously been implicated in communication.
   - Benzodiazepines: These are generally prescribed as antianxiety medication and may be helpful when stuttering is considerably affected by anxiety.

- Antidepressants: Medications such as selective serotonin reuptake inhibitors (SSRIs) and serotonin and norepinephrine reuptake inhibitors (SNRIs) help minimize some of the emotional suffering that results from stuttering.
- Botulinum toxin injections: There is evidence that its application helps decrease muscular tension and allows for precise control of the vocal folds (Abramovitz et al. 2017).

C. *Virtual Reality Therapy*

Virtual reality (VR) therapy is one of the most effective and modern approaches that allow creating realistic speech situations with certain limitations. This therapy entails pointing the patient to a computerized environment and coming up with scenarios that resemble true-to-life scenarios. The primary benefits of VR therapy for stuttering include:

- Controlled exposure: VR also enables the clients to confront what makes them anxious about speaking situations in a protected zone. For instance, they can speak in front of an audience or speak with other people without the actual environment affecting them and, consequently, become less sensitive to such situations.
  - Customizable settings: Another advantage of using VR is that therapists are able to modify the scenario with reference to the person's needs, meaning that the VR therapist is able to increase the levels of difficulty in the interactions, as well as the types of interaction according to the VR client's progress.
  - Desensitization: When the individual is exposed to stuttering in the virtual environment, he or she practices or works through managing it there and eventually gains more confidence and fluency over time.
  - Enhanced engagement: The use of VR makes therapy more fun and thus encourages patients to adhere to the set therapy schedules consistently.

D. *Use of Artificial Intelligence (AI) in Stuttering Treatment*

AI is becoming an increasingly valuable tool in the treatment of stuttering, offering several advanced methods to enhance therapy outcomes.

(a) *AI-driven diagnosis and monitoring*: Computer programs for artificial intelligence can be employed to map patterns of speech, diagnose stuttering, and monitor the progress of therapy. These systems utilize several large databases that allow for highly accurate identification of stuttering events and the type and degree of feedback of stutters in the subject's speech. Such continuous monitoring can assist the therapists in how they respond to the patients since they would have the flexibility to change their plans as needed (Liu et al. 2022).
(b) *Personalized therapy plans*: AI can assist in the identification of the correct approaches to treatment that are personalized to address the peculiarities of each patient. AI

algorithms for therapy sessions help suggest the best exercises and methods given the patient's results from their sessions (Zhao et al. 2021).

(c) *Virtual assistants*: Real-time interactions with people can be facilitated through practicing with AI-supported virtual assistants. For illustration, applications such as ChatGPT can mimic dialogues through which certain people can rehearse speaking in diverse settings and get instant feedback on their flows (SpeechIRL 2023).

(d) *Enhanced engagement and accessibility*: Therapists have to be fully engaged to recommend the application of AI in the delivery of therapy since it may increase the accessibility of therapy for more patients. Mobile applications and online portals based on AI provide patients with games, simple mental exercises, and online communities of like-minded people who can help patients adhere to techniques learned in therapy outside of the clinic (Smith and Smith 2020).

6.8 Key Roles of Time and Tension in Stuttering Therapy

Stuttering is a speech disorder that has numerous causes and is related specifically to two components: time and tension. Yaruss (2001) found that these factors have a huge impact and contribution on stuttering and thus have a major role to play in stuttering management as well.

6.8.1 Time and Stuttering

With regard to stuttering, time relates to the pressure and speed with which speech is generated. When people feel pressured to speak or are in a hurry, their speech production system can be overburdened. This pressure can cause a disturbance in the harmony of speaking, leading to stuttering.

6.8.2 Tension and Stuttering

Stuttering is characterized by physical tension as well as an emotional sense. Muscles involved in speech production, for example, the lips, tongue, and vocal cords, may get tense and lead to choppy and/or dysfluent speech. Anxiety or fear that is associated with speaking can also worsen these physical symptoms, thus increasing the frequency of stuttering.

6.8.3 Techniques That Address Time and Tension for Stuttering Management

1. Easy onset and gentle voicing: These techniques assist in decreasing physical tension because they enable a gentle approach to the commencement of speaking and the use

of a soft voice. This does not stress the vocal cords and muscles of speech in the same way.

2. Prolonged speech: Slowing down speech helps the individuals to control their speech muscles in a better way and helps them to construct words properly and thus there are less chances of stammering.
3. Light contacts: This technique involves generating speech sounds with the least contact between the articulators as this minimizes the tension that may cause speech difficulty.
4. Diaphragmatic breathing: It helps to maintain a constant flow of air, which assists in the smooth delivery of speech and prevents muscle strain.
5. Rate control: Slowing down the rate of speech assists the speaker in being very keen on how they articulate their words and minimizes the pressure and rush that may worsen the stuttering.
6. Voluntary stuttering: This technique is quite simple and involves intentional stammering to help alleviate the fear and stress connected to it. Thus, people can develop the habit of stuttering on purpose and, thereby, decrease their sensitivity to fear and minimize the level of tension.
7. Cancellations: This technique is based on the premise that the client should stop at a word that has been spoken with stutter, take a deep breath, and then try to speak the word without stutter. This minimizes the physical and psychological stress that is felt during the occurrence of stuttering.
8. Pull-outs: This technique entails systematically moving out of a stuttered word or phrase to the correct one to control and lessen tension during speaking.
9. Chunking and pausing: Dr. Yaruss also stresses the strategy of chunking and pausing to control stuttering to a great extent. Chunking is the process of dissecting speech into smaller and more easily manipulatable pieces, while pausing gives the speaker time to collect their thoughts and decrease speech anxiety.
   - Chunking: Breaking down the longer sentences into chunks is another way of decreasing the load and effort on the working memory and the motor speech production. This way, the child does not develop tension that can make them stutter while speaking.
   - Pausing: Pausing alleviates the stress and the urge to go on with the speech, hence lowering the chances of stuttering.

6.9 Treating Various Subsystems of Speech Production

As mentioned above, speech production is a multifaceted process that implies the interaction of several subsystems. Briefly, these subsystems include:

1. *Respiratory system*: Provides the amount of airflow needed for speech. It affects the lungs, diaphragm, and any other muscles that are used in breathing.

2. *Phonatory system*: This is the part of speech that involves the larynx or voice box and the vocal cords, which vibrate when air passes through them.
3. *Articulatory system*: Comprises of the tongue, lips, teeth, and the palate which are responsible for modifying the airflow to produce different speech sounds.
4. *Resonatory system*: Comprises the oral and nasal cavities, which alter the quality of the sound produced by the vocal cords.
5. *Prosodic system*: It involves elements of speech that include the rhythm, intonation, and stress which add to the natural flow of speech.

Various subsystems of speech production need to be treated to cure some of the speech disorders such as stuttering. All these subsystems perform specific functions in the generation of speech, which is both smooth and easy to comprehend; disruption of any one of these areas results in disruption of speech. Benefits of treating each subsystem in speech therapy include:

1. *Improving coordination and timing*: A well-coordinated and synchronized working of all the subsystems is crucial for production of an efficient speech. For example, the respiratory and phonatory systems need to be coordinated to produce constant airflow and proper vibration of the vocal folds. To minimize the occurrence of stuttering and lessening their impact, the issue of coordination can be tackled (Bothe 2004).
2. *Enhancing fluency*: The methods targeting specific subsystems can enhance speech fluency immediately. For instance, diaphragmatic breathing exercises change the pattern of airflow and help in getting rid of breathiness or jerkiness in speech. Also, light articulatory contacts reduce the amount of muscle tension, which in turn facilitates the flow of speech (Craig et al. 2003).
3. *Reducing physical and emotional tension*: The physical tension in the articulatory and phonatory components of speech can be helpful in relieving the burden of stuttering. Furthermore, handling these conflicts can minimize the psychological stress, which often worsens the oral communication problems (Smith and Weber 2017).
4. *Facilitating generalization*: By addressing several subsystems, therapy can promote the transfer of the skills acquired during the sessions to everyday communication practices. This approach enables the enhancement of one area to benefit the other aspects of speech and communication (Kent 2015).

6.9.1 Breathing and Stuttering

Stuttering is a clinical condition that is defined as an abnormality in speech fluency and timing that significantly interferes with communication, impacting academic, occupational, and social functioning. Stuttering is often accompanied by irregularities in airflow during speech, making breathing techniques a critical component in managing the disorder.

Stuttering is also characterized by the constriction of the vocal folds, and thus, the airflow and speech output are affected. This may be a total lack of breathing or prolonged periods of breathing during the time of stuttering. Stuttering research also shows that individuals who stutter have reduced airflow during speech, and this affects the control of the larynx muscles and, consequently, the volume of air in the lungs prior to speech production.

Breathing is arguably as vital to speaking as fuel is to a car. Just as a car requires an adequate amount of fuel to run efficiently, speech also requires a constant and sufficient supply of air. Breath, if not managed well, can cause communication problems, just like how the absence of fuel can affect the working of a car.

Zocchi et al. (1990) reported that severe stutterers show disjointed respiratory muscles, therefore producing erratic fluctuations of subglottic pressure (PSG). This lack of control interferes with normal speech production, which indicates respiratory muscle incoordination, which could be one of the primary causes of stuttering. Therefore, the knowledge and regulation of respiratory processes are beneficial to the control of stuttering. Here are some of the techniques that are employed in the treatment of stuttering through the modification of patients' breathing patterns:

6.9.2 Diaphragmatic Breathing

Diaphragmatic breathing, commonly referred to as abdominal or belly breathing, is the process of using the diaphragm muscle to control the breath in speech. This technique ensures that there is a smooth and continuous flow of air necessary for proper speaking.

Breathing also plays a very crucial role in the production of speech since it is the source of energy. Thus, appropriate breath control is important. Breathing problems or breathlessness can also affect the timing of the speech and cause stuttering of words. This way, breathing ensures a constant and rather smooth flow of air that is crucial for continuous and normal speech. For example, diaphragmatic breathing involves putting a hand on the stomach and breathing in and out slowly with the focus on the movement of the stomach. To support speech, when speaking, following the pattern of breathing is beneficial: inhale and exhale, inhale, and exhale.

6.9.3 Regulated Breathing

Regulated breathing (RB) is a behavioral treatment method that aims at correcting the airflow abnormality by teaching breathing patterns that are relatively incompatible yet are related to stuttering. Hence, the aim is to obtain a particular breathing pattern that is related to the flow of speech.

The literature shows that RB is beneficial in the treatment of stuttering. Different researchers have shown that stuttering frequency and speech fluency are greatly reduced after RB treatment. Azrin and Nunn (1974) found that stuttering was reduced by 94% the day after one 2-hour treatment session with a retention of the benefit for at least 1 month. Williamson et al. (1981) reported a significant decrease in stuttering, facial muscle activity, and increased speaking rate with positive effects observed at 3 months' follow-up.

Ladouceur and Saint-Laurent (1986) observed that stuttering was decreased from the pre-treatment to posttreatment phase and at the 1- and 6-month follow-up evaluations. RB encompasses several components:

6.9.4 Awareness Training

The first process of RB is awareness training, where individuals are informed of the times they stutter and the feelings that are attached to it. This involves:

- *Response description*: The client chooses to stutter intentionally and gives a very precise verbal account of the motor activities and the physical perceptions of the act of stuttering.
- *Response detection*: The identification of stuttering events is done by the client on their own, although this is done in conjunction with a clinician who gives feedback.
- *Situation awareness*: Learning about particular words, events, situations, or people that are likely to cause stuttering.
- *Anticipation awareness*: Identifying predisposing factors and somatic indicators of stuttering as a way of prevention.

6.9.5 Relaxation Training

The relaxation training intends to target the physical component of the stuttering problem. Techniques include:

- *Relaxed posture*: Sitting and standing positions that are easy to assume to help relax the muscles of the chest and abdomen.
- *Diaphragmatic breathing*: Instructions for diaphragmatic breathing to teach the proper way of breathing while using the diaphragm for steady airflow.
- *Self-directed relaxation*: Learning relaxation procedures to decrease muscle tension.

6.9.6 Competing Response Training

Competing response training is based on the idea of performing activities that are opposed to stuttering, mainly dealing with breathing strategies. Techniques include:

- *Diaphragmatic breathing during speech*: The client stops speaking, tries to use diaphragmatic breathing, consciously relaxes chest and throat muscles, thinks about what needs to be said, and then continues to speak after a small exhalation.
- *Gradual increase in speech duration*: At the beginning, the output will be in small chunks, and then as the student gains more confidence, they are nudged to increase fluency.

6.9.7 Motivation Training

Motivation training relies on proper utilization of the competitive response. Techniques include:

- *Inconvenience review*: Using the previous setbacks in stuttering as a way of encouraging change.
- *Social support*: Getting the family and friends to praise the individual and to remind him/her to use the competing response.
- *Public display*: Motivating the clients to engage in situations where they are likely to stutter and efficiently apply the competing response.
- *Generalization training*: Generalization training is used to check if the treatment gains made are sustainable in other environments outside the clinic. Techniques include:
  - Symbolic Rehearsal: Describing different situations that may lead to stuttering and at the same time showing how to perform the right competing responses.
  - Positive Practice: Slowly building on the duration of fluency by pausing after words or phrases to take in a regulated breath.

Thus, RB seems to be a powerful and efficient approach to treating stuttering, as there is a considerable amount of empirical evidence for the treatment's effectiveness. Nevertheless, to be identified as a well-established treatment, further studies should be performed to overcome the mentioned methodological shortcomings such as the need for replication in randomized control trials and monitoring in longer follow-ups. Future research needs to establish the factors that are involved in RB and compare the effectiveness of this strategy with other treatments for fluency.

6.10 Contradictory Viewpoint by Dr. Yaruss on Using Breathing Techniques

Yaruss (2021) opposes the idea of practicing breathing patterns for a significant amount of time to cure stuttering. Breathing and stuttering could be compared to the fuel system of a car. However, overemphasis on breathing is similar to focusing excessively on only the fuel while overlooking other vital components of the car.

Yaruss claims that it is an unhelpful approach to concentrate on the breathing strategies alone because it does not bring significant results, even in the short term to those who stutter. Instead, Dr. Yaruss suggests that the focus should be on the fact that stuttering is caused by related tension, timing, and avoidance behaviors, which should be the primary focus of stuttering management.

Yaruss's approach is quite specific in this regard, stating that breathing exercises are generally not helpful for controlling stuttering. Hence, the goal of therapy should be aimed at making the affected individuals accept their stuttering and the feelings that come with it, thus reducing the physical and mental stress. This approach aims at helping the clients get a better, more natural way of communicating, especially those with speech disorders.

6.10.1 Modified Airflow Technique

One of the most powerful techniques that can be used involves modifying the airflow which is considered to be fundamental in speech production to enhance the fluency of the speech. The rationale for this technique stems from the fact that stutterers are known to have uncoordinated breathing and rather tense speech muscles. The above problems are specifically targeted by the modified airflow technique, which teaches client-controlled breathing and the smooth initiation of speech.

The Technique Helps to:

- *Reduce tension*: Initiating speech using a steady flow of air can reduce muscular tension and thus decrease stuttering.
- *Improve coordination*: The techniques enhance the coordination between breathing and speaking, thereby improving fluency.
- *Promote fluency*: The focus on continuous phonation in this technique helps in smooth transition from one sound or word to another, leading to more fluent speech.

6.10.2 Phonation and Stuttering

Various studies on the neurophysiological basis of stuttering have pointed to the larynx and phonation as being the key areas in speech. The larynx, referred to as the voice box, contains the vocal cords, which are used in the act of producing sound. The two vocal folds must vibrate to open and close at the right time for speech to be clear. Stuttering is characterized by impairment in the coordination of the two speech subsystems; hence, the speech of individuals who stutter is not fluent.

Phonation is the act in which sound is made by the vocal folds through the vibration of the air passing through them. In stuttering, the preparedness of vocal folds to vibrate or initiate sounds, especially in vowels, is also impaired. This stage, known as prephonatory tuning, involves the neural preparation of the laryngeal muscles to adduct (close) vocal folds together with the proper tension, just before voice production. When this tuning is disturbed, the vocal folds can either close too tightly or remain open, causing stuttering like blocks and speech interruptions (Smith and Weber 2017).

Numerous neuroimaging studies have indicated that people who stutter present abnormalities in the brain's structure and functioning in areas that are implicated in the planning and execution of the motor aspects of speech, including the motor cortex, the premotor cortex, and the basal ganglia (Chesters et al. 2018). These areas are involved in the planning, coordination, and control of the onset, tempo, and pattern of speech motor activities. This is because the control of neural signals in the vocal folds in the larynx can be disrupted, which may lead to stuttering.

The basal ganglia and cerebellar pathways' participation may also point toward the motor control and learning problems as being associated with stuttering. These areas of the brain are involved with the coordination of movements and the ability to modify movement in response to perceived errors, thus suggesting that stuttering could be due to defects in these processes.

The Speech Therapy Techniques Which Focus on Treating Phonatory Issues in Stuttering Are as Follows:

1. *Easy onset and gentle voicing*: Enabling people to start with phonation in a softer manner, to minimize the closure of the vocal cord.
2. *Laryngeal relaxation exercises*: The Valsalva maneuver is a breathing technique that involves forcefully exhaling against a closed airway. This can be harmful to the body, especially the laryngeal muscles. Thus, to avoid this, it is suggested to calm down and produce speech in a relaxed manner. To avoid the Valsalva maneuver and reduce tension in the laryngeal muscles, it is suggested to relax and calm down.
3. *Voluntary stuttering*: Helping children who stutter in speaking with ease by minimizing fear and anxiety.
4. *Biofeedback*: It is a process whereby the patient is provided with visual or audible feedback to facilitate control of the vocal folds. This can involve the use of visual aids of the vocal fold vibrations as well as auditory feedback.

6.10.3 Articulation and Stuttering

Articulation refers to the movement of the tongue, lips, jaw, and other speech organs that help to create sound. Right articulation is essential for speech to be fluent, and disturbances in articulation can lead to stuttering. The articulatory parameters that affect speech fluency are:

6.10.3.1 Rate of Speech

Definition: The rate of speech is the speed at which a person speaks in terms of words per minute (WPM) or syllables per second (SPS). It is imperative to address the rate at which one speaks in fluent communication.

Impact on Stuttering: A faster rate of speech can tire the motor control system that is required for proper speech production, thus increasing the frequency of stuttering occurrences. Consecutively, a very slow speech rate may also negatively affect the perception of speech and increase the cognitive load.

Techniques that Focus on the Rate of Speech for Stuttering Management Include:

- *Pacing*: Other physical aids that can be used include pacing boards, metronomes, or even digital applications. Pacing allows speakers to control the speed of their speech and not rush when they are speaking; thus, they will not stutter.

- *Chunking and pausing*: Dividing speech into phrases and inserting short pauses will also be very useful when it comes to speech rate control. This technique is helpful for motor planning and decreases the cognitive load for the task of speaking quickly. Research has shown that pacing and chunking make it easier to speak fluently since they give the speaker a guide and slow down the rate at which they speak (Höbler 2022).

6.10.3.2 Precision of Articulatory Movements

The role of the articulatory system is to produce correct and coordinated movements of structures for sound production. Movements that are poorly coordinated or inaccurate not only result in mispronunciations but also a breakdown of speech. Articulation entails a well-coordinated use of the lips, tongue, and jaw supported by their interplay at the appropriate time.

Techniques that Focus on Precision of Movements for Stuttering Management Include:

- *Light articulatory contacts*: As described above, talking softly with minimal contact between articulators helps to reduce the tension which usually results in stammering. Thus, through the elimination of the force of contact, speakers can come closer to producing transitional elements of sound. According to the present research, mild contact pressures may prevent stuttering occurrence by improving phoneme transition (Van Borsel 2018).
- *Phonemic drills*: Subsequently, it helps to practice the difficult sounds or words initially in isolation and then in the context of the sentence.

6.10.3.3 Resonance

Resonance refers to the kind of sound produced due to the vibrations that take place in the tract of the voice. Appropriate resonance is important when one wants to attain a good clear voice and a natural flow of speech.

- *Voice exercises*: The following exercises are suggested due to their ability to address resonance, which is defined as the sounds that are produced when an open and unobstructed vocal tract is used. Different approaches, like singing the hum-oh method and vocalization, are used to build up the voice. For example, the speaker hums while singing with his or her mouth slightly open and concentrates on the sensation in the facial mask area, which includes the nose and the cheeks.
- *Biofeedback*: One should also observe that the application of visual or auditory feedback as far as the regulation of resonance is concerned could also embrace significant efficacy. For example, spectrographic displays are employed in giving feedback on the voice resonance to the individuals in real time. Biofeedback has been used effectively in differently abled speaking individuals with stammering by helping them attain improved vocal health, hence clear speaking (Bunton 2018).

6.10.3.4 Prosody and Stuttering

The prosodic system is the attribute of speech that pertains to rhythm, stress, and intonation. These elements enrich the text and make it closer to a spoken language. Prosody involves several key components:

1. *Pitch*: The high or low frequencies of the voice.
2. *Stress*: Emphasis given on certain syllables or words.
3. *Rhythm*: The timing and flow of speech sounds.
4. *Intonation*: The variation in pitch across phrases and sentences.

Prosody is a critical component of verbal communication as it helps in transmitting meaning, emotion, and the speaker's intentions. Stutterers experience distortions in the prosodic components of speech which further results in communication barriers. Stuttering can get worsened by prosodic disruptions like incorrect stress, improper rhythm, and improper intonation. The impact of prosody on stuttering includes:

- *Disrupted rhythm*: Inaccurate timing of speech can increase the cognitive pressure and may lead to errors.
- *Abnormal stress patterns*: Stress placed at the wrong places can also make the speech sound unnatural and can cause hesitations and repetitions.
- *Intonation issues*: If pitch variation is not uniform, then the speech can sound monotonous or irregular and this affects fluency.

Recent research has also focused on the need to incorporate the prosodic features in stuttering treatment so that the patient can achieve more natural and fluent speech (Bunton 2018; Van Lieshout et al. 2020).

6.11 Various Techniques to Improve Prosody in Stuttering

Several therapeutic techniques focus on enhancing the prosodic elements of speech to help manage stuttering. Here are some effective methods based on recent research:

6.11.1 Rhythmic Speech Training

- *Metronome training*: Applying a metronome to practice can help an individual to maintain a certain speed when speaking. This helps to control the rate of speech and decrease the variability in speech which in turn improves fluency. Bunton (2018) concluded that the rhythmic speech training enhanced the speech fluency and naturalness of people who stutter. Metronomes and pacing boards were used to control the rate of speaking as well as the rhythm of speaking.

- *Pacing boards*: Pacing boards are another tool that can be used to control the rate of speech by giving a visual or touch sensation for every syllable or word that is said.

6.11.2 Stress and Intonation Practice

- *Contrastive stress drills*: These exercises include repeating sentences of different stress to help in fluency of the speech. For instance, "I *want* to go" versus "I want to *go*."
- *Intonation contours*: It is also helpful to pay attention to the rise and falls in the sentences when speaking, to add more pitch variation. This enables the individuals to make better and proper use of their speech. Van Lieshout et al. (2020) found that through the imitation of stress and intonation patterns, there is a possibility that the severity of stuttering may be decreased since speech becomes more fluent and expressive.

6.11.3 Choral Speaking

Group Reading Speaking in unison can also help in the coordination of speech tempo and stress, that is, in controlling the rhythm of delivery. It fosters a situation where not much emphasis is placed on the verbal output of a particular subject, hence increasing the possibility of prosodic features to emerge.

6.11.4 Changing the Duration of Sounds

- *Delayed auditory feedback (DAF)*: There are devices which send speaker's voice through their earphones with a time lag (say half a second or so). Such devices can aid speech fluency by reducing the speaking rate and encouraging the speaker to use more natural prosody.

For this reason, the application of speech therapy techniques to reduce the severity of stuttering is very important in the improvement of fluency and communication skills. These techniques are intended to enhance the coordination of speech motor gestures, the timing, and precision of the movements, involved in the different subsystems of speech production. Methods that include gentle onset, light contact of the articulators, diaphragmatic breathing, as well as rhythmic speech drilling have been seen to greatly lessen the severity of stuttering and enhance fluent speech.

Nonetheless, the significance of such techniques cannot be overemphasized since they offer people who stutter with methods that can assist them in modifying their speech and, in turn, decrease stuttering. Nevertheless, it is crucial to understand that these strategies must be carried out only by SLP. SLPs are educated and experienced in stuttering and are able to devise treatment plans that are appropriate for each client. They can check if the techniques are adequately employed and alter plans and interventions according to the subject's achievements and performance.

Supporters of the child in therapy include teachers, parents, and other members of society. They can encourage and motivate the client to apply the techniques in their daily life and help the child feel comfortable with their fluency in a nonjudgmental atmosphere that decreases the emotional and mental toll of stuttering. However, they should not try to conduct the therapy on their own and attempt to lead it. Inexperienced people may inadvertently encourage the negative use of language or raise the levels of stress, which, in turn, may worsen the stammering.

Thus, speech therapists, teachers, and parents can develop a coordinated approach to help children with stuttering manage their speech. The unique competence of SLPs complemented by the constant encouragement from teachers and parents ensures that the methods of speech therapy are effectively applied to people who stutter. This teamwork guarantees the patient the best services that strive to have them achieve fluent and confident speech.

6.12 Management of Stuttering in School

Stuttering is a severe condition that can hinder a child's learning process in school, and his or her ability to engage in class and with other students and achieve satisfactory results. School is a part of a child's life where communication plays a significant role in education and interpersonal relationships. Therefore, children who stutter might face certain difficulties. Thus, the successful management of stuttering in schools cannot be done without the involvement of SLPs, teachers, parents, and the students.

All the individuals involved in the child's life have a responsibility of ensuring that the child is supported and included in the communication and learning processes. The best practice in the management of stuttering in schools is where there is teamwork. This implies that SLPs, teachers, parents, and any other relevant personnel like counsellors or psychologists should be in constant communication and collaboration. All the aspects of the child are considered in this approach from speech to emotional and social spheres.

To achieve fluency, the schools could make a big difference to the educational and social achievement of children who stutter by adopting an integrated approach. This is a very effective management plan as it not only assists in minimizing the effects of stuttering on academic achievement but also ensures that the student enjoys a positive and inclusive learning experience in school.

6.12.1 Role of Educators

Stuttering is a condition that should be identified at an early age, and this makes teachers play an important role in stuttering identification and management. Since teachers are a direct contact for children on a daily basis, they can easily identify possible symptoms of stuttering, arrange for evaluations, and assist with the application of treatment methods at school environment.

6.12.2 Early Identification of Stuttering

6.12.2.1 Recognizing Early Signs

Apart from home situations, teachers are usually the first to observe changes in a child's speech production and fluency. This is important since early identification of the disorder is crucial for better results. Teachers should be aware of the common signs of stuttering, like:

1. Repetitions: It refers to the use of words, syllables, or sounds that are repeated with time, for instance, "ball, ball, ball."
2. Prolongations: Prolonging of one phoneme within a word more than once (e.g., *ssssnake*).
3. Blocks: Silent periods or hesitations in the child's speech where it appears that the child is having difficulty coming up with a sound.
4. Physical tension: The overt signs of tension or difficulty in the speech organs including the face muscles during the speech process.
5. Avoidance behaviors: Some of the strategies include not using some words or finding oneself in certain situations or not even speaking at all to avoid stuttering.

6.12.2.2 Early Referral and Collaboration

When educators notice some of the mentioned potentials of stuttering, it is important to refer the child to SLP for an assessment. Thus, cooperation between teachers, parents, and SLPs are crucial for the child to get the required help. Teachers can facilitate this process by:

1. Communicating observations: Reporting on the specific aspects of the child's speech, language use, and behaviors to the SLP and parents.
2. Coordinating meetings: These include convening meetings between SLP, parents, and teachers to address the issues at hand and map the way forward.
3. Providing continuous feedback: Providing feedback to the SLP periodically, concerning the child's progress and any noticeable changes in the classroom.

6.12.3 Assessment of Stuttering

The standardized evaluation of stuttering is done by an SLP; however, teachers have an active participation in the assessment process. For instance, teachers can share with the clinician important information concerning the child's speech and language abilities in different contexts, thus contributing to the assessment. Educators can assist in the assessment process by:

1. Observing speech in different contexts: Understanding the way the child's stuttering varies across different situations, such as during classroom discussions, group activities, and one-on-one interactions.
2. Documenting frequency and severity: Keeping a record of the frequency and severity of stuttering episodes, including specific examples and contexts in which they occur.
3. Identifying triggers and patterns: Identifying the child's stuttering and determining factors that may worsen the stuttering, including stress, fatigue, and specific speaking conditions.
4. Supporting classroom-based assessments: Help in conducting assessments within the classroom by allowing SLPs to observe the child in the classroom and even engage him in certain activities.
5. Administering informal assessments: Some of the tasks included providing support in the collection of speech samples, including reading passages to assess the child's speech.
6. Interpreting assessment results: To work with SLPs to interpret assessment results and understand implications to classroom management.
7. Monitoring progress: Teachers can help by observing the child periodically and recording his/her speech and communication behaviors to evaluate the success of the applied interventions and to modify them if necessary.

6.12.4 Generalization of Treatment

A major difficulty in stuttering interventions is having the children apply the techniques they have learned in therapy to real life. Educators play a significant role in this process by:

1. Integrating speech strategies into classroom activities: Adapting speaking techniques like speaking slowly, starting easily, and stopping at the right places can be helpful. Also understanding the use of speech strategies like slow speech rate, easy start, and pauses while in classroom activities and discussions helps in achieving better results.
2. Providing consistent feedback: Providing feedback to children to encourage them to use and improve their speech strategies in the right manner.
3. Modelling effective communication: Providing good models and demonstrating effective communication techniques, such as speaking slowly and clearly, help in achieving fluency faster.

Teachers can also play a big role in ensuring that the children who stutter are put in a comfortable position in the class to aid their normal speech. This can be done by:

1. Encouraging open communication: Enabling the students to share whatever they have in their mind without the fear of being corrected by their peers.

2. Modelling respectful listening: Exhibiting patience and encouraging active listening, especially when a student is explaining something, help with better speech fluency.
3. Reducing time pressure: Avoid putting pressure on speaking quickly or respond immediately to a question asked.
4. Organizing structured speaking activities: Frequent scheduling of tasks like show-and-tell, telling of stories, and debating so that the children can rehearse their speech strategies in a safe environment.
5. Facilitating peer interactions: Promoting peer interaction and group activities so that the child can use the identified speech strategies with other children.
6. Facilitating real-life conversations: To support CWS, educators should encourage the child to use the strategies when speaking in natural situations. This involves talking to strangers like guest speakers or other teachers, overcoming stage fear, having open discussions by providing safe environments, and encouraging students to express their thoughts and opinions, without being teased or mocked.

6.12.5 Supporting Emotional and Social Development

Stuttering affects the emotional and social aspects of a child and he or she may become frustrated, embarrassed, and lonely. Educators can support the emotional and social well-being of children who stutter by:

1. Fostering a positive classroom culture: Creating a healthy learning environment for all students so that they will be respected in the classroom.
2. Building self-esteem and confidence: Creating chances for children to develop their self-esteem and confidence through positive experiences and encouragement.
3. Encouraging peer support: Educating other children to accept their fellow students by explaining what stuttering is and making them more acceptable to the student who stutters.

6.12.6 Educating Others: Teachers, Peers, and School Management

To help children who stutter feel comfortable in school, the other teachers, peers, and school administration should be informed about stuttering. Educators can:

1. Conduct awareness sessions: Organize class meetings to inform the other students about stuttering, what it means and how they can help the students who stutter.
2. Promote empathy and understanding: Promote tolerance and understanding by telling students to accept and be tolerant of children who stutter.

3. Engage school management: Collaborate with the school's authorities and fellow teachers to guarantee that there are necessary measures that will help students who stutter. For example, they can have access to speech therapy, and they might not be required to do presentations during class.

6.12.7 Collaborating with Parents and Caregivers

Cooperation with parents and caregivers is crucial for the generalization of the treatment into everyday life. Educators can facilitate this collaboration by:

1. Communicating regularly: Reporting to parents/caregivers from time to time on the child's progress and any issues they may be experiencing.
2. Sharing strategies and resources: Modelling and providing materials for boosters at home for the parents and caregivers to use.
3. Involving parents in school activities: Inclusion of parents and caregivers in schools to acquaint them with school activities and events for them to feel part of society.

Thus, the real-life applications, peer education, and school engagement can assist teachers in guiding children who stutter and transform them into confident speakers. Thus, educators are not only responsible for providing students with academic knowledge, but they also have a great potential to create a tolerant atmosphere for diverse communication. Thus, being proactive, compassionate, and knowledgeable, teachers can help children who stutter and shape their futures for the better. This book depicts how teachers play a crucial role in identifying and dealing with stuttering, hence enabling these children to voice their ideas and excel in various facets of their lives.

6.12.8 Prevention of Stuttering in School

In the current social context of India, children are admitted to school at a very young age, mainly at the age of two with children 2.5 to 3 years of age being typically common. Due to the increased rates of parents working full-time, schools have become a cardinal part of children's lives and children now spend a lot of time in schools with teachers. This extra time spent by children in the school environment can thus allow the teachers a special chance to contribute toward early detection of stuttering.

Teachers are likely to be the first to recognize that a child has a speech or language problem as they spend more time with the child on a day-to-day basis. Their task is broader than teaching and guiding students, which allows them to create conditions that prevent the onset of stuttering. Since the first few years of a child's life are spent in school, educators have the potential of helping students achieve smooth and correct speech and thereby prevent stammering.

Furthermore, the first grades of school are important for speech and language development. This is the stage at which teachers can shape children's communication patterns and offer early management strategies to avert normal nonfluencies (NNF) from deteriorating into persistent stuttering. Thus, identifying the indicators of stuttering and the use of preventive measures, teachers could greatly impact the speech development of their students and their overall health.

Thus, the importance of teachers in the prevention of stuttering becomes even more significant when discussed within the given context. They work at the basic level of monitoring and comprehending speech dysfluencies and, thus, play a crucial role in the improvement of children. Thus, understanding specific strategies and techniques that teachers can use to prevent stuttering is very crucial, especially among children who are in their early years of education.

Various practical ways of preventing stuttering from worsening significantly in a young child are described below:

6.12.9 Classroom Management Techniques

- Structured routines: Set up a routine that the students and the teacher can follow in class to ensure that the children feel safe. For instance, a common schedule of activities in the morning may alleviate the level of anxiety and co-related dysfluencies. Thus, routines help to cope with unforeseen situations and stress, which may deteriorate the stuttering (Bloodstein and Bernstein Ratner 2008).
- Flexible questioning: It is advisable to use both the open-ended and the close-ended questions. Some broad questions that help the child speak more are "What did you like most about the story?" while some direct questions which may give the child some reliefs are "Did you like the story or not?" Thus, offering different kinds of questions can meet the needs of the child with different comfort and communication ability and take the pressure off the child.

6.12.10 Speech-Friendly Classroom Activities

- Turn-taking games: Use games involving turn-taking, for instance, the "Pass the Story" game whereby a student adds one sentence to a story. This makes the children to be able to speak without the feeling that someone will interrupt them. Another example is the game named "Talk Tokens" in which the students are required to speak in turns using tokens. Turn-taking decreases the competition for who gets to speak and children can give their full attention to the task of speaking without being interrupted (Yairi and Seery 2015).
- Show-and-tell: Promote daily show-and-tell which will help children to speak in front of their peers without fear of being laughed at. For instance, a student can come to class

with a toy which is dear to him/her and explain to the class about it for a few minutes. Organized chances to speak in a supportive environment increase the level of confidence and decrease the level of fear that is linked with speaking (Guitar 2014).

6.12.11 Supportive Communication Techniques

- Active listening: Listen carefully to what the child is saying and convey interest in what he or she is saying. Carry out gestures such as nodding and ensure making eye contact to show one is listening. For instance, when telling a story, listen and make actions and questions that depict active listening. Active listening affirms the child's attempt to make themselves understood and erases the possibility of aggression from the child (Craig and Tran 2005).
- Reflective listening: Paraphrase what the child has said to show that one comprehends what the child has said, and this will encourage the child. For example, if a child says, "I went to the zoo," one can respond, "Oh, you went to the zoo? That must have been fun." Reflective listening helps in affirmation of the child's statement and encourages him or her to express themselves more (Manning and DiLollo 2025).

6.12.12 Collaboration with SLPs

- Regular meetings: Meet with the SLPs at a fixed interval to review each child's progress and identify changes that may be required regarding the strategies to be employed, for instance, a monthly status meeting to assess the outcomes of the interventions and modify them if necessary. Such a structure helps to avoid discrepancies and inconsistencies in the implementation of the strategies which in turn increases the efficiency of the interventions (Yaruss et al. 2006).
- Integrated goals: Collaborate with SLPs to coordinate the implementation of speech therapy objectives into day-to-day lessons in the classroom. For example, particular speech exercises can be integrated into the daily schedule of a classroom. The process of incorporating therapy goals into the daily routines enhances the application of what has been learned and ensures the skills are transferred from one context to another (Fraser 2010).

6.12.13 Professional Development

- Workshops and training: Enrolling in seminars and other forms of learning related to stuttering and speech disorders helps in being aware of the new techniques and approaches, for example, a workshop on the contemporary practices for working with students who stutter. Lifelong learning enhances the teacher's capacity to teach effectively and to know the most current strategies for teaching and working with students (Reardon-Reeves and Yaruss 2013).

- Resource utilization: Expand the knowledge about children who stutter with the help of materials provided by SLPs, for example, handouts and videos, for instance, observing an instructional video about ways of supporting pupils with a stutter during the classroom lessons. It is important to note that professional resources help in increasing the teachers' knowledge and the ability to apply proper strategies (Onslow and O'Brian 2013).

6.12.14 Preventing Normal Nonfluency (NNF) from Becoming Stuttering

Normal nonfluency (NNF) is a condition that is usually seen in young children, and if proper care is taken, it does not lead to stuttering. This can be done in the following ways:

6.12.15 Parental Involvement

- Modelling calm speech: Suggest to parents to speak slowly and calmly at home to their children. For example, parents can describe the everyday actions in a slow and simple way. For example, the parent can say, "Now we are putting on our shoes." Children tend to copy the speech of the people who take care of them; thus, using proper and slow speech can minimize the dysfluencies (Bloodstein and Bernstein Ratner 2008).
- Positive reinforcement: Parents should be encouraged to appreciate the effort the child is making in communication as opposed to the actual output. For instance, parents can tell their children, "I enjoy listening to the stories you tell," instead of correcting them for a stutter. Positive reinforcement increases children's confidence and decreases their level of anxiety and thus they are more willing to speak without fear (Guitar 2014).

6.12.16 Home-School Collaboration

- Consistent strategies: Both the home and school environments should employ similar measures to support the child's speech depending on the case: For instance, if the teacher employed a pacing board in class, the parents could also employ the same at home to supplement the teacher's efforts. Thus, a similar environment helps to generalize the learning and does not cause confusion for the child (Yaruss and Reardon-Reeves 2007).
- Family workshops: Establish sessions for parents and caregivers to attend to learn strategies for promoting their child's speech development to avoid the advancement of NNF to stuttering, for instance, a workshop where the parents are shown how to make the

home environment supportive of speech. This is because through educating the families, they will be in a position to support and understand the child, leading to better results (Fraser 2010).

6.12.17 Early Intervention Programs

- Screening and assessment: Screen the children on a regular basis to determine which ones are at risk of developing stuttering, for example, the initial speech screenings performed at the beginning of the academic year. Due to this, onset can be detected before the disorder evolves to NNF and then to stuttering as pointed by Yairi and Seery (2015).
- Speech therapy integration: Schedule the children that are at risk for speech therapy sessions in school time, for instance, arranging the speech therapy lessons at school time to avail the child the required assistance at a specific time. The stability of therapy sessions is crucial because it assists in avoiding the intensification of speech dysfluencies, and this is due to the reason explained by Onslow and O'Brian (2013).

6.12.18 Classroom Strategies

- Relaxed speaking opportunities: Develop tasks that are casual and do not require the students to feel stress. For instance, the child is allowed to read in front of the class, in small groups, or directly to the teacher before reading in front of the whole class. Lifting pressure off speaking lessens stress and thus enhances the rate of speaking (Guitar 2014).
- Encouraging self-pacing: Encourage them to regulate their speech depending on the rate they want. Tips such as taking a moment of silence between words will assist in regulating the rate of speaking and avoiding repetitions or prolongation of words, for example, asking children to take a deep breath before they start speaking a sentence. The strategies that are used in managing the speech of children assist in minimizing the instances of stuttering (Bloodstein and Bernstein Ratner 2008).

6.12.19 Monitoring and Feedback

- Regular observation: Monitor the child's speaking habits and record it. Inform the SLPs of the child's performance to modify the plan of intervention, for instance, identifying any cases of dysfluency at any point during class lessons and activities. Enhanced monitoring enables one to make alterations of the strategies used in order to suit the child's changing needs (Reardon-Reeves and Yaruss 2013).
- Immediate feedback: Give quick and soft responses to the attempts that the child is making. For example, if a child with a stutter happens to stutter, one should say, "You're

doing good, just keep on talking." This kind of affirmation and feedback has an immediate positive effect on the child and reduces the effect of the dysfluency (Yairi and Seery 2015).

6.12.20 Preventing Development of Negative Feelings and Emotions

1. Create safe spaces: Setting up child-friendly environments to report any form of abuse without being shamed. This could be a specific section in the class where they can express themselves without fear of being reprimanded, for instance, a "quiet corner" to help children who want to practice speaking in a more pressure-free setting. Offering a comfortable environment decreases the level of stress and creates a good environment for speaking.
2. Open communication: Help children to express themselves on the matter of speaking. Alleviating their fears and anxieties may assist in lowering their stress levels, for instance, assigning a certain time of the day where students can express themselves and their emotions to their fellow classmates. It breaks the barriers that may be present in children and enables them to openly express themselves, hence alleviating the anxiety of talking.
3. Positive reinforcements and celebrate efforts: Thus, it is important not to focus on the child's fluency but to encourage him or her and celebrate the efforts that he or she has made. Encourage and acknowledge their efforts to speak even if what they say is not perfect, for instance, providing a child with a sticker or positive words as a result of contributing to a discussion in class. Positive reinforcement has a positive impact on a child's self-esteem and powers their level of nervousness, which makes them want to speak more (Guitar 2014).
4. Empathy and understanding: Promote the culture of tolerance and endorsement of other people's feelings among fellow students. Increase awareness with classmates to demystify the condition and decrease the negative backlash of the condition, for example, having a group discussion in the class regarding stuttering and how one can assist fellow students who stutter. Based on the reviewed literature, asking other students to join the campaign also assists in building a supportive environment for children who stutter because they do not feel alone (Yaruss and Reardon-Reeves 2007).
5. Encouraging expressive arts: Some of the activities that could be included are drawing, painting, or even telling a story which helps the child to create. The above activities assist in diminishing concentration on verbal communication and increase confidence, for instance, a "storyboard" project in which children draw out their story and then tell it. Creative activities are helpful in giving an individual a different way of expressing themselves, thus does not put pressure on verbal communication.
6. Encouraging expressive arts: Some of the activities to include are drawing, painting, or tale-telling, which are all ways through which children can be creative. All these activities help in minimizing the reliance on the spoken word and increase confidence, for instance, a "storyboard" activity where children both draw and narrate their story to the

teacher. Thus, creative activities are a way of self-expression which helps to solve communication problems and relieve pressure on verbal communication.
7. Resilience building through coping skills: Strategies like telling yourself positive things and deep breathing are useful, for instance, role-playing to speak in different contexts in the following scenarios. This can assist a child to design ways of dealing with real-life speaking situations that they may encounter. For instance, to mimic the real-life situation, the child could be taught how to order food in a restaurant.
8. Peer buddies: Assign the children who stutter with supportive peers so that they can get the support that they require when they are expected to speak, for instance, having a peer to assist the child in any group activity that he or she may have difficulty in.
9. Counsellor involvement: Ensure that school counsellors are included in offering comfort to the children and/or coming up with measures that the children can use to cope with the feelings that they may have regarding stuttering.

In conclusion, the management and prevention of stuttering in school cannot be done without the teachers, parents, and speech-language pathologists. Thus, schools can minimize the effects of stuttering on the learning process and social life of children by providing suitable conditions, applying effective measures, and using timely help. It is the result of cooperation between parents, teachers, siblings, friends, and all other people who are around children who need proper help to overcome stuttering and work on their fluency.

6.12.21 Steps to Manage stuttering in School

Step 1: Managing Stuttering by Identifying It at the Right Time
Stuttering can affect learning and social interaction in school among children in a very great manner. All tasks that require the use of speech, oral reporting in the class, reading out aloud, or engaging in group discussions can provoke anxiety and worsen the fluency of speech. Communication may also be a problem as there are possibilities of mocking or being embarrassed. Teachers also help in the management of children who stutter through reinforcing acceptance, time, understanding, and even patience from the fellow learners. With the help of SLPs, ways to manage communication can be planned, which boosts the child's morale and increases his or her desire to be involved. Including stuttering in schools as a topic of discussion is beneficial since children who stutter can comfortably learn and interact with other children in school.

Identifying Stuttering in School Settings
Various school scenarios can act as triggers for stuttering, including:

- Speaking in front of the class when teachers are asking questions.
- Reading out aloud in the class.
- Speaking or making presentations at the school assemblies.
- Conversing with fellow students in a casual manner.

- Participating in competition or other sporting activities.
- Navigating disciplinary actions.
- Dealing with other students in the class.
- Interacting with people or going to people one does not know.
- Reciting poems or telling stories.
- Group discussions and activities.

Step 2: Managing Stuttering by Providing Right Support

To the teachers, when working with students who stutter, it is important to help the child rather than the speech issue. To ensure that all the children, especially those who stutter, are comfortable in class, it is important to promote an accepting atmosphere. This fosters an environment within which they can easily speak and participate without fear, a situation that may help foster their communication skills. For this purpose, it is crucial to enhance the awareness of the educators about stuttering and their perception toward it should be positive.

The Power of Empathy

Empathy can be defined as the ability to put oneself in the other person's shoes and feel what he or she feels, which is vital in supporting students who stutter. Thus, empathy will enable the educators to get a better understanding of the difficulties these students encounter. This knowledge contributes to the formation of the class atmosphere that is characterized by trust and acceptance, which, in turn, makes the students more willing to share their thoughts. While sympathy can be described as an understanding of another person's pain, empathy is a feeling that creates a basis for support.

In the long run, the educators' responsibility does not stop at the conventional teaching and learning processes. To this end, teachers should support their students, as well as learn about stuttering, in order to positively influence their students' lives. It is equally advantageous for students who stutter, and for all the rest of the class, fostering tolerance and acceptance of each other.

Self-Exploration

Self-exploration is defined as the process of studying a topic in its entirety, and it is most important in the area of stuttering. It is quite common to have incorrect beliefs and prejudice in a subject area that one has no knowledge about. Through this process, educators can remove these barriers and fully comprehend the nature of stuttering from the stutters' perspective. This process is crucial in creating a culture that will enable students who stutter to be accepted and therefore supported.

To comprehend stuttering on a deeper level, one needs to go beyond the surface and discover the problems and issues that people who stutter encounter. Self-exploration helps educators to:

1. Break down misconceptions: Without appropriate understanding, it is quite possible to misunderstand the behaviors and requirements of students who stutter. Self-exploration helps the educators to erase the wrong information with the true information.
2. Build empathy: Learning about the real-life situation of people who stutter is very important in gaining true understanding or empathy to be able to support them.
3. Enhance support strategies: Improving the awareness of teachers and educators will help them to choose proper approaches to teaching and supporting students who stutter.
4. Promote inclusivity: Aware teachers are in a better position to create an equal learning environment in the classroom and make all the students to be accepted and welcomed.

Methods of Self-Exploration

1. Watching videos and documentaries: Videos and channels on YouTube and TED Talks are available to know about people who stutter and their stories. These videos are beneficial for teachers as they allow them to watch real people who stutter and their struggles and successes.
2. Listening to podcasts: Many of them include interviews with people who have a stutter, speech therapists, and professionals working in the area. These discussions help to present different opinions and ideas about the everyday lives of people who stutter.
3. Reading books and articles: Teachers can turn to books, articles, and blogs by people who stutter or speech therapists. These resources offer information on the psychological and emotional side of stuttering to give general information about the condition.
4. Engaging with personal stories: It has been through autobiographies, blogs, and interviews that readers get a close look at what it feels like to stutter. These stories shed light on how these people can find ways to overcome their situations, thus making people become more aware of their struggles.

Being reflective has many advantages to the trainers and this book has discussed the same. It also increases awareness and thus allows teachers to have a better relationship with students who stutter. This book also highlights successful people who stutter, which is encouraging for the students as well as the educators. In addition, the book provides the educators with speech therapy techniques and strategies to help students with disabilities. Specifically, knowledge about stuttering makes it possible to dispel the myths and prejudices and contributes to the creation of a tolerant environment at school.

Step 3: Applying Empathy in the Classroom

In view of this, it is crucial that teachers of students who stutter avoid being merely sympathetic but instead be empathetic. Empathy can be defined as the ability to perceive, as well as respond to, the emotions of other people. This is very influential in the classroom setting. While sympathy is the ability to understand another person's pain without having to experience it firsthand, empathy goes beyond that by promoting relationship and support.

Encouraging Open Dialogue

- Safe space for discussions: It is therefore important for teachers to help the students feel comfortable when they are in a class so that they can discuss stuttering. This could be done through scheduling common class discussions where the students can express themselves. To this end, teachers may use such conversations as telling the students stories of their own learning experiences about stuttering.
- Classroom activities: Organize events such as "Ask Me Anything" forums in which students who stutter can discuss their experience and respond to questions from other students. This is useful in desensitizing others on the issue of stuttering and creating a good appreciation of the condition.
- Inviting guest speakers: Have speakers come in occasionally to share their stories including those of SLPs or people who stutter.

Modelling Patience and Active Listening

- Demonstrate patience: Whenever a student who stutters is speaking, teachers should not get impatient with him/her. This entails not rushing the student so that they can complete what they are saying, not finishing their words or sentences for them, and making sure that one's eyes are in the normal range of the student's while having the conversation.
- Active listening exercises: Include activities that will help the learners to develop active listening skills. For instance, students can be asked to work in groups of two and try to listen to each other without interrupting and then, paraphrase what the other person said.
- Role-playing: Here are some examples to discuss and model active and empathic listening in role-playing. For instance, divide students into pairs and make one student explain something to the other student while the other student is supposed to listen attentively.

Avoiding Interruptions

- Classroom norms: Devise class rules on how students should conduct themselves when in the class, especially when communicating. State that it is incorrect to cut off another person when they are speaking and for students who stutter.
- Visual reminders: Some of the things that can be used include posters and signs that encourage patience and active listening. These can be used as reminders for the students to take turns and to listen attentively to their peers' answers.
- Silent cues: Instruct the students to make signs when they want to speak next, for instance, raising of the index finger. This takes the burden off the students who stutter to rush through their speech.

Celebrating Progress

- Acknowledgment of efforts: Ensure to appreciate and applause students who stutter from time to time. This can be through an oral endorsement, an award, or recognition

during class meetings. Accept any positive change in the communication, whether it is a gradual one.
- Sharing success stories: Give examples of people who have learned how to handle their stammering and come out successful. Mention the achievements of famous people who have stuttering, for instance, Winston Churchill or Joe Biden, to encourage the students.
- Peer support: Have the students appreciate the efforts of their colleagues, especially when they are improving. Introduce a "Kindness Wall" in which students are encouraged to write kind messages, things they like about other students, their progress, etc.

Understanding Empathy Over Sympathy

Teachers who are searching for information about stuttering have to forget about sympathy and turn to empathy. Empathy goes a step further than compassion in that the teacher can put himself or herself in the shoes of the student who stutters. It enhances the environment that is needed by the student to build confidence and improve his or her communication skills.

Step 4: Managing Stuttering Using Speech Therapy Techniques in Real Life

Gaining control over stuttering in real-life conditions requires that certain procedures that are learned in speech therapy be adapted in order to enable the affected persons to communicate in a more smooth and confident manner. For the educators, the application of these strategies must be done with a certain level of sensitivity to the comfort levels of the student. It is therefore important that these strategies are done in a very careful and polite manner so that the students do not feel that they are being pointed out or picked on.

Teachers are very critical in assisting students who stutter to regulate their speech. Such support should be offered either covertly or at least in a manner that will not make the student nervous about the procedure. Shouting out the disability in the presence of everyone in the class can be counterproductive if the student is not prepared or willing to do so. The main purpose is to facilitate the student in a manner that is considerate and also empowering.

Guidelines to Use When Trying to Implement Therapy into Practice:

1. *Encouraging Natural Speech Patterns*: Teachers are encouraged to be themselves in their own classrooms. No, they are not speech therapists, and they DO NOT have to be one when dealing with a child who stutters. They are another source of support, and they should always bear in mind that they are an intermediary between the child and the world. Hence, they should ensure that they make the speech native-like (with or without the techniques).
   - *Avoid overemphasizing techniques like breathing*: According to Dr. Yaruss (2021), even though breathing techniques are incorporated in stuttering treatment, there is little evidence on how manipulating breathing may assist the individuals who stutter in their day-to-day lives. On the contrary, the family members, and teachers, by

pointing at the specific breathing patterns make the child more aware and worsen their speech. He observes that normal and spontaneous breathing is adequate in the majority of cases for speech production. When a student is asked to "breathe" or told to "breathe from the diaphragm," it adds undue complexity to the speech, and attention to the breathing, which may worsen the stuttering.

It is therefore important that the teachers should concentrate on the natural way of talking. The teacher should not look away when the student who stutters starts to talk and should not make the student feel embarrassed by looking at him or her in the face and waiting for him or her to produce words without making a fuss about the stuttering. Thus, the students will not feel as much pressure to change their breathing and stay calm.

2. *Reducing Avoidance Behaviors*:
   - *Address root causes*: It helps to know and treat the physical discomfort and actions to avoid that are related to stuttering rather than certain methods. These problems mainly arise from people's dislike of stuttering itself. Teaching people to accept and tolerate stuttering can lessen the anxiety, fear, and avoidance that leads to the problem of speaking.

To design an effective classroom environment, teachers should encourage participation without making students feel pressured. For instance, allowing the student to present in small groups or even to one person before involving the whole class can help the student to gain the confidence needed to perform in front of the whole class and avoid avoiding the activity.

3. *Normalizing Speech Variations*:
   - *Undoing misdirected focus*: Strategies such as paying less attention to breath control, slowing down of speech, and other forms of speech deviation are also vital in demystifying natural speech. This must be done in a very gradual way and in a very gentle manner so that the child is using the techniques but not relying on them exclusively. The aim is to make these techniques the way of communication and not the way of "annoying communication." Thus, teachers may help to neutralize the attitudes to speech variations by telling the students about popular speakers who stutter. One way is to point out to the student that stuttering is a form of speech, and thus, there is no need to stress to fit the standard way of speaking.

Practical Approaches:

- *Modeling and Reinforcement*: Students can be taught to only speak calmly and slowly without being told directly to do so by the teacher. Thus, the student can watch without being directly addressed and then copy what has been said or done.
- *Positive Reinforcement*: One can get motivated by celebrating the small wins and progress made so that they can gain confidence. This way, students will be appreciated for the effort they put into their work rather than the results of the work.

4. *Referral to Healthcare Providers*:
   - *Identifying genuine difficulties*: However, where there are true problems with breath support or use of other strategies, correct medical and/or physiotherapy referrals are necessary. This ensures that any other health complications are well taken care of by the doctors. Teachers should take cognizance of the fact that certain speech difficulties may require attention from parents and medical practitioners and should therefore report any such occurrence.
   - *Supporting children at every aspect*: One must be patient and have interest in handling children who stutter. Creating a patient and tolerant attitude helps students to share their thoughts and ideas with each other without feeling ashamed or being laughed at. Teachers can gain the trust of these students, and therefore develop a better relationship with them, if they listen to them, watch them, and interact with them in class.
   - *Recognizing your own worth*: Teachers have a critical part to play in the lives of children who stutter, being in regular contact with the SLPs. Even though SLPs give specific instructions, teachers monitor and evaluate the child's communicative behavior in the classroom and other natural contexts. It is therefore important to put into practice measures that enhance the child's communication in all forms and his or her health on a daily basis. Teachers should take credit for the wonderful progress that the child has made and feel confident in their input. This encourages them to keep on creating a conducive environment for children who stutter to learn, to overcome any barrier that may be in their way and be successful. Above all, it can be said that a happy and positive teacher brings out a successful student.

5. *Implementing Effective Communication Practices*:

To support a child who stutters, there are a set of guidelines that one has to consider. It is advisable not to fill in the gaps but instead just wait for them to say something; one should just remain quiet and let them speak at their own pace. Telling them to try and slow down or take a breath may not work at the time and may place further stress. It is important that one does not prompt the child to use speech tools all the time as he or she requires time to build up his or her own mechanisms of how to handle stress. They should be handled just like any other child, wherein they are given the chance to contribute to the class discussion but with consideration of their disability. Understand that some days may be difficult and, in such cases, try to use less words, be patient, and seek the child's help to find out what they want.

6. *Fostering a Supportive Environment*:

These include ensuring that one looks at the child in the eyes and ensures that the child has enough time to complete saying what he or she has to say. To model wait time, the teacher should take some time to answer a child's question, say two seconds, and also reduce the amount of talking done in a particular time to give the child time to answer. Ensure that nobody speaks over each other, thus promoting courtesy and making sure that all the students, especially those who stutter, feel included. Encourage children to have positive self-esteem and encourage the children to express themselves and talk about the differences in the ways people communicate to embrace diversity and ensure that the children who stutter are comfortable and have confidence.

7. *Empowering Participation and Turn-Taking*:
   The attitude of students who stutter and their willingness to communicate should be considered. Defining certain gestures, such as a thumbs-up or clapping signals, the child will be able to show that he or she is ready. This helps the child to participate at their own capacity without been rushed by other students or the teacher. Encourage the students to take turns in speaking, for instance, by using an object of discussion or adhering to a particular order of speaking, in order to give all the students an equal chance to express themselves. This practice helps students to be more patient, to listen to their peers, and to be more considerate of other people's feelings, which makes the learning environment better.

8. *Promoting Content Focus and Personality Development*:
   Educating students who stutter on how to inform their classmates that the content of the message is more important than the way it is delivered assists in fostering a positive attitude of the class toward the child. Through this approach, students will be able to embrace their fellow students' opinions and feedback, hence promoting tolerance. Understanding that communication is not only spoken, teachers should also give children a chance to express themselves with various tasks. Promoting children's involvement in arts, sports, and leadership activities gives them confidence and boost up their morale to discover their talents and potential.

9. *Collaborating with Parents*:
   Involvement of parents is very essential in the overall management of children who stutter. This makes parents and teachers work hand in hand to address the progress, difficulties, and ways of handling them that the child is facing. There is a good opportunity for teachers to share information with parents, exchange experiences, offer advice, and talk about the child's development. Thus, parents and teachers can guarantee that the child gets all the necessary support that is needed at a particular stage of development.

10. *Classroom Inclusion*:
    Stuttering should not be an issue that would make one set low expectations for a student. Encourage the student who stutters, address him or her calmly and patiently, and give them time to respond. The content of the message to be sent back to the sender should be focused on showing that one is listening. Share required adjustments with the student during individual meetings, and be sensitive to the student's requirements but not overprotective. Do not stigmatize stuttering; approach it like any other issue to foster a positive environment. Avoid talking to the child about the speech problem in front of other people as this would breach the child's rights to dignity and comfort. Implementing all these strategies in the classroom will help the children who stutter feel welcome and comfortable in the classroom.

6.13 Managing Preschool Children in Classrooms

To help preschoolers who stutter, teachers and other caregivers have a great responsibility. Thus, they can use fluency reinforcement, corrective feedback, and response cost and other evidence-based practices to make the classroom a welcoming and encouraging place. Thus, this approach does not only develop fluency but also confidence and proper communication skills of a child, which helps in the growth and development of a child. Thus, it is possible to distinguish a few effective techniques that are grounded in evidence and can be easily applied by teachers to help preschoolers who stutter. These include:

6.13.1 Fluency Reinforcement

Fluency reinforcement is the technique of using positive reinforcement for fluent speech; this has been a fundamental technique since the 1970s. This method involves praising children to some extent, helping them speak fluently, and therefore promoting the right behavior.

- Principle: Positive reinforcement rewarding of desired behaviors is done to ensure that the behavior is repeated.
- Application: The following can be used to incorporate this technique in the classroom: positive verbal reinforcement and offering rewards for speaking in full sentences.

Classroom Activities

1. *Smooth Speech Stars*: Design a star chart to put in the classroom and give the student stars every time they speak fluently. For instance, during circle time, each child who speaks without stammering is awarded a star. At the end of the week, they can cash in their stars for some prize, for instance, stickers or some more time on the play set.
2. *Fluency Treasure Hunt*: A treasure hunt can be arranged in which children get clues for every fluent speech. For instance, during a story, the teacher can give a cue to a child for every three smooth sentences that they make. The clues take the child to a small treasure chest containing goodies such as pencils, small toys, and healthy snacks.

6.13.2 Fluency Reinforcement Plus Corrective Feedback

This means praising the child when he or she speaks without stuttering while offering mild correction when the child stutters. This approach seeks to boost the treatment outcomes by treating both the normally functioning and the dysfunctional speech.

- Principle: Thus, it is possible to work on effective speech as well as speech with mistakes by using reinforcement with feedback.
- Application: The child is made to practice fluency reinforcement while at the same time, the educators give feedback from time to time in a classroom setting.

Classroom Activities

1. *Story Time Feedback*: In story time, the teacher praises fluent speech and offers slight correction in case of stuttering. For example, when a child speaks fluently, the teacher can encourage them by saying, "That's good, you are speaking fluently." However, when a child stutters, the teacher can help by saying, "Let's try that again, and this time, take your time."
2. *Peer Support Circles*: Organize subgroups where students can count on each other's encouragement and constructive criticism. For instance, in a group activity, the children say good job for clear speech and if a child stutters, the other children politely offer a chance to speak again at a slower rate.

Classroom Activities

1. *Token Economy*: Children get tokens for speaking fluently and lose tokens for stuttering. For example, during show-and-tell, a child will be given tokens for each grammatically correct sentence they utter. The tokens can be traded for little gifts or certain rewards.
2. *Speech Store*: Develop a "speech store" where children will be allowed to purchase items for use with tokens they will get for speaking fluently. For instance, during a lesson, a child gets a token for every correct and understandable sentence that they construct. By the end of the week, they can redeem their tokens to get items such as coloring books or toys from the speech store.

6.13.3 Response Cost

Response cost entails systematic arrangement of reinforcing and punishing behaviors that help to make fluency desirable and yet children still get to face the implications of stuttering.

- Principle: Thus, positive reinforcement of good behavior and negative reinforcement of undesirable behavior in the form of mild consequences.
- Application: Rewards for smooth talking and remove the tokens for the opposite but do not give the child an adverse feeling.

6.13.4 Modelling Fluent Speech

Children who stutter need to be given activities that model normal speech to enable them to learn how to speak normally. When teachers and parents speak clearly, calmly, and fluently, the child will have something to imitate. This includes:

1. Speak slowly and clearly: To assist the child, one must break the language down into shorter phrases and try to enunciate every word as best as possible to be imitated by the child.
2. Pause frequently: Remember, if you are using phrases, or even sentences, it is useful to pause so that the child does not feel under pressure and the child can be taught how to regulate speech.
3. Use simple language: The teacher should use simple and brief language which the child will be able to understand and even mimic.
4. Maintain eye contact: Here, one can make the child interested by making eye contact and gestures to show that the child is being understood, and the child is being given an audience.
5. Be patient and encouraging: The child should be placed in an environment where he or she will not be fearful to practice speech and language.

Classroom Activities

1. *Fluent Reading Circles*: Ask the children to read in small groups and the teacher should read a passage slowly and in a correct manner. Every child afterward reads a sentence or two, following the teacher's smooth reading.
2. *Interactive Storytelling*: Hold a storytelling session where the teacher will initiate a story and then the child will take over the storytelling while using the same speech.

6.14 Implementing Speech Therapy Techniques in Classroom

6.14.1 Implementation of Concept of Speech Machine in Classroom Activities

Introducing the speech machine and its parts to the students is significant in enabling them to understand how speech is produced, especially to the students who stutter. Speech-language pathologists (SLPs) are the professionals who provide therapy and interventions to children who stutter. However, there is also a part played by the teachers in enhancing these ideas in the classroom in a more practical and interesting way. Thus, teachers can explain the ideas about the speech mechanism in detail and with the help of practical tasks and comparisons that students will easily comprehend. It also helps the students to understand how speech works and at the same time equips the students with the ability to use the insights on communication.

Help children to understand the parts of speech production by illustrating to them the various stages of producing the speech from the respiration to the articulation. For students who are stuttering, this knowledge will go a long way in helping demystify the speech process and therefore reduce anxiety when speaking. It also allows for the application in real life of many of the techniques that are used in speech therapy. Thus, teachers, through these ideas, contribute to the day-to-day practice of SLPs. Their participation makes sure that the child is constantly motivated and praised, which is very crucial in the development of the child.

Activity 1: Learning About the Speech Machine by Identifying Speech-Related Body Parts

I. *Initial Discussion*:
- *Ask the child*: Begin by asking the child, "What parts of your body do you use when you speak?"
- *Create a basic list*: Help them list primary parts involved in speech, such as the lungs, voice box (larynx), and mouth.

II. *Expanding the List with Details*:
- *Discuss function*: Explain how each part contributes to speech. For example, the lungs help with breathing, the voice box (larynx) with phonation (sound production), and the mouth with articulation (forming words).
- Add detailed parts: Expand the list to include:
  - Muscles of the chest wall and abdomen for breathing.
  - Muscles of the larynx and vocal folds for phonation.
  - Muscles of the tongue, lips, and soft palate for articulation.

Activity 2: Drawing the Speech Machine Followed by a Discussion

I. *Guided Drawing*:
  (a) Help the child to make drawings of the body parts that are involved in the process of speaking. Describe how these parts operate during speech process.
  (b) Divide into categories: These three areas should be of particular interest:
    (i) Respiration: Sketches of the lungs, diaphragm, and chest muscles.
    (ii) Phonation: Illustrations of the larynx and vocal cords should also be included.
    (iii) Articulation: Depictions of the tongue, lips, teeth, and soft palate.

II. *Interactive Learning*:
- Engage in drawing yourself: Support the child by making your own basic sketches to help them copy. This makes the activity more engaging and thus safer than the conventional, tangible ones.
- Discuss each part: After the drawing, explain to the child in simple language and in simple terms the function of each part in speech production.

Activity 3: Using Analogies to Further Understand Speech Mechanisms

I. *Lily Pad Analogy*:

Rationale: Words in speech are like lily pads floating on the water. Stuttering is like a lily pad on the water, which shakes for a while.

A teacher can use words like lily pads on water during a lesson. As for stuttering, it is like a lily pad that shakes and then again becomes stable. Explain that techniques make the words "float" without sticking and then stuttering becomes a concrete and solvable problem.

II. *Bumpy Road Analogy*:

Rationale: Using a bumpy road, for example, children can see stuttering as part of the road, a part that is not smooth but can be overcome.

A teacher can use the analogy of a bumpy road when explaining stuttering to the students in class. As a rough road does not block the way to development, the occasional stammer will not interfere with communication and will promote coping with challenges.

III. *Garden Hose Analogy*:

Rationale: This can be compared to a kinked garden hose to show how airflow can be affected when it comes to speech. As with any hose that has become tangled and in consequence has stopped flowing, there are methods that can be used to enable the free flow of speech.

A teacher can use a garden hose to explain to the learners how kinks can restrict water movement. Connect it to disorders which are induced by problems with airflow in speech. Tell them that techniques are like unkinking the hose to make the speech smooth again. This analogy creates a vivid image in the reader's mind, thus making the importance of techniques easily understandable.

IV. *Blown-Up Balloon Analogy*:

Rationale: This is evident by comparing speech to a blown-up balloon which shows the effect of tension on fluency. Similarly, when one lets the air out of a balloon, the tension is reduced, and techniques reduce speech tension.

A teacher can use a balloon to show tension. Tell him or her that speech is like a swollen balloon that can become taut. Teaching methods such as letting the air out can help the speech to be more relaxed. This analogy is useful in explaining the concept of tension in speech to the children.

(a) Balloon as lungs (for respiration): A balloon may depict the lungs. When you blow into the balloon, tell the child that this is the same way that we breathe in, and our lungs get filled with air.

(b) Controlled release: Another activity involves having the student blow air into the balloon and then slowly releasing it. This activity can help the student understand the role of airflow in speech.

(c) Vibration demonstration (for phonation): Slowly shaking the balloon as one releases the air from it can seem to reproduce the work of the vocal cords. Describe to the class that as air moves over our vocal cords, they vibrate to make sound just like the balloon did.

(d)Shaping the air (for articulation): One can blow into the balloon and then let the air out with different techniques. This can help to illustrate how the tongue, lips, and mouth form words.

V. *Traffic Light Analogy*:

Rationale: Just as traffic signals control the traffic with "Go" and "Stop," speech has "Go," smooth speech, and "Stop," stuttering. The analogy is that red does not mean the operation has to come to a complete halt.

A teacher can use the traffic light analogy while explaining communication. Tell them that both green and red moments are inevitable during speech. In the same way that people can be trained to wait for a red light to change to green, students can be trained to move from red to green in speech.

VI. *Finger to Thumb Analogy*:

Rationale: The use of the finger and the thumb to make a ring stands for clear speech. Separated finger-thumb signifies stuttering. This links them in some way, in a way that speech flows.

A teacher can encourage the use of signs for smooth speech by demonstrating the finger-thumb join. Depict the "finger-thumb apart" for stuttering. Tell them those techniques assist in connecting them, to enable them to speak fluently.

Practical Tips for Teachers Using Analogies

1. *Simplicity*: Select age-appropriate analogies. Make them understandable so that the readers can easily comprehend.
2. *Engagement*: Include activities that have to do with the analogy for the students to be more engaged.
3. *Personal Connection*: Promote the class participants to come up with the examples they have in mind regarding the analogy so the class atmosphere is permissive.
4. *Consistency*: Review analogies after some time to ensure that the learner has well grasped the concepts being put across.
5. *Positive Framing*: In a positive way, explain that there are problems which can be solved and there are ways to solve them.

However, as helpful as these analogies are in providing a way of thinking about the process, it must be pointed out that they should be employed in the context of a speech-language pathologist's assessment of a child's specific requirements and prospects. Therefore, by employing these powerful and interactive learning tools and examples, the teachers can easily explain the speech machine and its parts to the learners and thus make them be able to understand how speech is produced and controlled. This approach not only enhances the learning process but also enables the students to apply these ideas to enhance their interpersonal communication skills.

6.14.2 Implementation of Fluency-Shaping Techniques in Classroom Activities

Stuttering management techniques are immensely helpful means of assisting people who stutter to attain a normal and more manageable flow of speech. These techniques alter the process of speech production to promote fluid speech. Thus, in a classroom, teachers can contribute to using these techniques in daily practice, which will help SLPs in their work. As was discussed in the previous sections, these techniques include the following:

1. *Easy onset and gentle voicing*: This kind of approach includes starting every speech softly and gently to relax the vocal cords. Gentle voicing is a relatively quiet, calm, and devoid of strain in the voice during speaking. For instance, Sarah, a student who stutters, wants to read a text in the classroom. Sarah's teacher provides her with a tip, "Sarah, let's begin this paragraph with a gentle airflow to ensure that the speech is smooth. If you were to imagine that you are blowing a gentle breeze at the start of every sentence, then that will assist you and me to speak in a more fluent manner." As Sarah enforces this tip, she finds that her speech is not only more fluent but also more confident. A child who stutters will not like to be constantly reminded of the speech strategies that he or she should use. Hence, using these techniques in class activities or even when practicing with the student can result in better implementation and confidence.
2. *Prolonged speech*: This entails prolonging the duration of certain sound or syllable. Hence, the rate of speech can be adjusted to enable the control of the articulation process and minimize on stuttering. When the students are in a class and the teacher wants the students to express themselves regarding their favorite hobbies, the teacher can use the prolonged speech technique to help the students develop fluency. For instance, David is a student with a speech impediment, and as class assigns them to give the title of their favorite book, his teacher says, "Okay class, let us now practice on the way we speak, let us speak slowly and elongate" and then to him, "David, let us begin with prolonged speech technique." Others then say, "Daaaaviiid, teeeell uuusss abooout yooouuur boooook." This is useful in making sure that everyone is involved and using fluency strategies, as the environment is more accepting of everyone's participation.
3. *Light contacts*: This includes light contact of the articulators (lips, tongue, teeth) when making sounds. This decreases the tension in the muscles, which in turn makes for better speech output. For instance, during a class exercise, Priya, a student who stutters, is asked to present her opinions. The teacher then teaches the whole class saying, "As we argue… let us gently touch the tongue and lips when making sounds to ensure that all of our speech is clear and flowing." This makes it easier for Priya and her classmates to present their arguments with more ease.

4. *Modified airflow technique*: This technique entails managing breath prior to and at the time of speaking in a bid to guarantee a fluent flow of air while speaking.
5. *Rate control*: This means controlling the rate of talking and going slowly to bring down stress and tension, which in turn minimizes stuttering.

A detailed description of Classroom-Based Techniques is given in Table 6.1 which provides guidance on ways in which children can be helped in overcoming their fluency problems.

6.14.3 Implementation of Stuttering Modification Techniques in Classroom Activities

Stuttering modification techniques are aimed at the reduction of the severity of stuttering and to assist the person to avoid stuttering or to minimize embarrassment when it does occur. These techniques entail identifying and manipulating the stuttering behaviors in one way or another. To apply these techniques in a classroom, teachers have to design certain activities and ensure they consult with SLPs on the same.

Identification of Stuttering Areas

Note: This aspect is very sensitive and should be done in private with the teacher and the child to preserve the privacy of the child. Feeling like a victim of bullying, teasing, and mocking is very typical for people who stutter. In order to not let the child experience such bullying and develop even more negative emotions, one has to talk to the child directly. Moreover, the teacher should ensure that the child is comfortable to discuss issues with speech or stuttering. If he or she does not want to, then this issue should NOT BE RAISED. To identify the areas of stuttering, one must determine the words, sounds, or situations that lead to the occurrence of stuttering. This is very important in the formulation of interventions to be taken to handle the issue of stuttering. An example of teacher-led activities for identification of stuttering is provided in Table 6.2.

Note: It should be done with permission of the student, and the student should be aware of the process that is being followed to make him or her comfortable. This step should not be done without checking with SLP and/or psychologist as this directly has to do with the child's stuttering and may be too much to handle for the child. It entirely depends on the level of stuttering and the child's state of mood. Also, the child's preparedness to cope with various events is equally important. Desensitization is a process of desensitizing the student to the fear and anxiety that is attached to stuttering by gradually taking the student through speaking situations which he or she may have fears about. So this should be done only when the professionals involved and the child consents to it and when the child is ready. Table 6.3 outlines a range of structured classroom activities designed to help students with stuttering gradually become more comfortable and confident in their speech. These activities focus on reducing anxiety and desensitizing students to challenging speaking situations through methods like gradual exposure, role-playing, supportive group

Table 6.1 Classroom-Based Techniques for enhancing fluency skills using fluency-shaping techniques

Technique	Classroom-based activities	Description	Implementation
Easy onset and gentle voicing	Reading aloud in pairs	Pair students to read out sentences or short paragraphs one at a time where they have been instructed to use easement onset and gentle voicing.	Offer students set of interesting materials, for example, short story or an article for reading. Tell them to read their materials aloud making sure they start slow and keep a soft tone all the way. Support and promote each other by giving positive feedback on how the technique is being used.
	Soft-spoken discussions	Introduce group discussions in which students are to softly and gently speak to one another.	Select an exciting discussion topic that will engage students by bringing points which will interest them. In the classroom setting, make the learners form groups and debate on various topics using easy onset and gentle voicing. This is because if deprived of variation, then the topic tends to get boring, and the parties involved get out of spirit of making the debates interesting.
Easy onset and gentle voicing	Gentle voice presentations	Provide students with short presentation assignments during which they are to practice easy onset and gentle voicing.	Teachers can say to each student, "I expect a 7- to 7-minute presentation on any subject of their selection." during their presentations, one should ensure that when forming a sentence, he or she starts off softly and speaks gently. As a part of it, discuss their performance concerning the usage of the technique as well as possible improvements and further practice.
	Calm conversation circles	Introduce groups of students to discussions where they start their comments with an easy onset.	Put the students into groups of four or five at round tables and write some phrases for them to discuss. Remind them to focus on "sinking the voice into their chest and attempting to start the sentences softly" and advise them accordingly. Most importantly, keep the conversations fresh and engaging, e.g., offering questions like "what hobby do you enjoy and why?"
	Voice warm-up exercises	Warm up the voice every morning with exercises concentrating on easy onset and gentle voicing.	Take the lead in easily practiced vocal warm-ups, for instance, humming or saying phrases with minimal vocal intensity and minimal pressure. Advise the students to perform these exercises early in the morning so they will have the kind of speech that is calm and relaxing, e.g., plain words such as "good morning, nice to see you" or "how are you?" make sure to use phrases that one uses in day-to-day conversations for better understanding.

(continued)

Table 6.1 (continued)

Technique	Classroom-based activities	Description	Implementation
Prolonged speech	Slow reading sessions	Schedule reading sessions in which the students read the text aloud and pronounce each word with much emphasis.	Give students a passage to read or use in a study. It is helpful to use a timer to encourage them to read slowly and stretch out each word. Select texts that will capture students' interest as well as their attention to work on prolonged speech.
Prolonged speech	Extended storytelling	Students narrate a story or an incident that occurred and in so doing ensure that their narration is slow.	Provide a storytelling prompt. Teach students to tell their story in a slow and draggy manner to the extent that each syllable and word is pronounced. The format of the practice session should not be informal to help them feel at ease while practicing.
	Pacing partner practice	Assign students in pairs to speak slowly to each other, and while doing so, use pacing guides.	It is suggested to give each pair a pacing tool which can be a finger tapping the table for each syllable, for example. Engage them to practice slow and calm way of speaking to each other with the right tone. Swap pairs frequently so that each student has an opportunity to deal with a variety of students.
	Slow and steady debates	It can be done through debates where the most important point is to pronounce the words as slowly and as clearly as possible.	Decide on the subject to be discussed in class and then form two groups. Instruct them to speak for their side slowly and clearly, making their voice strong. Give them feedback on the way they have utilized prolonged speech and remind them of the need to better in the next round.
	Stretching syllables exercises	Include activities where students try to stretch syllables in frequently used words and phrases.	Stress the use of diagrams to show directions of expansion of speech sounds. Advise them to try and elongate each syllable as much as possible and in a perfectly smooth manner. The list of simple words and phrases to be practiced are as follows: *Words starting with /h/*: 1. Happy 2. Hello 3 .Heavy 4. Hold 5 .Help *Sentences starting with /b/*: 1. "Bring the book here." 2. "Better be on time." 3. "Big balloons are fun." 4. "Bright skies make me happy." 5. "Blue birds are singing." *Phrases starting with /k/*: 1. "Keep it safe." 2. "Can you help?" 3. "Call me later." 4. "Kicking the ball." 5. "Catch the cat." More such words, phrases, and sentences can be created based on the child's preferences.

(continued)

Table 6.1 (continued)

Technique	Classroom-based activities	Description	Implementation
Light contacts	Articulation stations	Organize specific articulation exercises; some of which should be aiming at using very light contacts.	Set up different stations all around the room, and in each of them, instruct the kids to practice different articulation exercises. Rotate students gradually through the stations, encouraging them to vocalize sounds while using light touches on different body areas to enhance their awareness of each sound. Shout, encourage, and correct students during their performance at a particular station for them to perform better. *For example*: 1. *Station for /m/ sound*: At this station, students say words like "moon" and "mouse" while placing their index finger on nasal bridge to feel vibrations on nose associated with the /m/ sound, reinforcing nasal resonance and sound production. 2. *Station for /s/ sound*: For words like "sun" and "sand," students receive light touches on their open lips to feel the airflow when producing the /s/ sound, promoting better feedback. This approach uses tactile cues to help students understand articulation through gentle physical prompts, enhancing their phonetic awareness.

(continued)

Table 6.1 (continued)

Technique	Classroom-based activities	Description	Implementation
Light contacts	Soft sound games	Suggest games, for example, where students have to come up with some sounds with the help of full-body contact, but not heavy ones.	Arrange games like whispering a word or gently, rhythmically patting out the syllables of a word to be guessed. Light contacts should not be boring or tedious. So make it fun and make practicing such contacts enjoyable. Praise those students who managed to use light contacts correctly and remind them in case they were not able to do it properly. Example: The games have names such as whisper, quiet, and gentle, by where students give soft answers to words mentioned in the game.
	Gentle tongue twisters	Teach the students some tongue twisters with an important note on only light contact with the tongue.	Ask students to repeat the tongue twisters five times using light contacts: Use prompts such as "slow and smooth" to prevent the speaker from tense and broken speech. Use it as a game to see who can say the twists in the tongue twisters most clearly. Example: For /b/: Betty Botter of course, bought some butter, but she stated that the butter has become bitter. For /g/: Gary collected good green grapes on the garden.
	Soft speaking partners	Group students to employ light contacts to engage in the practice of conversations.	Group the students and give them some topics or questions that they have to discuss. It will be useful to tell them that they should avoid full physical contact such as handshakes when speaking. It is also important to rotate the partners from time to time to allow the students to get acquainted with different partners.
	Interactive sound charts	Make charts of sounds that are made with little or no stomping and let the students play these.	For sound that requires light contact, use charts and diagrams to explain the different issues. Let the students trial these sounds and guide them when their articulation of the sounds is not correct. Suggest to them to use the charts during practice and prepare questions based on the information contained in the charts.

(continued)

Table 6.1 (continued)

Technique	Classroom-based activities	Description	Implementation
Modified airflow technique	Breath control exercises	To prepare students for PT or exercise time, start with respiratory exercises to enable the student to regulate airflow.	While the students prepare for their physical training session, they must be guided through exercises such as deep breathing and the exhalation of air in a controlled manner. One can try to use diagrams of the lungs in an endeavor to make people aware of the process involved. Do not forget to recommend that they should do exercises of this kind as often as possible.
	Controlled breathing read-aloud	Have students participate in specified reading loud sessions while emphasizing proper airflow.	Provide books and ask them to read in turn, and in the meantime, think about their breathing. Schedule a particular time and tell the students to time themselves when commenting on their breathing so as to set a pace. Example: The book can be "the cat in the hat" by Dr. Seuss. Students then read, focusing on maintaining steady airflow.
	Airflow synchronization activities	Integrate lessons that involve the pacing and breathing of the students when they are speaking in classroom.	Encourage students to use timekeepers such as a metronome or rhythmic clapping to ensure that they stay acoustically in rhythm with their breathing when speaking. Start with a simple base sentence and gradually build on it step by step. Example: Some of the tips to generate conversation topics are "tell me about your favorite food." students converse, counting their breaths: "I like pizza (I say this while pretending to inhale and exhale, in, out, now I release and inhale)."
Rate control	Timed speeches	Make the students deliver short speeches with an emphasis on the rate of speech.	Instruct them to use timers that will assist them to control the rate at which they speak.
	Slow conversation practice	Buddy slow-talking learners with faster speech learners.	Give them some ideas and tell them to kindly answer as many as they can so that each answer is elaborate.
	Paced reading aloud	Develop the strategy on reading aloud with a major emphasis on rate control.	Employ pacing guides or signs that will remind the students to walk slowly and at the same pace as the other students.

(continued)

Table 6.1 (continued)

Technique	Classroom-based activities	Description	Implementation
Rate control	Controlled discussion groups	Organize group discussions with specific instructions for the students; that is, they are to speak at a certain pace.	Bring changes in the topics to be discussed to make the conversation more interesting and stress slow speech.
	Slow and steady storytelling	Have students retell a story particularly in terms of the speed of speaking.	Tell them to spread out their words and relax on each phrase that they are saying.

Table 6.2 Teacher-led activities for identifying and supporting students with stuttering

Teacher-based activities for identification of stuttering	
Private conversations	It is advisable to arrange for frequent one-on-one meetings with the student in order to let the student share his/her experiences of stuttering. These are the sessions you should use in identifying the patterns and triggers.
Stuttering journal	Suggest the student to write down when and where he or she stutters the most and do it in the form of a diary.
Trigger mapping	Make a concept map of situations that make a person stutter. Below is a list which may help you to underline the most frequent conditions or terms which create problems: 1. Public-speaking situations 2. Answering questions in class 3. Introducing oneself in a group 4. Speaking on the phone 5. Meeting new people These situations often create pressure or stress, which can increase the likelihood of stuttering. Identifying these triggers helps in developing strategies to manage them effectively.
Reflective discussions	Discuss with the student their emotions and experiences during the times they stutter.
Personalized feedback	Suggest real-time solutions and interventions in the areas of stuttering that were pointed out as a way of assisting the student to find ways of coping with these situations.

Table 6.3 Classroom-based activities for desensitization of stuttering

Classroom-based activities for desensitization of stuttering	
Gradual exposure	Ensure that you make time and set a specific time to meet with the student to discuss the stuttering. These are the sessions where one should be able to recognize the patterns and triggers.
Role-playing	Organization of the speaking skills activities in which the student will engage in speaking in different situations. Some of which are role-play, such as pretending to order food at a restaurant or having a conversation with the principal, making a self-introduction to a new classmate, dealing with a bullying school senior, having a conversation with a father who is furious over marks on a test, and so on.
Supportive group activities	Engage the students in group exercises that require each of the students to introduce himself or herself to the rest of the group. Make sure the therapeutic environment is nonjudgmental.
Positive reinforcement	Praise the child every time he or she speaks or tries to speak without putting emphasis on the stuttering aspect. The corrections and the feedback that should be given should be documented and must be told to the child personally.
Relaxation techniques	Use stress-decreasing strategies like deep breathing or mindfulness exercises right before the speaking activities to minimize the anxiety. Apply this for all the students in the class.

exercises, and positive reinforcement. Additionally, techniques like relaxation exercises are integrated to create a stress-free and encouraging environment that promotes better communication skills.

1. *Modification Techniques*

The techniques of modification are particular methods of changing the pattern of the stuttering. Table 6.4 describes these techniques in a step-by-step manner.

(a) *Cancellations Technique*: Cancellations are built on postponing the next word after a stutter, thinking about the stutter, and then saying the word without stuttering.
(b) *Pull-Outs Technique*: Pull-outs are when you "catch" a child when they are stuttering and then gradually letting the child speak slowly without pressure and with ease.
(c) *Preparatory Sets*: Include anticipating a stutter and performing practice and preparation until the word is said smoothly and without a hitch.

2. *Voluntary Stuttering*

Voluntary stuttering is the deliberate stuttering on a word to minimize fear and tension that is related to stuttering (Table 6.5).

3. *Stabilization*

It includes the strategies used in the maintenance of fluency in different speaking contexts. Stabilization activities in classes of other teachers are important to build on the learned strategies and techniques. The activities include:

Table 6.4 Classroom-based techniques for enhancing fluency skills using stuttering modification techniques

Classroom-based activities for modification of stuttering	
Story creation and performance	This is an activity of coming up with a story as a class and acting it out while applying the stuttering modification strategies. Activity: Step 1: Preparatory set: Here, as the class writes a story as a group, every learner will spot what they deem as difficult words and thus mentally ease themselves to deal with them cooly. Step 2: Pull-outs: In the rehearsal, if a student is in problem with any word, then with pull-outs, the student can shift easily. Step 3: Cancellations: During performance, students will undergo a successive and intense process for a particular word which will be pronounced with less difficulty the second time. Example: Devise an imagination journey of a fantasy world. Every student composes and sings their verse and uses various skills to avoid stuttering while speaking.
Interactive speech games	Speech games that are play based and engaging where clients imitate words and phrases and, in the process, use stuttering modification strategies. Activity: Step 1: Preparatory set: Before beginning the game, students decide upon the expected difficulties in the text and get ready psychologically. Step 2: Pull-outs: In the game, on some occasions, if a learner is stuck on a word, then pull-outs will be in use. Step 3: Cancellations: After a difficult word, students stop, think, and then pronounce the word with ease. Example: Engage the students in a game of "speech charades," in which they will act out words or phrases the instructor has said and rehearse the techniques informally.
Classroom debate and reflection	Involve the students in a formal debate in groups on a theme that has connection with the stuttering, and then have reflective session where students have to practice stuttering modification strategies. Activity: Step 1: Preparatory set: In other words, before the debate, the students name the probable difficult words that may be encountered. Step 2: Pull-outs: While delivering their speeches, students employ pull-outs to address speech issues to do with fluency. Step 3: Cancellations: As a result of a daunting word, they take time to think before resaying it in a fluent way. Example: Stage a debate over an issue such as "should students be required to wear uniforms to school?" then after the debate, conduct a postdebate discussion on speech techniques used during the debate.

(continued)

Table 6.4 (continued)

Classroom-based activities for modification of stuttering	
Interactive story maps	Make distinguishing story maps that will let the students perform the stuttering modification strategies in a moving map manner. Activity: Step 1: Preparatory set: Making the difficult word choices easier for students, the story map assists the students in the following way: Among the most important aspects of learning connected with the help of the discussed tool, the students are to identify the main difficult words, and as students go through the story map, they are to prepare for the main difficult words. Step 2: Pull-outs: While navigating, if the student is in doubt of a word, they use the pull-out. Step 3: Cancellations: It has been observed that they spend time after a demanding word, and they pronounce it gently in the next trial. Example: Story maps should be applied for adventures or historical journeys where the students describe each step in the journey as well as their techniques.
Creative arts and speech integration	Teachers can perform speech practice overlaying creative arts inclusive of a presentation, which includes use of stuttering modification techniques. Activity: Step 1: Preparatory set: During the planning of their performances, students recognize difficult words and get ready psychologically. Step 2: Pull-outs: In the presentation, if a student is in a fix as to how to pronounce a certain word, they use pull-outs. Step 3: Cancellations: Following a challenging word, learners walk, make a pause, and pronounce the same word fluently. Example: Activities like "speech and art," whereby the students paint objects and exhibit them before their group, using techniques of stuttering modification when describing them

Table 6.5 Classroom-based activities for enhancing fluency skills using voluntary stuttering

Classroom-based activities for voluntary stuttering	
Role-playing with empathy	Lead students to a game in which they have to stutter on purposes, for example, for 1 hour. Turn it into a competition in an effort to cut on the amount of stigma that people with stutters encounter. Raise awareness of such issues, draw attention to the challenges, and make other children to know and even feel for such situations.
Hot and cold (strength and weakness discussions)	Introduce the concept of strengths (hot) and weaknesses (cold) of all students as a way of making other students understand CWS and have empathy toward them. Emphasize on the fact that everyone faces some or the other kinds of difficulty in their lives.

A. *Cross-class presentations*: Make the students present in different classes, and while doing so, they should use the techniques they have learned to enhance their fluency.
B. *Interdisciplinary projects*: Get other teachers to develop a project where students can apply their fluency in a certain subject.
C. *Peer teaching*: Empower students to explain a topic to other students of different classes to enhance their verbal fluency.
D. *School announcements*: Get students to make school announcements allow them to practice their fluency skills in a setting where they are expected to perform.
E. *Extracurricular activities*: Promote the extracurricular activities where the students can practice the use of their speech techniques in different settings.
F. Pausing and chunking

Pausing and chunking refers to dividing the speech into smaller sections with intervals and thus lowering the speaking pace. Table 6.6 presents a variety of engaging classroom

Table 6.6 Classroom-based activities for developing pausing and chunking skills to enhance speech fluency

Classroom-based activities for pausing and chunking	
Timed reading game	This game utilizes the need for a clock in reading by making the students read in segments with breaks between segments to be able to increase their reading speed and fluency.
	Game setup *Materials*: Clock or watch, short articles, or passages.
	Instructions: 1. Divide the class: Divide them into small groups in order to be safe. 2. Reading passages: Distribute to each group a different passage that they must read as a team. 3. Set the timer: Give a signal in the form of a time signal to indicate the number of minutes that they can take (e.g., 2 minutes). 4. Timed reading: Each student reads his passage aloud with normal pause at a punctuation point or in between two meaningful ideas. 5. Feedback: At the end of the specific time, give them feedback on their speed of speaking and time taken to make pauses.
Phrase segmentation relay	In this relay race game, students are awarded to break down sentences into phrases and pause as they recite each phrase.
	Game setup *Materials*: Rectangular strips of paper which can be numbered, a large whiteboard, or chart paper.
	Instructions: 1. Prepare sentences: On the paper, students should write long sentences in order to cut after the selection of the subject. 2. Divide the class: The learners should divide into groups. 3. Relay race: Each pair of students in the team competes to be the first in writing one phrase from the resultant sentence on the board and hold the writing pen before the next student comes in. 4. Completion: The first team to segment let alone writing his or her sentence wins.

(continued)

Table 6.6 (continued)

Classroom-based activities for pausing and chunking	
	Example: Major groups of words such as routine sentences like "the quick brown fox jumps over the lazy dog" can be soused into "the quick brown fox/jumps over/the lazy dog.
Group discussion carousel	This active classroom exercise helps the students to speak in chunks and also switch between their ideas. *Game Setup* *Materials*: Discussion prompts and timer. *Instructions*: 1. Arrange seats: Arrange chairs in circular or carousel manner. 2. Discussion prompts: Issue each group with a discussion topic. 3. Timed rotations: Tell the student(s) to set a timer for 1–2 minutes. Students talk about the topic and the ideas; they express themselves in pieces and there are silences after every few words. At the end of the timer, they switch the prompts in the rotation. 4. Feedback: Comment on their pauses and their use of chunks mentioned in the guidelines. Example: Examples of the kind of questions that elicit chunked responses include "What is your favorite book and why?" or "Tell me about your dream vacation."
Speech maze adventure	This activity makes speech practice into a game in which students are to go through a series of mazes while practicing pausing and chunking. *Objective*: The first group to navigate the maze and complete all the speech challenges wins. This activity promotes teamwork, enhances speech fluency, and makes learning fun. *Game setup* *Materials*: Largely open area, materials that can be used to create markers (masking tape or chalk), maze with different checkpoints, and cards with scenarios. *Instructions*: 1. Create the maze: It is possible to use masking tape or chalk and draw a maze on the classroom floor for instance. Divide the maze into several zones, at each of which the students have to perform speech activities. 2. Scenario cards: For every checkpoint, put a scenario card that has a sentence or a phrase that the students must read with the use of pausing and chunking. 3. Navigating the maze: Put the students into small groups. The task is for one student from each group to go through the maze and at each checkpoint, perform a task. 4. Speech challenge: When a student gets to a checkpoint, they take a scenario card and read the sentence focusing on using pauses and dividing the sentence into parts. 5. Feedback and progress: The student is expected to finish the particular task at each checkpoint and then receive feedback from the peers or the teacher and then proceed to the next checkpoint. *Example scenarios*: Checkpoint 1: "Describe your favorite holiday in three sentences." Checkpoint 2: "Explain how to make a peanut butter and jelly sandwich." Checkpoint 3: "Talk about your pet or a pet you would like to have."

(continued)

Table 6.6 (continued)

Classroom-based activities for pausing and chunking	
Pausing at a chunking theater	This activity entails the students to act out short scenes or plays by which they have to apply and practice pausing and chunking in reciting the lines. *Objective*: It enables the students to practice the practice of speaking and speaking fluency while at the same time being creative in their speech delivery, in a way that can help them afford public speaking. *Game Setup* *Materials*: Short skit ideas, objects used in the skit (optional), and space required to perform the skit such as a stage area or any other area marked for performance. *Instructions*: 1. Script selection: Choose or develop brief scenes that are provocative and suitable for children. Make the scripts somewhat long so as to make room for practicing break time in sections. 2. Assign roles: Teachers should assign roles to the students so that each of them will take an equal portion of the monologue and practice their pausing and chunking. 3. Rehearsal with focus on pausing: Before the performance, teach students the necessity to divide words into smaller segments and such things as pauses. Offer recommendations as to where to breathe and how to stress out certain fragments of the dialogue. 4. Prop and costume integration: Props and costumes should be utilized to make the performance more interesting. That also makes the students feel more at one with what they are doing, in this case their roles. 5. Performance: Organize group debates where students have to stage their skits in front of an audience. 6. Suggest to the audience that they need to focus on the "listened-for tempo and rhythm," the student's ability to pause, and segment the material when presenting it. 7. Feedback session: Subsequently, it is advised that one debrief the students and the teacher where students share their impressions and thoughts on the issue of pausing and chunking and what worked well and what did not during the performance. Example Skits. A short play regarding an ordinary day at the seaside where each of the students describes an activity, for instance, sandcastle construction, swimming, and having a snack. A dramatic play scenario in which students portray astronauts that have come back from the space mission and have to explain what they have seen and gone through.

activities designed to help students practice and improve their pausing and chunking skills in speech. These activities, such as timed reading games, phrase segmentation relays, and speech maze adventures, emphasize breaking speech into manageable parts, enhancing fluency, and creating natural pauses during communication. Through creative exercises like pausing at a chunking theater and group discussion carousels, students learn to apply these techniques in fun, interactive, and meaningful ways, fostering confidence and clarity in their spoken language.

6.15 Managing Teenagers in Classrooms

The management of stuttering in teenagers includes the following: physical treatment, which deals with the physical part of speech, and the psychological treatment, which deals with the effects that stuttering has on the individual. It is thus important for formulating a comprehensive strategy that will assist the teens to deal with the emotional and social aspects of stuttering.

Enhancement of speech naturalness is still a major goal of stuttering treatment for teenagers. Some of the techniques including easy onset, light contacts, prolongation, pausing, and speech rate control are specific to each teenager and can be quite useful in their daily communication.

It is therefore very crucial to manage physical tension when it comes to stuttering. Strategies such as progressive muscle relaxation, diaphragmatic breathing exercises, and block modification strategies (as mentioned prior) encourage a more relaxed manner of speaking.

Emotional Well-Being and Stuttering Management

Treatment for teenagers also includes psychological aspects because stuttering affects not only speaking. CBT is quite useful in this regard as it assists adolescents to change their perception and build a better self-esteem. Below are classroom-based examples of CBT techniques:

1. *Cognitive restructuring*: For instance, in a classroom setting, if there is a student like Rohan who stutters, the teacher might assist in changing the student's perception toward public speaking. It is recommended that before a class presentation, the teacher should explain to Rohan to recognize such negative thoughts as "I will embarrass myself" and replace them with helpful ones, for example, "I know I am prepared and ready to do it." As a strategy, teachers can encourage students to write and post on the so-called "Positive Thought Wall" their positive beliefs about themselves and their abilities. This fosters a good culture and at the same time assists in building up the positive attitude in the individual.
2. *Exposure therapy*: The teacher can build up the level of speaking activities to perform, to help the students develop their speaking skills. For example, Asha, a student who stutters, may first read a sentence in front of the class, then speak in front of small groups of people, and finally facilitate a class discussion. This gradual exposure to public speaking allows to prevent anxiety related to speaking in public. Hold "Confidence Circles" and have the students present to one person and gradually increase the group size up to the entire class.

3. *Behavioral experiments*: The teacher can assist Priya, who has a speech impediment, to try out what she is afraid of regarding stuttering in front of her peers. Thus, by asking her classmates questions or by discussing the subject of stuttering, Priya discovers that her classmates are quite tolerant unlike what she thought before. Organize a "Fact and Fiction" task in which students are invited to list some myths about stuttering and other students post comments that would help to break the stereotypes.

6.15.1 Managing Bullying and Teasing at Teenage

Children with speech difficulties, particularly stuttering, have to endure the problem of stuttering and bullying at the same time. This is a rather sad state of affairs that often has a negative effect on their emotional and mental health. Stuttering, which is an easily noticeable and hearable peculiarity of their speech, can become a reason for bullying and mocking from classmates who do not know what to do with such a student. This bullying increases anxiety and fear, which has the potential to worsen the stutter, and this makes it a cycle of speech problems and low confidence. To counter this, it is important for teachers, parents, and other children to create an environment where such variations in speech are not only tolerated but also accepted. Prevention of bullying and spreading information about stuttering and understanding it could help children who stutter to feel comfortable in expressing themselves. Thus, the child who stutters is supported, and at the same time, the class fosters an atmosphere of tolerance.

Bullying is one of the worst things that can happen to children, and it can cause a lot of emotional harm to the child and may lead to tragic outcomes. We as educators have a duty of ensuring that all students, including those who stutter, are well protected and comfortable in class. It is for this reason that knowledge of the nature of bullying and its influence on children who stutter is important. Here are six essential steps for a comprehensive intervention program to address bullying effectively:

Step 1: Building Stuttering Awareness: It is for this reason that educating children about stuttering is important so that they can curb unwanted reactions which CWS may receive from others and to help them have confidence and control over their speech. When students are aware of what is happening in stuttering, they will not be easily annoyed when they are speaking. Include lessons and activities that define what stuttering entails, the causes of the condition, and how it interferes with communication. For instance, teachers can arrange group activities such as watching videos, inviting speakers, or carrying out group assignments on stuttering.

Step 2: Recognizing and Addressing Bullying: Illustrating the concept of bullying to children makes them know that it is not their fault to be bullied. They should realize that not every remark made about them about their speech is malicious. Some people may just be interested to know more, which creates a chance to explain what stuttering is to other people. Group activities and debate can assist students to identify the right response to bullying cases. Educators can simulate situations and make the students face teasing or bullying situations in a secure and simulated manner.

Step 3: Fostering Positive Self-Perception: Encouraging children who stutter to have a positive outlook on their speech and raising the children's self-confidence can help them not to be affected by bullying. In this way, we are also able to minimize the intensity of stuttering as well as the impact that it has. Some of the strategies include "Self-Esteem Journals" where students write positive things about themselves and/or "Achievement Boards" where students display their achievements.

Step 4: Developing Appropriate Responses: Teaching children how to make the right responses to bullying is one of the most crucial processes. Factual information about stuttering can help to prevent incidents and to calm down aggressive behaviors. These are responses that teachers can facilitate in students through role-play exercises. For example, students can rehearse saying that "I stutter from time to time, but I am getting better" or "Stuttering is just a part of the way I communicate."

Step 5: Educating Peers: Helping the children who stutter to explain to their peers and classmates about stuttering and bullying can help to make others refrain from being spectators. Peer education promotes the culture of tolerance and understanding among learners and thus creates a culture of togetherness. Teachers can encourage peer education by having "Stuttering Awareness Days" during which the students who stutter explain to their fellow students about stuttering.

Step 6: Involving Parents and Caregivers: It is therefore important that the parents and caregivers of the children who stutter be educated on what stuttering is, what therapy entails, and what bullying is. It is important to understand that only by joining our efforts can we reduce the potential harm from bullying and contribute to the improvement of the children's lives. It is recommended that teachers should arrange for workshops and meetings for parents in order to exchange ideas and experiences to support the child.

6.15.2 Strategies to Promote Acceptance and Handle Teasing

To promote acceptance and handle teasing related to stuttering, educators can implement the following strategies:

1. *Open discussions*: Encourage the class to talk about stuttering to create the class's awareness of the students who stutter so that they won't make fun of him. Ask students about their questions and emotions to raise awareness of acceptance.
2. *Famous personalities*: Explain to students that there are many people who stammer and who are nevertheless successful. Telling their stories can make others develop compassion and may make students understand that stuttering does not affect one's capabilities or prospects.

3. *Discuss emotions*: Describe difficulties and feelings in connection with stuttering. Open discussion encourages the students to voice out their opinions and to encourage their classmates.
4. *Address gender-specific issues*: Make the classroom setting safe for students to share their own personal barriers and experiences and those that may be linked to gender in relation to stuttering.
5. *Weekly strengths and weaknesses*: Determine a certain day of the week that everyone will bring out their strengths and weaknesses. This practice assists the students to value the uniqueness of individuals and fosters a positive attitude in the classroom.
6. *Diversity examples*: It is important to explain what we mean by diversity. Here are some examples that can help to illustrate this concept. For example, using backpacks to compare and contrast people in the class will enable the children to accept and appreciate diversity. Similarly, showing different physical stature of people to denote how we are all similar (humans) yet diverse in our appearances and nature.

The above strategies, if put into practice, will help the teachers to ensure that children who stutter are integrated and welcomed in the learning institution. Improving their interpersonal communication and promoting their health leads to their success in the learning process. It is, therefore, possible to make every child who stutters to feel accepted and confident to express himself or herself by creating awareness, understanding, and prevention.

6.16 Targeting Oral Presentations: The Most challenging Tasks for Children and Teens with Stuttering

It is very challenging to stutter during oral presentations, and this is a big problem for students who do not have a smooth way of speaking. This is especially the case in situations where communication must be as unambiguous and assertive as possible, which is why stutterers can be extremely anxious. The anxiety of speaking in public and the uncertainty of stuttering only makes the task even harder. Students may feel anxious due to the fear of being judged by their audience, and this may make them stutter more often or with more intensity.

This cycle of anxiety and dysfluency influences not only the presentation of the student but also his or her confidence and motivation to participate in the next public-speaking activities. To overcome this issue, there is a need for a caring approach by both teachers and fellow students in order to ensure that learners can express themselves without the fear of being judged. This could mean allowing students to complete the task in a different way, such as through a different form of assessment, giving them more time to prepare for the task, or allowing them to use aids such as Power Point presentations or written notes. Most importantly, developing a culture of understanding and tolerance can, to a great extent, help to reduce stress and allow the students who stutter to handle oral presentation tasks with much ease and minimum anxiety.

To support children with stuttering during oral presentations, educators can employ specific strategies:

1. *Confront stuttering openly each time, even if the class is already aware*: Thus, educators who do not hide the child's stuttering make it less a shameful issue so the student does not fear their speech.
2. *Develop an order and organize tasks for presentations*: Laying down certain guidelines as to how oral presentations ought to be made can greatly help in managing stress and anxiety in those students who stutter. Giving the students a guide on what to do and how to do it can make them feel more at ease and sure of themselves.
3. *Provide practice opportunities*: Students need to practice their presentation in order to gain confidence and to have a feeling of their fluency strategies. Suggest that they practice in conditions that are less stressful for them, for instance, with another person or a few people at a go.
4. *Consider the audience size*: Ask if the student wishes to present it in front of the class or if the student feels more comfortable presenting it to the teacher. Having choices can prevent or minimize tension and make the situation less stressful.
5. *Reduce or remove time limits*: Time pressure, however, can worsen the fluency of some students who stutter. One can remove or extend the time limits of oral presentations to reduce stress on students and give more attention to the content they want to deliver.
6. *Liberation through saying "Yes, I stutter"*: In the context of a classroom where communication is the foundation of teaching and learning process, it is crucial to discuss about stuttering through a classroom presentation. This is not just an effort to transfer knowledge; it is an effort to create a culture of tolerance and acceptance.

It educates the students about stuttering through a presentation that aims to decrease the students' ignorance on this speech disorder. It defines what stuttering is, its causes, and the implications of the condition. This knowledge is important in breaking the misconceptions that are always related to stuttering to eliminate the stigma related to it. It is therefore important to tell students that stuttering is a communication disorder and not a sign of lack of intelligence, emotional instabilities, or any other form of disability that may make the fellow student a burden in class.

Furthermore, such presentations are of significance for the students who stutter because it can be liberating for them. It validates them and informs them that their situation is known and recognized. This acknowledgment can greatly enhance their confidence and self-image, allowing them to contribute more easily to group discussions and other class activities. This can be a good chance for the teachers to teach the students on issues of empathy. In this way, students can recognize the difficulties that fellow students who stutter go through and thus are able to be more patient and accepting, which are qualities that are important in society. Some tips which can also be included in the presentation are not completing the person's sentence as well as not avoiding their gaze during the presentation.

Further, this initiative can create a platform for talking about other matters of interest, for example, tolerance and acceptance of the diverse. This course contributes to the educational mission of the school, which is to equip the student for life in a diverse society, accepting and tolerant.

It also demonstrates inclusiveness, because a lesson on stuttering was also delivered by the student who stutters. It shows that students who stutter are not invisible, and their concerns are considered in the course of study. This approach not only helps students who stutter but also improves the general educational process of all the students in the classroom.

Make sure to reassure that the child is prepared for these presentations. It is important to check for the willingness of the child who stutters for the presentation, since not all children would be comfortable in presenting to their fellow classmates as someone who stutters. Watch the child's level of readiness and see the decision to present as a way of working on their thoughts and feelings about stuttering, as a part of the therapy.

Addressing Negative Emotions

- If the child has been teased or feels negative emotions, first, it is necessary to do desensitization to eliminate anxiety, shame, and guilt.
- This is why it is important to explain the presentation to teachers and parents, even if the child has not yet been exposed to teasing for the purpose of skill building.

Involvement of the Child

- Include the child in the preparation for the presentation, asking them what they want to talk about and how much of the presentation they want to make and how much the SLP should make.
- For children who have unpredictable speech management skills, they should be allowed to read only brief passages or lines which they have rehearsed several times or read aloud with other children.

Age-Appropriate Discussions

- Adapt the content to the child's age and cognitive/developmental abilities.
- Children in kindergarten, up to second grade level, can comprehend concepts on bumpy speech and the feeling of being bullied.
- Students of the third and fourth grade should be able to understand the advanced explanation of stuttering, speech production, therapy, and the effects of bullying.

General Tips for Oral Presentations

1. *Plan*: Before that, it is important that the presenter decides what information he or she will be presenting to the audience. Make sure that your ideas and the main points are presented logically and coherently.
2. *Know Your Audience*: Think about who will be in the audience when you are giving your presentation. Consider what there is that they may be interested in and how you can relate with them.

3. *Practice, Practice, Practice*: Make sure you have good practice of your presentation so that you do not make mistakes. Rehearse before a mirror or with your family and friends to help you with the actual delivery. The more you do it, the more you will build your confidence.
4. *Use Visual Aids Wisely*: Use of pictures or props in the presentation can make the presentation to be more enjoyable. Make them easy and accurate to the subject you are writing about.
5. *Engage Your Audience*: Begin your presentation with a catchy and engaging beginning. Here are some ideas; start with a story or a question to make everyone listen.
6. *Maintain Eye Contact*: Gestures should be done when speaking and the speaker should look at different sections of the room. It is also acceptable to look at the notes, but, at least, try to look at the audience.
7. *Speak Clearly and Confidently*: Breathe in and out and try to control your speech. Take a break from speaking when you need to draw a breath and ensure that you stress in the appropriate areas.
8. *Handle Questions Gracefully*: It is advisable to be ready for the questions from your audience. If a word eludes you for a moment, do not be in a rush; take a moment and try to remember it. Sometimes, it is good to seek assistance in case of difficulty, for instance, in this case.
9. *Manage Nervousness*: Some amount of nervousness is completely normal. As people, we all know that sometimes we can get nervous. Breathe in, relax your muscles, put on a nice smile, and give it all you have.
10. *Conclude Strongly*: End your presentation and provide a conclusion as well, for a good presentation. State your conclusions and express your gratitude to the audience for their attention.

Using the steps described above, a child can become a self-confident and effective presenter. As a reminder, it is okay to have some setbacks at some point in the process. The more a child rehearses, the less the child will be afraid of speaking in front of a group of people.

6.17 Training Students to Educate Teachers About Stuttering

Counselling children who stutter requires making people aware of the condition, and the students themselves are usually the most effective campaigners. It helps to educate the students to address their teachers regarding the condition and, in the process, prepare the children to face their communication struggles boldly. A good approach that has been found to work is to have the students write letters to their teachers explaining who they are and what stuttering is not. This is because a student-led letter to teachers enables children who stutter to convey their experiences directly to their teachers; this builds confidence and awareness in the children and their teachers. This process enhances both the content of the letter and the development of the students when developing and delivering the letter.

Crafting the Letter

1. *Personalized insights*: Begin by asking your students the following question: "What would you like your teachers to know about stuttering?" The students should be encouraged to think about different areas of discussion which include facts about stuttering, personal mechanisms used to cope with the stutter, emotions, and other non-stuttering interests.
2. *Structuring the message*: Assist the student to structure and present their ideas in a brief letter, handout, or informative packet. This step can help them in passing important information or messages to the audience but in their own style.
3. *Distribution and impact*: It can either be done by hand delivery, through phone, or even through email to all the teachers, support personnel, principals, and any other personnel that have direct contact with the child.

Key Elements to Include in the Student-Led Letter

The following are features that should be in the student-led letter:

1. *Factual understanding*: Promote students to spread the right information regarding stuttering to help in changing the perception of society. The following are the things that teachers should know regarding the phenomenon known as stuttering: prevalence, physiological basis, and effects on communication.
2. *Personal narratives*: Encourage the students to discuss other parts of their life apart from their stuttering. Listing the likes and dislikes, hobbies, and interest makes the student more real and more recognizable.
3. *Classroom dynamics*: Cooperatively develop the strategies that can help in supporting CWS in the classroom. Students and teachers should cooperatively develop strategies that can help everyone calm down in stressful situations like an oral exam. This can be done by working in teams or groups. The groups must include children with stuttering who can suggest techniques that can help them relax and speak better. These suggestions allow teachers to foster an environment in which viable communication and better interaction among classmates can occur.
4. *Therapeutic progress*: Emphasize the student's process and development in speech therapy. Emphasizing the milestones helps teachers to understand the therapeutic procedures and objectives.
5. *Access to resources*: At the end of the letter, include information about resources from stuttering organizations, websites, and references that can help teachers and to support their further learning.

Implementation Tips

- Initiate with an outline: Begin with the outline in order to make writing easier and to have a clear structure.

- Encourage expression: In the letter that each student should write, the student should use his or her own words. Promote originality but, at the same time, ensure that the work is correct.
- Fact-check: Make sure that whatever you are saying is factual and does not cause harm to the subject.
- Regular revisions: Revise the letter as the student progresses in understanding and, as such, reflects in the letter.

Alternative Communication Approaches

- Face-to-face discussions: Schedule meetings with students, teachers, parents, and facilitators with the purpose of having a one-on-one conversation.
- Electronic communication: Employ emails and other forms of digital content to outline some of the major facts about stuttering and other occurrences.
- Visual aids: To improve the understanding of the topic, it is advisable to use visual aids such as charts, diagrams, or even informative posters.

6.18 Empowering Students to Develop Positive Emotions

Emotions greatly determine how people are able to view or actually experience stuttering. Negative emotions, beliefs, and perceptions about speech may cause the development of other behaviors, which worsens the condition of stuttering. This book states that while developing and managing stuttering, emotions are crucial where teachers have a significant say in the affairs of a student. It is important to know the feelings of the students who stutter so that educators can be of help to them.

Educators have a special chance to help students who stutter not only in the classroom and not only by using the standard techniques. Here are some innovative techniques to consider:

1. *Technology-integrated communication*: As much as possible, incorporate technology into the classroom setting. Allow students who stutter to make use of speech-to-text software for writing tasks or when making presentations. There is also a possibility of using the applications that demonstrate graphics and visualizations of speech habits for the same purpose.
2. *Drama and role-play*: Provide the students who stutter with drama or role-play exercises that allow them to try various speaking behaviors or personas. This can however be a very useful method of looking at speech without the constraints that are normally present.
3. *Mindfulness and relaxation techniques*: This should be taught to the students so that they can have a way of dealing with anxiety when speaking. Some relaxation techniques that can be done before making a presentation including breathing exercises and

short relaxation techniques in the form of guided meditation. The particular methods of Mindfulness-Based Exercise Program (MBEP) are demonstrated in further sections.

4. *Peer mentorship programs*: Allocate students who stutter with partners who will understand, accept, and support them. This can foster unity, and people may be able to relate to one another in some way or the other.
5. *Creative expression workshops*: Hold group meetings that totally engage the participants in other forms of production such as writing, drawing, or singing. This can help students to freely express themselves creatively and at the same time help in boosting their self-esteem.
6. *Public-speaking clubs*: Teachers should help students who stutter to join or create speaking organizations in which they will practice the act of speaking in public. Some of the activities could be debate, poetry recitation, or telling stories.
7. *Collaborative learning projects*: Develop group assignments that help the individual speaking skills of the students in the class. It can assist students who stutter to feel appreciated not only for the message that they are delivering but also for the efforts they make in the process.
8. *Virtual reality simulations*: In individual counselling rooms, use of VR can help simulate speaking environments for practice. Here, VR can help students to increase their level of confidence when it comes to speaking in public.
9. *Feedback through games*: Include educational games in which feedback about communication can be given in the course of the game. This can be helpful in learning communication skills because it will be more fun and not seem like learning.
10. *Parent-educator workshops*: Organize seminars that can help the teachers and the parents with how to manage and support the students who stutter and ensure they receive the same treatment from home to school.

Such techniques when incorporated can help in establishing a safer and welcoming environment for students who stutter, which assists in their psychological well-being.

6.19 Encourage Students to Work on Self-Development

Self-development of students who stutter can be promoted in ways that are not limited to conventional speech therapy. It covers the promotion of self-acceptance, the enhancement of self-advocacy, and the introduction of new methodologies to address the students' emotional and social development. If the educators work to make the environment safe for these students, they will be able to build self-esteem, tenacity, and communication skills. Here are some key strategies to promote self-development in children who stutter:

A. *Cultivating Self-Acceptance for Children Who Stutter*

In the context of the present study, the process of self-acceptance for the child who stutters, especially at school, is substantial. Focusing on that manner of speaking is not only about coping with the stutter; it is about how to live successfully with it. Centrality of educators is not in doubt in this process, but more innovative strategies than the conventional ones are called for.

1. *Creative expression through arts*: Let the children who stutter use different modes of communication such as artwork, music, or drama. Thus, these outlets can become ways for expressing oneself and for feeling and thinking, which can contribute to the feeling of success and self-esteem.
2. *Personalized communication projects*: Engage the child in activities that would enable him or her to express self through the means that he or she would prefer; it could be a presentation, a written documentation, or a digital documentation. This kind of approach recognizes and values their different modes of communication.
3. *Peer-led support groups*: Set up the so-called "buddy groups" in which children can talk about what happened to them, with their peers, in a protected manner. This peer support is very vital in the aspect of promoting self-acceptance.
4. *Storytelling and role models*: Read and tell stories from books where the characters have a stutter and present the characters in a good light. It is also effective to have guest speakers who stutter come and talk to the children as they may inspire them.
5. *Interactive and inclusive learning games*: Design activities that will enable students to learn while playing and interacting with their peers where the performance of the game does not depend on the students' speaking skills. This can be useful in creating the sense of a community among the students.
6. *Fostering a growth mindset*: Children who stutter should be encouraged to foster a growth mindset by explaining to them that things such as speaking are learned and can be developed over time.

B. *Creating a Speech Notebook for Stuttering Management in the Classroom*

Stuttering is a condition that can be supported in the classroom by having the child complete speech notebooks. These are the notebooks that are very handy in enhancing the learning and teaching process of both the learners and the teachers, respectively. Usually used in speech therapy, teachers and parents can also effectively utilize speech notebooks to generalize and enhance speech management.

1. *Supporting documentation*: Speech notebooks contain information about the subjects, activities, and achievements concerning stuttering and their management, which is useful for monitoring the students' progress and working with parents and teachers.
2. *Flexible and creative use*: Some of the suggestions include using inexpensive and flexible materials, such as ruled-line paper or binders. Have students create a step-by-step guide for managing stuttering.
3. *Home and school integration*: Permit the notebook to be sent home for the purpose of practice and documentation as the students can show their work to their families.
4. *Highlighted and accessible content*: For special pages, one can use colored paper and use page flags for important assignments. Make sure that entries are both from the

teacher's and the student's side; this way, there is flexibility in the amount of written content to be submitted.

5. *Engaging and fun entries*: Promote enjoyment and creativity on the notes to be taken in the notebook. Apply them as a review and as a refresher when students have forgotten some of the information learned.
6. *Organized content*: In the inside covers, one may depict the anatomy and physiology of the speech system. Notes from the classes, thoughts of the student, the tasks that are to be done, and questions for the parents and teachers can also be added to the inside pages. It is possible to include reference information, progress checklists, glossaries, and special pages at the back.

C. *Empowering Children with Stuttering to Self-Advocate* Stuttering affects the child's social interactions and experience in a negative way. Since teachers are in a position of authority, they have a great responsibility of ensuring that these children are protected, helped to speak up for themselves, and encouraged in schools.

6.19.1 Empowerment and Building Confidence

1. Understanding stuttering: Explain to the children on the basics of speech production as well as the complexities of stuttering in order to create a feeling of mastery.
2. Therapy process awareness: It is necessary to label the reasons for the use of certain therapy techniques that help children to become active problem-solving individuals.
3. Content over fluency: Stress on the content than on the language; children should be allowed to speak without being much concerned about their grammar.
4. Support networks: Teach children to tell someone—any family member, friend, teacher, or another person who stutters—that they are not the only one who stutters.

6.19.2 Empowering Self-Advocacy and Educating Others

Self-advocacy is the ability to speak for oneself and this is one way of ensuring that one is empowered to speak for himself or herself.

1. Teaching about stuttering: The children can teach the parents, teachers, and peers about the condition and therefore create awareness and acceptance.
2. Sharing experiences: Make the children explain to others regarding their situations with stuttering that others may be aware of the struggles they go through.
3. Seizing teachable moments: Teach children to educate people in real-life situations and thus lead them to effective and positive behaviors.

Thus, we ensure that children are comfortable to share their experiences and struggles that they have with stuttering within a comfortable environment. Cooperating with SLPs and engaging parents can help the child to learn to speak up for himself or herself. This dedication to children with stuttering is therefore a sound foundation for empowering children who stutter as they build their self-esteem and develop resilience. It is the basis for raising awareness, tolerance, and acceptance in society.

6.20 Helping Students Manage Stuttering During the Holidays

The holiday season and other special days, characterized by relaxation, change of schedule, and increased social contact, can be both good and a tough time for children who stutter. The lack of fixed tutoring and school schedule may cause the child to feel more stressed, and fluent and nonfluent moments may be more frequent. Some of the complications that can worsen stuttering include family gatherings, traveling to new places, and even interacting with unknown people. But with good strategies and assistance, parents can assist their children to cope with this condition in the course of the festivities.

We know that children who stutter are facing some specific difficulties during this period, and being teachers, we can only imagine how it is for them. A teacher's role also involves preparing the parents on how to manage their children in the right manner. Below are some useful guidelines for parents to enable their children to go through the holiday season confidently and comfortably:

1. *Manage Excitement Levels*

Holidays are meant to be fun and lively, and they indeed can be so for all children, but the child who stutters may easily get overstimulated. Parents should ensure that things remain as calm as possible and the time that is spent together is fun-filled. Make sure to inspire the parents to ensure that the child is in a comfortable environment where he or she can express him or herself with ease and free from pressure or even much stimulus. This balance can assist in decreasing anxiety and manage communication in a better way for the child.

2. *Encourage Relaxing Activities*

The festive time is usually very stressful and may increase the pressures on children who stutter in terms of communication. It may be helpful to recommend that parents try to include some low-stimulus, low-pressure activities into their holiday program. Some of the activities which are available for children include reading, puzzles, or crafts, and these activities help in soothing the children in order to reduce speech stress. These activities not only give the child a sense of comfort but also assist the child to have a schedule to follow.

3. *Fostering Understanding and Acceptance*

Holidays are a time when the child may have to spend time with extended family and friends, within whom there may be little awareness of the child's stutter. Empower parents on the possible insensitivity and make the conversation about stuttering as transparent as possible. Tell them to make others aware, telling people that stuttering is a part of their child, and that people should accept it rather than make fun of it. This can lead to a more accepting environment for the child to be in.

4. *Embrace Variations in Stuttering*

In the course of the holiday, children may experience fluctuation in their stuttering due to alterations in their schedule, changes in setting or environment, and alterations in their social interactions. It is for this reason that parents need to understand these fluctuations and to assure their child that it is quite all right. Knowledge of these changes could also create a positive and acceptable perception toward them to make the child comfortable and confident in his/her communication.

5. *Take Strategies More Seriously*

It is thus important that the parents continue to remind the child what he or she has learned in speech therapy. It is possible to use quite effective measures, for example, speaking more slowly, stopping, and practicing breathing. Tell the parents to use these strategies often and to teach their child to apply them in different contexts, including home, with relatives, and when interacting with strangers.

6. *Provide Emotional Support*

This can be highly problematic for children who stutter, as they lack the structure of a school environment and the support of teachers. The parents should be there to give emotional support to the child during this period. Remind the parents to listen to what the child has to say and assure them and encourage them. Having a positive and supportive home environment can make the child more confident and assist them in social situations.

Parents should also follow through on informing other relatives who are within the family about the condition. Easy to understand information and steps to take when faced with a person who stutters can go a long way. Suggest that parents involve other family members in creating a conducive environment for the child and make him or her feel welcomed.

7. *Incorporate Routine and Structure*

Although, during the course of the holidays, children are supposed to be free from the normal schedule, some form of schedule should be observed. Put forward the idea that parents should stick to certain schedules like eating times and the time the child should sleep in order to create some form of stability. This can make the child to be comfortable and not stressed, thus reducing the rate of stuttering.

8. *Prepare the Child for Social Interactions*

Travelling and getting to meet new people is quite rampant during the holidays. Teach the children what to expect in such situations and how to act in such a way that they are not taken advantage of.

This preparation will assist the child to have confidence and reduce the anxiety they may have when they are asked to speak in a new environment.

6.21 What NOT TO DO to Manage Stuttering at School

Managing stuttering in school is a delicate process and requires careful and accepting handling. Here are some crucial actions to avoid:

1. *Avoid interrupting or finishing sentences*: Do not interrupt or finish the student's sentences when a student who stutters is talking. This can lead to more anxiety and frustration among the students. Let the child express himself or herself to the full extent by giving him or her sufficient time to do so.
2. *Do not correct or criticize speech*: Do not correct or criticize the manner in which a student uses language. Many people experience a rise in the consciousness of stuttering when they are being corrected, and since this increases stress, the stuttering only gets worse.
3. *Refrain from offering unsolicited advice*: Examples of the most frequent recommendations, including "Slow down," "Relax," or "Take a deep breath," may be rather ineffective. Such suggestions can bring a child more pressure and increase his or her awareness of their speech, for instance.
4. *Do not isolate or single out*: Do not make the student feel as if he or she is the only one in the class with the problem of stuttering. However, do not exclude them from speaking activities but at the same time, be very considerate of their feelings.
5. *Avoid pressuring to speak publicly*: It is advisable not to compel the students to present their work in front of the class if they do not wish to. Stress can make the person experience more stuttering and anxiety more than usual.
6. *Do not mock or imitate*: It is also wrong to copy or to make fun of a student who stutters. This is very cruel, and it can greatly harm their self-esteem and create doubts in them.
7. *Avoid negative reactions*: Some reactions that can be seen include impatience, frustration, or even sympathy. These may harm the self-confidence of the student. To this, one has to remain very patient and supportive and make sure that the child feels comfortable.
8. *Do not use stuttering as a teaching moment for the class*: It is improper to make the class emulate the student's stuttering without the student's permission. Speaking about their stuttering without their consent is embarrassing to them.

9. *Do not make assumptions about capabilities*: One must not conclude that a student who stutters is either not intelligent or is not willing to contribute to class. Stuttering is a fluency disorder, not an intelligence disorder.
10. *Avoid excluding from group work*: Make sure that the students who stutter are not excluded from group activities and discussions. The process of exclusion makes individuals feel isolated and can also affect the social improvement of a child.
11. *Avoid calling on the student unprepared*: Do not call on a student without warning him or her to do so. Let them volunteer or have them come prepared.
12. *Avoid forcing oral presentations*: It is not advisable to make the students do oral presentations, especially if they feel that they are being compelled to do so. Suggest other means of submitting the assignments like written assignments or one-on-one presentation.
13. *Do not ignore the stutter*: Not paying attention to the stutter at all can also be rather counterproductive. If the student introduces the issue, you have to accept it positively and make sure that the student has the freedom to express himself or herself.

6.22 Management of Stuttering at Home

Parents play an indispensable role in managing their child's stuttering. Parents are crucial in the management of their child's stuttering. They are also useful in the identification of the patient, assisting in therapy, and to ensure that the strategies learned are put into practice in day-to-day life.

6.22.1 Prevention of Stuttering

Preventative management of stuttering therefore encompasses the development of conditions that will not lead to the occurrence of the disorder. The cause of stuttering is not fully known but it is thought that it is caused by genetic, neurological, and environmental factors. Some of these environmental factors are beyond the child's control. However, parents can play a part in buffering the child from such factors and decrease the chance of the child stuttering. Prevention is not about the complete prevention of the occurrences; it is about creating environments in which the child can learn how to speak effectively. Stuttering in young children can be normal and is usually seen as the child is learning how to speak. It is characterized by intermittent repetitions, omissions, and pauses, which are a normal aspect of learning how to speak. Though these dysfluencies are quite general, certain measures can be taken to prevent them from becoming regular stuttering. Below are some guidelines of what parents should and should not do to help their child develop fluent speech and avoid stuttering.

Dos

1. *Encourage slow and relaxed speech*
   - Model calm speech: Make sure you enunciate your words when addressing your child and do so calmly. Relax the language and the tempo of the presentation so that the child does not get tense or feel that there is too much pressure on him/her.
   - Create a calm environment: Family members should model good speech and should avoid rushing through words or talking fast. Also, they are suggested not to overreact to a child's speech by listening to other people's judgmental viewpoints. Make sure that all the interactions that are held within the home environment are held in a nonaggressive manner. Do not talk fast or act on other people's words.
2. *Promote open communication*
   - Listen attentively: To make your child feel that you are eager to listen to what he or she wants to say, ensure that you listen to him or her carefully. Try to make and keep eye contact; don't speak while the other person is still talking.
   - Allow time to speak: Ensure that your child has all the time that he or she requires to complete the thoughts that he or she is expressing. Let them say whatever they want to say and at their pace.
3. *Encourage positive speaking experiences*
   - Praise efforts: Praise your child when he or she tries to express him or herself. Encourage the efforts as well as the achievements of the targeted group despite how little they are.
   - Engage in daily conversations: Speak to your child on a daily basis about the events of the day, activities, and emotions, without having to pressure them into doing it.
4. *Monitor and adjust communication demands*
   - Simplify language: Make sure you use simple language that a child of that age will be able to easily understand. This makes it easier to understand the user and for the user to be able to convey what they need to say.
   - Adjust expectations: Have a set of expectations when it comes to your child's speech. Do not anticipate that the student will speak without making grammatical errors and instead analyze what the student is saying.
5. *Foster a positive emotional environment*
   - Validate emotions: Child psychology suggests that you should validate your child's feelings. If they complain about speaking, it is advised that you encourage them and help them.
   - Encourage play and relaxation: This is because play and rest are important sections of a child's life as they will help in reducing stress and other related vices.

Don'ts

1. *Avoid criticizing or correcting speech*
   - No negative feedback: You should not ridicule or correct your child's speech. Do not make comments that may focus on their fluency problems or make them be conscious of them.

- No finishing sentences: Do not complete sentences for your child; let them come up with the words on their own. Permit them to finish their ideas on their own.

2. *Reduce time pressure*
   - No rushing: Do not force your child to answer quickly in a conversation or respond to your questions urgently. Allow them to take their time to express themselves as and when they want to do so.
   - No high-pressure situations: Reduce those conditions that most likely make your child feel pressured, such as being expected to speak in front of many people or being questioned.
3. *Avoid comparisons*
   - No comparing: It is also important not to compare a child's speech to the speech of other children, including siblings. Childhood speech development is individual and comparing them might only lead to an increase of pressure on the child.
   - No highlighting differences: Do not point out variations in speech stumble. Pay attention to factors such as the positive aspects of their communication.
4. *Avoid overloading with questions*
   - No bombarding with questions: Do not ask many questions at once. Do not ask your child another question until he or she is ready to answer the first one.
   - No complex questions: Do not ask questions which have several parts or are rather complicated for your child to answer in full.
5. *Reduce exposure to stressful situations*
   - No high-stress activities: Do not immerse your child in activities that may trigger stress since this will worsen the dysfluencies. Exposure to new or stressful conditions should be done in stages and with a lot of scaffolding.
   - No negative reactions: It is best not to have negative reactions to the child's speech dysfluencies. Be patient and reassuring even if the person is having difficulty expressing himself or herself.

Proactive Strategies for Preventing Stuttering in Children

Apart from handling normal nonfluency, here are some things that parents can do to prevent the occurrence of stuttering. These strategies are not restricted to interactions during the speech production but are aimed at promoting a general environment that is conducive for normal speech and healthy emotional functioning. Here are some points on how parents can prevent stuttering:

1. *Encourage expressive activities*

   A. *Art and music*
      - Art projects: Encourage your child to draw, paint, or do some crafts. For example, you could involve them in making a collage. These activities may also help the child in expressing himself in a different manner, thus alleviating the pressure on speaking.
      - Music and singing: Promote singing and other musical activities. Singing can help with rhythm and flow to give the child a fun way of practicing his or her speech.

B. *Drama and role-playing*
   - Drama activities: Make your child engage in drama and role-playing acts. Role-playing may be used in order to gain confidence and fluency in speaking.
   - Storytelling: Promote storytelling in your child. This can be done using puppets or teddy bears or even using story telling techniques.

2. *Foster strong parent-child bonds*

   A. *Quality time*
   - Dedicated time together: It is also recommended that you should take some time and play with your child in activities that the child likes to do alone. This enhances affection and serves as a foundation for the establishment of good communication standards.
   - Positive interactions: See to it that all your communication with your child is full of positive affirmation, hugs, and motivation. Positive result is the absence of stress and the development of confidence.

   B. *Consistent routines*
   - Daily routines: Make sure to have a schedule that is regular and that the child knows what is expected of them when. Expectation helps in minimizing anxiety which is of great benefit in speech development.
   - Bedtime rituals: Encourage relaxation activities like reading a story or a recount of the day's events before sleeping. This can create a comfortable place to practice and think which can be a useful tool.

3. *Promote physical well-being*

   A. *Healthy lifestyle*
   - Balanced diet: Make sure that your child is taking a balanced diet that contains all the nutrients that are required in the body. Malnutrition affects the growth of all parts of the body including the brain which is used in speech.
   - Regular exercise: Counsel the patient to be physically active on a daily basis. Stress is also known to be reduced through exercise and this in turn enhances general health, thus improving speech fluency.

   B. *Adequate sleep*
   - Sleep schedule: Keep to a routine so that the child gets enough sleep to enable him/her to have a good day. Loss of sleep can enhance stress and also alter the ways of communication.
   - Sleep environment: Establish an environment that is conducive for sleep in order to have a good night's sleep. This includes a dark and quiet room as well as having a set time for going to sleep.

4. *Address emotional and psychological needs*

   A. *Building resilience*
   - Teach coping skills: Help your child to know how to manage stress and anger. Some of the strategies include controlled breathing, imagery, and positive thinking.
   - Problem-solving skills: Promote the use of problem-solving skills and critical thinking skills. This makes it easier for your child to face some difficulties on his or her own and helps to lessen stress.

B. *Engage in mindfulness and relaxation practices*
   - Mindful communication: Take note of nonverbal communication and be fully present when talking to your child. This makes them free to express themselves and, therefore, helps to ease communication barriers.
   - Relaxation techniques: Coping skills such as progressive muscle relaxation can be taught to the child to enable them to manage physical tension and stress. Employing the use of imagery to assist your child to picture himself or herself speaking the language to be learned without any difficulty at home as well as in different scenarios can also help.

5. *Encourage social interactions*

- Arrange playdates: Engage children in activities with other children daily to enable him or her to practice his or her social skills and communication.
- Group activities: Engage your child in group activities, for instance, sporting activities, clubs, or any other classes. The other way is socializing, for instance, in group discussions that will enable them to practice how to talk in front of people with less pressure.

6. *Encourage independence and responsibility*

A. *Age-appropriate tasks*
   - Assign responsibilities: Make your child to have some responsibilities and tasks that are suitable for his or her age. Doing tasks by themselves will improve their confidence and their perception of their capabilities.
   - Decision-making: Encourage your child to help with decision-making, for instance, in the selection of clothes to wear or the activities to do in the family. This fosters the spirit of individualism and confidence because the child is able to come up with the answer independently.

B. *Problem-solving opportunities*
   - Problem-solving games: Involve your child in activities that will involve him to solve some puzzles or play games that need logic. Games that involve solving puzzles, strategy games, group assignments, and projects are interesting and fun.
   - Encouraging exploration: Let your child meet new people and try new things. It can develop flexibility and competence in dealing with different issues that may occur.

6.22.2 Early Identification of Stuttering

It is the parents who are usually the first to notice their child's speech and therefore are in a suitable place to observe early signs of stuttering. This is with a view to ensuring that the person is attended to as early as possible since this has been seen to have a positive impact on the results. Some of the various signs that parents should look for in their children include repetition, prolongation, blockage, tension, and so on.

If parents have any idea that the child may be stuttering, then they must keep a record of the occurrences so as to inform the healthcare provider. This can include:

1. *Frequency and duration*: Recording the frequency of the stuttering and the duration of the same.
2. *Context*: Realizing at what times stuttering is likely to occur (e.g., at home, at school, when a child is happy or nervous).
3. *Associated behaviors*: Documenting any physical actions or affect displayed during the time when the person stutters.

6.22.3 Seeking Professional Help

Parents' awareness of the fact that their child needs assistance from a speech therapist is essential in this case, and only they can make the decision. They are the most suited to monitor their child's language and interactions on a day-to-day basis and therefore know when the child needs help. It is advisable to seek the services of an SLP in order to get a comprehensive assessment and a treatment plan unique to the individual in question. Thus, parents have to assess the knowledge and the attitude of the potential SLPs to meet the needs of their child. Apart from the SLPs, parents may also consult other professionals such as psychologists or counsellors if the child has emotional or psychological issues that are as a result of stuttering. In this regard, taking the right decision and engaging the right professionals, parents can give the child the best chance to get the most effective help, encompassing both the speech disorder and its psychological consequences. This helps with the appropriate management of stuttering and at the same time assists the child to build confidence and cope with the situation when they are communicating. Parents should:

1. *Consult with SLPs*: Share your concerns with child's SLP to make sure that the child gets the early treatment as soon as possible.
2. *Collaborate on evaluation*: Perform the assessment by sharing your observations and present any issues that you think needs to be addressed.

I. *Creating a Supportive Home Environment all through the management process*

This is an aspect of the management process that can be maintained throughout the lifetime of the subject. Home environment plays an important role in a child's confidence and their ability to communicate including a child who stutters. Developing such an atmosphere is a process that requires deliberate efforts on the part of parents and other family members, the effort being toward cultivating an atmosphere of pressure-free communication. Here are detailed strategies parents can implement to foster a supportive atmosphere at home:

A. *Encouraging open communication*
   - Creating a safe space: Children should be encouraged by parents to share their thoughts and feelings at home since homes should be safe places for children. This makes the child to feel that the adult is open to listen to what they have to say, and their opinion is important, making them feel valued.
   - Active listening: Parents should listen to the child without interruption and give him/her full attention when he/she is talking. It involves things such as

making eye contact, tilting the head occasionally, and saying things like "I get it" or "Please continue." All these give the child a feeling that they are being heard.

- Nonjudgmental responses: Do not ignore the child's verbal output, but do not correct them either, telling them that they are wrong. Do not interrupt them in the middle of a conversation and correct them which may make them nervous and discourage them from speaking. Rather than concentrate on the manner of speaking of the other person, one should concentrate on the content of the message being passed across.
- Encouraging expression of feelings: It is helpful to enable children to express themselves on how they feel, for instance, if they are frustrated or worried about stuttering. Empathize with them and empathize with their feelings by explaining to them that you understand what they are going through.

B. *Modelling calm speech*

- Demonstrating slow and clear speech: Parents should also imitate slow and clear speech, and this will help in easing the pressure on the child to produce speech. Talking slowly and using short pauses can also work as a model for the child to mimic and thus stay calm.
- Using simple language: Avoid the use of complex and compound sentences when talking to the child. This can be of assistance in decreasing the level of complexity and ensure that the conversation flows smoothly.
- Avoiding interruptions: Be a good model of communication by not interrupting people when they are speaking. This makes the child to understand that it is not wrong to take time when talking and that nobody will interrupt them.
- Regular practice: Ensure you apply speech therapy strategies and skills in your day-to-day life in your natural interactions. This reinforcement also assists in the enhancement of these strategies as the child's general mode of interaction.
- Avoiding time pressure: Avoid making the child feel that he or she has to respond quickly or has to speak faster than what he or she can.
- Creating a relaxed environment: Make sure that the home is a peaceful place to be, especially when speaking to people.
- Providing time to speak: Give the child enough time to give their opinion and not feeling pressured to do it quickly.

C. *Showing patience*

- Listening attentively: Listen carefully to what the child is saying and try to get the child to see that you are interested in what he or she has to say. This entails ensuring that the child is directly in front of the counsellor, both the counsellor and child has eye contact, and ensuring that there are no distractions such as phones or other gadgets.
- Allowing time: Let the child talk and try to set a realistic time limit for the child and do not interrupt them in the middle of the conversation or rush them up. This patience makes the child to have a relaxed mind and hence when speaking, the child is not under pressure.

- Avoiding corrections: It is important not to correct the child's speech at once when you hear the improper usage of words. Direct interventions can undermine the child's confidence and make them wary of speaking. Instead, attention should be paid to the message that the child is trying to get across.
- Positive reinforcement: Praise and motivate people for trying to speak, even if they do so with errors. Reward the child for the progress made and the small achievements that he or she makes; this will motivate the child.

D. *Additional strategies for creating a supportive home environment*

- Structured routine: Promote the child's verbal interactions by setting up a consistent schedule for activities that require verbal interactions such as mealtimes, story time, or bedtime. Steadiness makes the child to have a sense of belonging and confidence to handle various situations.
- Mindfulness and relaxation: Teach the family on how best to adopt relaxation and mindfulness in their everyday lives. Some activities such as deep breathing, yoga, and meditation will help in lowering the levels of stress and anxiety which could be an added advantage to the child's fluent speech.
- Educational resources: Ensure that everyone in the family gets to know about stuttering. As a result, knowing more about the disorder and the difficulties it brings will help the family members be more tolerant and supportive.
- Social skills development: Promote the child's social interaction and social skills in different contexts. Encourage them to engage in social activities like clubs, sports, or other organizations where they can engage with other children.

II. *Collaborating with Extended Family*

- Educating extended family: In particular, teach other relatives of the child about the child's stuttering and how they can help. This may involve parents' parents, siblings of the parents, siblings of the child, and other relatives who may be in a position to have frequent contact with the child.
- Setting expectations: The child's speech should be explained to other family members on how they should respond to him or her. Promote patience, prevent interference, and give praise.
- Involving extended family: Engage the child's extended family members in activities and measures that could help in the child's development of communication skills. This brings in a lot of support and understanding, thus creating a better forum for the same.

III. *Building a Supportive Community*

- School collaboration: Make sure that the school that the child attends is informed of the child's stutter and the best way to approach the child. Since teachers are responsible for student's behavior in class, having a way of communicating with them can assist in ensuring that the child is receiving the same message at home and at school.

- Community involvement: Join support groups for parents, stuttering associations, community centers, and other organizations to look for more support and information.
- Raising awareness: Join community and social activities that can help promote awareness on stuttering. Informing society can also assist in the reduction of prejudices and social exclusion of the child.

IV. *Promoting Positive Self-Esteem*

Stuttering is something that can decrease a child's self-esteem and confidence as a speaker. Parents can help build their child's self-esteem by:

- Celebrating efforts and successes: Acknowledging the child when he or she has tried to communicate and giving cheers for the milestones they make.
- Encouraging participation: To promote the child to engage in activities and engage in social interactions to increase self-esteem and social development.
- Focusing on strengths: Emphasizing the positive qualities of the child and making sure that the child knows that he or she is not stuttering.

V. *Collaborating with Professionals*

It is recommended therefore that professionals such as speech-language pathologists and psychologists, as well as support groups for stuttering, should be involved in the management of stuttering. Parents can support this collaboration by:

- Attending therapy sessions: Where possible, being present in the therapy sessions in order to know the strategies and the techniques that are being applied.
- Implementing strategies at home: Implementing speech strategies and exercises as advised by the SLP can be done at home in order to enhance the therapy.
- Regular communication: Some of the strategies include checking on the progress of the child by meeting the SLP, identifying any difficulties that the child may be experiencing, and discussing them with the SLP, and reviewing the treatment plan to ensure that it is appropriate for the child.
- Consult psychologists: Consult with a psychologist if the child has severe anxiety, frustration, or other emotional issues connected with the stuttering.
- Work with educators: Help the teachers to help the child in class and make sure that the child gets any form of help or adjustments he or she needs.
- Join support groups: Support groups that exist for parents of children who stutter can be helpful in order to share experiences and get ideas and support.

VI. *Implementing Speech Techniques during overall communication*

Parents can help their child practice and generalize speech techniques learned in therapy by:

- Using slow speech: Promoting the child to talk slowly and clearly and imitating this in one's own interactions with the child.
- Practicing pausing: Help the child to make pauses while speaking so as to help him or her to reduce tension and enhance fluency.
- Encouraging easy onset: Where the child is encouraged to have an easy onset of speech, that is, they are encouraged to speak softly.

- Engage in role-playing: In the class, simulate different speaking scenarios like placing an order in a restaurant or asking for directions in order to rehearse on speech strategies.
- Encourage storytelling: Encourage the child to narrate stories or experience in a casual atmosphere for the child to use his or her voice.
- Plan social activities: Offer the child to play with other children and to visit friendly gatherings so that the child can practice communication with peers.
- Talking to strangers: Perhaps, tempt the child to communicate with strangers, for example, shop assistants, and neighbors, to help him or her gain confidence in speech.
- Managing stage fright: Ensure that the child is allowed to talk in front of people like during family functions or school to overcome fear.
- Facilitating open discussions: Make sure that the child has an open platform to express himself or herself at home without the fear of being laughed at or punished.

VII. *Collaborating with School and Community*

Support cannot be confined to the home but has to be spread to all areas of life. Parents can collaborate with the school and community to support their child by:

- Engaging with teachers: Collaborate with teachers to ensure that classroom tasks are modified to help the child, for example, request teachers to permit the child more time and use praise.
- Involving school management: Promote the adoption of school policies and programs that welcome children who stutter, for instance, speech therapy services and campaigns to raise awareness.
- Building community awareness: Engage in community activities and activities that aim at creating awareness on the issue of stuttering with a view of ensuring that people who stutter are embraced.

VIII. *Promoting Self-Advocacy*

It is also instrumental in giving children the tools to seek for themselves the help they need to overcome their stuttering. Parents can promote self-advocacy by:

- Encouraging self-expression: Promote the child to tell what he or she wants or needs in certain circumstances.
- Teaching communication strategies: Encourage the child to learn ways of coping with stuttering in contexts of social interactions and learning, for instance, to request more time before responding in class.
- Supporting independence: Mothers and fathers should therefore help the child to learn how to reduce their stuttering and, if they cannot do it alone, to seek help.

IX. *Building Support Systems*

It has also been seen that establishing contacts can help to gain support and other useful information for both parents and children. Parents can:

- Join support groups: Attend support groups for parents of children who stutter so that they can share experiences with other parents who are going through the same experience.

- Engage with advocacy organizations: Reach out to support groups that are focused on people who stutter including the Stuttering Foundation or the National Stuttering Association.
- Seek professional guidance: Seek advice from professionals including speech-language pathologists and psychologists in order to deal with stuttering and promote the child's psychological health.

X. *Celebrating Progress and Success*

Learning and improvement are important as it helps the child to build confidence and motivation regardless of how much they have achieved. Parents can:

- Track progress: Record the child's progress of how well he or she is able to control the stutter and meet speech targets.
- Celebrate milestones: Rejoice at the accomplishments and achievements, for instance, gains around speech fluency or positive social interactions.
- Provide positive reinforcement: As a result, one should encourage the kid and praise them for their efforts and provide positive feedback.

6.22.4 Determining the Optimal Time to Begin Therapy for a Child

As for the parents of a child who stutters, they have many questions, including when it is the right time to turn to a speech therapist. It is, however, important to understand when to step in to assist a child in the right path of communication development. Here is a concise guide based on research insights (Yaruss and Reardon-Reeves 2007):

1. *General Guideline*: Approximately 6 months from the start of stuttering are usually allowed before commencing treatment. This is not set at a certain time but an approximate duration within which one should propose intervention for the child and family. The literature suggests that parents usually delay referral for an initial assessment of a child's stuttering for about 6 months.
2. *Timing of Therapy*: Therapy does not have a definite time when it should be initiated since there are different circumstances. Some professionals advise that early treatment is advisable if there is a high risk of the child to develop a persistent stutter or if the child or parents have raised the issue. Some could advice that one should wait for as long as 1 year. However, if one waits for a long time, for instance, a year, it may not be very good for the child since the child may develop speech anxieties, tension, and avoidances or have negative attitudes toward verbal communication.
3. *Parental Intuition and Observation*: In this case, parents are the first to recognize the signs of stuttering and what they observe is vital. Understanding ways and means of how a child speaks is vital as this is a step toward being preventive. When there is suspicion of a child's speech skill gaps, it is advisable to consult a professional for an assessment.

4. *Individual Considerations*: Therapy may be advised earlier for a child who has had a new onset of stuttering but is considered to be at high risk, for example, if there is a family history of stuttering or if the child has had negative responses to their speech. On the other hand, there is a possibility that therapy may be delayed beyond 6 months if there is no family history of stuttering, the child has normal language development, and the child has a good home environment.
5. *Balanced Approach*: This aspect involves determining when to commence with the therapy since it is a balance. In most cases, it is advisable to act as early as possible as soon as there is a warning sign or concern about the child's stutter.

Every child's case of stuttering is different and therefore treatment has to be personalized to fit the child in question. Encouragement, patience, and even anticipating the child's needs from the parents can greatly help in the child's communication process.

Step 1: Managing the First Stage of Denial and Acceptance
The process of coming to terms with the fact that a child has a speech impediment in the form of stuttering can be tough on parents. The first phase can be characterized by denial, during which the fact that the child has speech problems may be hard to swallow. This means that the child is likely to be in this phase longer and therefore needs support.

Step 1a: Understanding Denial and Its Impact
It is important to understand that denial is a common way of dealing with the first impact of a child's stuttering diagnosis. It can present itself as minimizing the impact of the stutter, saying it is only occasional, or that it will eventually go away. Although denial helps the child to avoid emotional pain in the short run, denying a child's problematic behavior in the long run hampers the child's access to the help he or she needs.

Tips for Parents
1. *Acknowledge your feelings*

One should not forget about feelings which include sadness, guilt, or frustration. These feelings are very normal and are to be expected. Being able to tell someone how you feel in a controlled way, for instance, when talking to a counsellor or to other people in a support group, can make the patient realize that these are normal feelings that other people also have in the same situation.

2. *Educate yourself about stuttering*

Knowledge is empowering. To this end, knowing the actual nature of stuttering is useful in demystifying it and thus reducing anxiety or a sense of powerlessness associated with it. Therefore, it is crucial to have information on where to access information regarding stuttering, its occurrence, signs, and cure. Only books, reliable websites, and workshops containing all the information should be used.

3. *Focus on the child's strengths*

Transforming the attention from what the child is not good at to what the child is good at can help to decrease the stress and the uncomfortable feelings a little bit. It is very important to value the child and to acknowledge his or her success and abilities. Positive aspects of the child can be emphasized to reflect more acceptance and understanding of the child's behavior.

4. *Accepting that it is okay to feel pressurized*

Reassurance that feeling pressured is a normal part of the process is necessary. This does not make one inadequate or uncaring. Discussing the pressures felt and validating these experiences is important. Talking about the pressures one feels and acknowledging them is useful. Learning how to cope with these pressures can be done through the use of coping mechanisms which include the use of mindfulness and stress management.

5. *Set realistic expectations*

Unrealistic expectations can lead to disappointment and frustration. Setting achievable goals for the child's progress is encouraged. It is recommended to set the goals for the child that are reasonable and attainable. The need to produce sound strategies for the child's speech therapy and the fact that progress may be slow and that each step achieved is worthwhile are something that must be grasped.

6. *Create a supportive home environment*

It is very important for the child to have good support at home because it can greatly influence the child's confidence and achievement. Some of the strategies include being patient with the child, encouraging the child, and not completing the child's sentences for him or her. This is to mean that such a nurturing home environment should be sustained.

7. *Seek professional support*

Professional help can assist the child and parents' management in the right manner by offering the right tools and techniques. People who practice speech-language therapy for stuttering should be sought out. Going to and observing the therapy sessions to know the techniques that are applied and how they can be implemented at home is helpful.

8. *Connect with support groups*

Contacting the other parents whose children have the same speech issue can help with emotional support and tips. Counselling or other support groups where one can meet others with similar challenges and learn from them is advised. This feeling of belonging may be very useful at the time of acceptance.

Step 2: Managing Negative Emotions

The second vital task practiced after denial is to regulate the existing feelings in connection with the stuttering of a child. When parents recognize and control their own emotions, it becomes less challenging for children who stutter. Besides, acceptance not only releases the parents from feelings of stress and anxiety but also contributes to the formation of the child's positive self-image and their success.

Step 2a: Understanding the Impact of Acceptance

To deeply understand the notion of acceptance and its effects, one must try to perceive the concept in its entirety. Approval is therefore central to the process of parenting for a child who stutters. While accepting a child who stutters, this relieves the child of unnecessary pressure, and the stuttering also becomes part of their new positive self-image. Children have very keen awareness and are very sensitive to their parent's responses to anything presented to them. When the parents accept the speech of the child, then it makes the child happy and could encourage the child to speak without much worry. This acceptance forms the basis of creating a conducive environment where the child feels wanted and accepted. Hence, therapy as well as daily communication is easier to be administered.

Step 2b: Ways to Manage Emotions Effectively

1. *Educate yourself and stay informed*: Knowing about stuttering becomes crucial if negative emotions are to be self-regulated. The more parents learn about the condition, the less it appears to be a fearsome illness to face. Information from books, focused workshops, support groups, and other related forums can go a long way in offering the right strategies for coping with the situation. The knowledge which they acquire helps parents face the child's stuttering with confidence and without stress.
2. *Practice self-care*: The care of a child with stuttering is very emotionally cumbersome. In this case, parents need to spend time on themselves or, in other words, pamper themselves and do something that would make them calm down a little. Exercising, taking up some hobbies, and going out with friends are good ways of breaking the cycle of emotions. When parents meet their own emotional needs, they are well poised to attend to the needs of their child appropriately.
3. *Seek professional support*: It is recommended that parents seek the help of therapists and counsellors who will help them contain the emotions that they may display when parenting a child who stutters. Counselling allows the professional to listen to those feelings of frustration, guilt, or sadness which are generally never expressed

to other people. Counselling can also enable parents to learn how to deal with stress and develop a positive frame of mind which is something that is also good for the child.

4. *Communicate openly*: This should mainly be able to reduce or get rid of most of the existing negative emotions within the family regarding stuttering. Stuttering should be explained to the child as often as possible since this will reduce embarrassment and self-consciousness. The involvement of the child in speech therapy entails the child to share his or her feelings and worries on the speech, which creates trust and support. Such an open conversation can also help in building the relationship between a parent and a child and develop trust.
5. *Focus on the child's strengths*: Changing the point of focus from learning dysfluencies to wellness of the child can do wonders to their emotional health. Learning of the child's achievements and accomplishments transforms the focus from the child's stuttering, further making the child to develop enhanced self-image. This makes parents and children to look beyond the stutter and embrace the child and focus on the other abilities.
6. *Use positive reinforcement*: There is nothing as efficient as positive reinforcement in dealing with negative emotions. Reinforcing the steps made by the child, irrespective of how small the steps are, gives the child the inspiration to work harder. Positive feedback helps in reaffirming the child to keep on practicing the speech techniques that are being taught and thus discourages frustrating feelings of inadequacy.
7. *Develop a support network*: Families should be able to find friends and other parents of children who stutter to find emotional support and advice. Discussing with people who understand the difficulties can alleviate the sense of loneliness and isolation. This sense of community is asserting, which helps the management of emotions in some way.
8. *Implement relaxation techniques*: It would be beneficial to include in the plan activities like deep breathing exercises, meditation, or even yoga to alleviate stress and anxiety. These techniques can be done alongside the child, meaning that it is a routine that can help both the parents and the children. Stress relief measures enable one to stay emotionally balanced, and the development of a favorable environment in the household.

Step 3: Managing Other Family Members

Having dealt with their reactions to the child's stuttering, parents need to consider other family members so that the child can be supported well. Other family members such as the brothers, sisters, grandparents, and other relatives are also involved in the life of the child, and their reaction to the child's stuttering will also influence the child's progress.

Family members are very important to the child for support. Parents, siblings, and other significant people in a child's life can help the child by accepting and acknowledging the child's stuttering. On the other hand, if the family members do not understand the child or are insensitive, then the child's anxiety worsens, and they do not improve. It is equally important therefore for parents to ensure that everyone in the family understands the child's situation of stuttering. Here's how parents can manage other family members to create a supportive and understanding environment:

Step 3a: Ways to Manage Other Family Members

1. *Educate the family*: Education is the first way to creating awareness in the family on how to embrace and accept the differently abled members. The parents should educate the child on what stuttering entails, the causes, the features, and the difficulties that the child might be experiencing. Giving them articles, books, or even websites to read will enable the family members to gain more knowledge about stuttering and the effects of it.
2. *Hold family meetings*: This is one of the reasons that it is imperative that a child's stuttering becomes an open topic of discussion within the family. These meetings are useful to clear up any misunderstanding or worries that may be there among the family members. This is a good time for parents to be able to describe how the child is doing in therapy and what interventions are being made so that everyone is aware.
3. *Encourage empathy and patience*: The family members should be encouraged to have and display patience with the child. Telling family members why they should not interrupt the child or complete his or her sentences can assist the family members to know how to effectively communicate with the child. This makes them feel that they are in an environment that supports listening and responding appropriately for the child.
4. *Involve siblings*: Siblings can have a very significant impact on the emotional development of the child. Siblings may be included in the child's speech practice, and this may be helpful. To foster positive sibling relationships, it is important to educate the siblings about stuttering and get them involved in supportive activities so that they can build positive sibling relationships and feel that they are working together as a team. Siblings need to be directed at how they can withstand without being too much of a shield for the child.
5. *Model supportive behavior*: First, parents should demonstrate the expected behavior to other members of the family. When people show patience and understanding and even reward good behavior, it helps others to follow the same set of behavior. Thus, when the parents and other family members notice such positive interactions, they are likely to follow the same pattern with the child.
6. *Address insensitive comments*: This means that any form of prejudice remarks or acts should be discussed as soon as possible in a polite manner. Parents should teach children why some words and actions are painful and how one can express themselves differently. This approach is preventive in nature, minimizes the chances of conflicts, and increases the level of support.
7. *Create a positive environment*: It is very important to create a positive and encouraging atmosphere in the home environment. The family should ensure that they encourage the child and celebrate any achievement that the child has made in his or her academics. This is because when the child receives positive feedback from several family members, it increases the child's confidence and encourages the child to practice the new speech skills that he or she has been learning.

Besides this, it is important that the family should communicate freely about stuttering. Family members should not only be able to express how they feel but also be able to ask questions. This openness makes people aware of the fact that stuttering is not a rare phenomenon, and everyone should accept it.

8. *Having a limit with extended family*: Other family members do not have to be in the child's life on a daily basis, but their support is also significant. It is important that parents explain the child's stuttering to other family members and acquaint them with the rules of how they should react. In this way, the users will be able to perform their activities in a positive and supportive manner.

Step 4: Generalization of Speech Therapy Technique at Home

Step 4a: Understanding Speech Production (Analogies)

Follow-up activities that are done at home are important in order to ensure that the child practices the lessons learned in speech therapy. These activities assist children with stuttering to comprehend the procedures of speech production and, therefore, increase their capacity to deal with and alter their speech in a nonthreatening context. Sustaining the practice at home helps them to build on these strategies and use them in their day-to-day interaction, thus making it easier and efficient. Some of the general and analogy-based activities that parents can use in order to enhance their children's knowledge and comprehension of speech production include the following:

1. *Breathing awareness exercise*

This is to assist children to comprehend the usefulness of controlling breathing in the process of speech.

- The child should be instructed to lie down on their back and the parent should put a book or a teddy bear on the child's belly.
- The book should be inhaled and exhaled as the person should focus on the coming in and out of the book.
- It is necessary to define the notion of controlled breathing in speaking.
- Only simple phrases or short sentences are recommended, and a focus on diaphragmatic breathing.

2. *Silent speech practice*

This is in order to enable children to concentrate on the movement of the mouth, tongue, and lips without having to produce any sound.

- The child should be made to face a mirror.
- Oral words or phrases should be read with one's lips, and at the same time, they must be asked to watch the movements of the mouth.
- It is possible to make remarks, for example, about how lips produce certain phonemes or where the tongue should be positioned.
- When the words are to be uttered, they should be conscious of their mouth's movements.

3. *Analogies-based activities*

(a) *Blown-up balloon*

This is to explain the significance of the control of breathing in oral communication process.

- It will be useful to explain what it means to speak "as if one were releasing air from a balloon slowly."
- A balloon should be inflated and then a small amount of air should be released as if the deflation is also gradual.

Parents should then explain how we must write and read sentences with words that should be let out slowly and evenly as if from a balloon.

Home Implementation

- The child should be encouraged to take a deep breath before he or she speaks, and the child should imagine that words are air coming out of a balloon that is being deliberately let go of.

The child should be taught to employ this technique when at home and feels that someone is putting pressure on him or her to speak.

(b) *Lily Pad Hops*

This is to encourage the child on how one should take time and space while making his or her presentation.

- The idea that one speaks as if they are a frog jumping from one lily pad to another with pauses in between should be explained.
- The child should use actual paper lily pads or those that are drawn on the floor. The child should have to hop over the lily pads saying a word or part of a sentence in each hop.
- This exercise assists in teaching the value of taking breaks and how to regulate the rate of speaking.

Home Implementation

- A basic path at home with paper pieces as lily pads should be designed. This can be practiced by speaking in short sentences, moving from one "lily pad" to another for each part of the sentence.
- The child should be encouraged to take brief pauses in the conversation, and each pause should be seen as a time to "disembark" on the next lily pad.

(c) *Thumb and finger opposing*

This is to show the harmony which is required in order to speak effectively.

- One has to explain the way speech organs should coordinate in a manner similar to the thumb and fingers to pick up an object.
- For infinitesimal items such as beads or buttons, one has to use the thumb and the index finger to pick them up and then with the other fingers.
- The relation between the tongue and lips as to how they should work to facilitate speech should be explained. Coordination can be practiced with words that demand it, for instance, "butterfly" or "tiger."

Home Implementation

- Tasks that demand coordination, for instance, when putting on shoes or dressing up, should be employed to teach the child the idea of coordinated movements.
- At mealtimes, the child should be encouraged to name the food in front of them, ensuring that they are able to coordinate their tongue and lips as they do so.

(d) *Traffic light speech*

This is for the purpose of explaining the structure and the rhythm of speech to the students.

- The traffic light analogy should be explained: Red means stop (do not continue), yellow means slow down, and green means go (speak).
- Speaking should be practiced with the traffic light cues:
  - Red: Take a moment and just breathe before you begin the next sentence.
  - Yellow: Pause slightly before enunciating difficult words to slow down the rate of talking.
  - Green: Tell the story at a normal speed.

  For the practice, it is better to use colored circles or even a toy traffic light.

Home Implementation

- At home, it is advisable to use a toy traffic light or colored paper circles to draw the child's attention during conversations.
- Family conversations should involve the traffic light system. The child should be informed to stop (red), take time (yellow), and speak easily (green) where necessary.

(e) *Garden hose*

This is to exemplify the fluent and coherent manner of speaking.

- The idea that speaking should be like water passing through a hose should be defined.
- One of which is to practice speaking in a way where there are no breaks or pauses in the speaking which is the same as water flowing through a hose.
- The real or a toy garden hose can be employed to model the smooth flow. The sentences should be rehearsed fluently with a view of ensuring that there are no gaps in between.

Home Implementation

- The class should use a real garden hose during outside play or garden time to explain how water moves without interruption; this is the same way that speech should move.
- It is recommended that the child should be made to speak in a fluent manner during day-to-day activities like describing what he or she is doing while, for instance, watering plants or while taking a bath.

Step 4b: Implementation of Fluency-Shaping Techniques at Home

These techniques are best practiced at home to create practice sessions that complement therapy as they are more effective for studying in a familiar and supportive environment. Practicing at home makes it easier to apply these techniques in everyday interaction and hence be useful. Table 6.7 highlights some pointers to assist parents in fluency-shaping techniques for children at home.

Table 6.7 Home-based techniques for enhancing fluency skills using fluency-shaping techniques

Technique	Home-based activities	Description
Easy onset and gentle voicing	Balloon breathing	Start blowing the balloon and show that one does not blow the balloon with force but gently. This supports children's views on the necessity of a soft approach when developing speech.
	Humming transitions	These are songs and the basic procedure is to begin with a hum and then sing a word. Another possible function of the hum is to minimize "startle effects" that might occur at the onset of speech.
Easy onset and gentle voicing	Singing to speaking	The song begins with singing of a certain phrase and this phrase is then spoken gradually till a speaking rate is achieved. This assists to mimic a more natural start of speech.
	Word relay	Build a non-stimulating and relaxed game when you say a word in a low-intensity onset and your child reiterate the word back.
	Gentle voice puppet show	To make the activity interesting, get your subjects to use the puppets. Let the puppets "speak" using easy onset and model this for your child.

(continued)

Table 6.7 (continued)

Technique	Home-based activities	Description
Prolonged speech	Syllable stretching game	Always use simple words and try to stretch all the syllables. Make it fun, and if possible, get another parent or your sibling involved and try to outdo each other by stretching the syllables right.
	Singing slowly	Write down the lyrics of a favorite song and then sing it with your partner at a rather slow tempo. Concentration should be given to stretching the vowels of each word.
	Storytelling with stretched syllables	Develop a story in pairs with a brother/sister or parent while rehearsing the slowed speech wherein one stretches the syllables as they tell the story.
	Stretchable sound hunt	Find a word with a stretchable sound for an object in or round the house or in a book and then attempt to say the word in the stretched syllable way.
	Timed syllable stretching	Start with a particular amount of time and dedicate that time to stretch all the syllables; the time should be gradually increased as the child gets familiar with the exercise.
Light contacts	Word repetition drill	Select a set of easy lexical items that share the same first phoneme, for example, /b/—Ball, boat, book. Consultative contact should be made with light pressure applied to the first sound of each object's name. Emphasize the fearful words, which are stuttered more often.
	Mirror practice	In front of the mirror, encourage children to say words aloud so they can see how the lips are moving and avoiding contact.
Light contacts	Phrase extension exercise	Let them initiate on one word and progressively develop into a phrase/sentence, and it is advisable to practice soft contact only on the first sound of the utterance.
	Record and playback	Let them practice the habits and record themselves and then listen to it and find out flaws made during the practice.
	Reading aloud	Choose their favorite magazine or even the homework assigned at school to read aloud using the light contact technique on the sound of letters of the first words of the worked-out material.

(continued)

Table 6.7 (continued)

Technique	Home-based activities	Description
Modified airflow technique	Balloon inflation exercise	Ask them to perform diaphragmatic breathing in the manner of pretending to blow up a balloon through the mouth to fill it up with air. Guide them by asking them to picture taking an actual balloon and inflating it up in the region of your stomach every time you breathe in.
	Guided breathing with a book	Lying down, put a thin book on your child's abdomen and instruct the child to breathe normally. The child should pay attention to the act of breathing and feel the movements in the book while they breathe.
	Relaxation to music	Incorporate diaphragmatic breathing techniques with playing some music. Breathe in tune with the music.
	Progressive muscle relaxation	When practicing diaphragmatic breathing, use it along with the progressive muscle relaxation by tensing and relaxing each group of muscles with focus on the breath.
	Breathing with visualization	When practicing diaphragmatic breathing, try and visualize a peaceful scene each time you are taking a breath.
Rate control	Metronome practice	Slow down the tempo of the metronome and invite the child to games: Snap finger, tap foot, nod head, and so on, aligning speaking with such rate. Slow it down at first and then add the heat gradually as they adapt to the slower rate of questioning. In between, stop the beats and make the child continue talking or performing tasks they are doing.
Rate control	Bedtime choral reading	Select a book that is enjoyable for you and the child. At night, it is best to read the text aloud to each other and the aim should be to do this slowly, more, or less in choral singing. This can be done through audiobooks also, where the child reads along a recorded voice reading the text.
	Pacing board	As a vacation task, make a pacing board with the slots for the words of a sentence that has to be learned. The child or the subject uses a marker to draw on the whiteboard. As they say a word, they ensure that they take a few seconds between each word. This visual cue allows them to keep a better pace.
	Mirror exercises	Stand the child in front of a mirror and tell them to pronounce slowly and observe the actions of their mouth. This is a typical form of visual feedback that assists the learners become more conscious of their speech rate and their regulation of the same.
	Record and playback	Film the child with a voice recorder or smartphone while the child is reading a passage or talking about an interest. Rewind the recording and find out if there was any time when speech was delivered at a fast rate. Organize repeated reading or repeating the passage aloud at a slower pace and recording and replaying it again for feedback. Other free software can be used to edit the recorded sound (delayed mode) and then the child can be made to practice the same

Step 4c: Implementation of Stuttering Modification Techniques at Home

The parents have a very active role to perform in order to help their child to deal with and propel him or her forward after formal speech therapy sessions. Their role is essential in the general maintenance of the learned skills from therapy, providing encouragement, and enable the child to effectively deal with issues which may result from stuttering. Practically, one of the major responsibilities of parents is to help their child to find out when and what exactly caused them to start stuttering and if there are any patterns. This process entails watching and recording the cases of stuttering and making records of situations, feelings, and/or specific words and sounds which have an impact on the process. From these patterns, the parent is in a position to assist the child put strategies in place with an aim of learning ways of handling the stuttering better. Aside from helping a child to speak fluently, the practice also helps to support the child because he or she no longer feels that stuttering is a "monster" which can never be defeated. Following identification, it is necessary to teach the child to desensitize various situations such that the child applies the speech therapy learned in all those situations. Listed below are various activities for all the stuttering modification techniques (Table 6.8):

Table 6.8 Home-based techniques for enhancing fluency skills using stuttering modification techniques

Technique	Home-based activities	Description
Identifying and accepting stuttering	Stuttering journal	Documentation in a developmentally appropriate calendar daily in which the child will document speaking incidents, and stuttering occurrences may reveal scenarios that cause the child to stutter. 1. Daily entry: Ask your child to write in a diary on the speaking activities that he or she engaged in, with a comment on the places or times when they stuttered. 2. Detailed description: They should describe what they were doing and who they met or spoke to at the time as well as the emotions felt at the time. 3. Review together: Then, at the end of each of the following weeks, all family members (father, sibling, grandparents, or others) can share their journal with each other and discuss frequent stimulus and trends. Example: Some of the things that happened today include, "today, I stammered when a teacher posed a question in class. I felt very uncomfortable because the teacher was observing keenly."
	Emotion and stuttering chart	Drawing of an emotions chart whereby one plots emotions alongside the stutters to determine which of them cause emotions. 1. Create the chart: Create a chart with the speaking situation column followed by date, emotions faced, and the degree of stuttering. 2. Daily updates: It is recommended to let your child complete the chart during the day. It is crucial to indicate what specific situations hindered the smooth flow of speech and how the child felt at the time. 3. Color coding: Adults are expected to choose different colors for different concepts. For example, red means nervous while blue means calm. Example: "I remember eating with my family and as much as I tried to speak, I rarely stuttered. While on the other hand, I was presenting before a class in school, and I stuttered bad."

(continued)

Table 6.8 (continued)

Technique	Home-based activities	Description
Identifying and accepting stuttering	Stuttering bingo	A fun and interactive game in which the child finds and highlights situations in a bingo card when he or she stutters. 1. Create bingo cards: Create bingo cards with different speaking opportunities such as talking on the phone or reading aloud or asking a question. 2. Identify stuttering: For every point you make at one of the listed situations, they are expected to place a check on the respective spot on the card. 3. Weekly review: At the end of the week, it is recommended to check the bingo card and identify all the situations that lead to stuttering. Example: "Talking to a stranger" could be on their bingo card 1 week along with "Reading aloud in class."
	Video diary	Using video diaries in the fourth act of therapy is helpful in that the child is able to notice what they are doing when there is stuttering on the video, and the child can also note what he/she is doing prior to and during the stuttering episodes. 1. Record daily videos: Help your child shoot a 1-minute video in the morning where you and he or she talks about their day or a particular subject. 2. Self-observation: The last activity again involves watching videos and making notes on any stuttering that is in the videos. 3. Discussion and analysis: It is important to describe in detail pre-, intra-, and post-stuttering situations, with reference to environmental and affective factors. Example: "You know people tend to stammer more when they are stressed so in today's video, I realized that I stammered a lot when speaking about my math test."
	Interactive storytelling	The carrying out of storytelling exercises that will help in the identification of stuttering cues in an entertaining manner. 1. Story creation: Encourage your child to write down or tell you in words what he or she feels, or what he or she dreams of the day, or to think of any dream scenarios. 2. Identify stuttering: Avoid timely focusing on stuttering when narrating stories. 3. Pattern recognition: Talk with them and come to understand what particular words, sounds, or situations cause fluency breaks.

(continued)

Table 6.8 (continued)

Technique	Home-based activities	Description
Desensitizing the stuttering situations	Desensitizing or using speech techniques with supportive family members	1. Story time: Alternate in reading the storybook aloud so as to enhance on the practices of speech therapy. 2. Dinner conversations: Participate in well-arranged dinners so that everyone will discuss one interesting event that occurred in the day. 3. Family games night: Play board games that involve following verbal instruction or games that involve storytelling. 4. Praise and feedback sessions: There should be time allocated for the family to praise the child with regard to efforts made in speaking. 5. Role-playing games: One of the best characters from a movie of a book can be enacted by a person where only speaking will be imitated.
	Desensitizing unsupportive family members	1. Emotion mapping: This can be done through an emotion map to explain emotions previously and after encountering unhelpful team members. 2. Mock conversations: Engagement of mock parent-child interactions where a friendly parent can act as the unfriendly one. 3. Calming techniques: Use relaxation exercises or mediation with each other before the agreed social activities. 4. Positive affirmation jar: Develop a positive affirmation jar for the child by having messages that should be provided when the kid receives negative words. (a) Fill the jar: On some papers, one has to write positive affirmations and words of encouragement. (b) Daily practice: Make it a point that the child will grab a slip from the jar in the morning so that he or she will have something positive for the day. (c) Reflection time: Finally, talk with them on how the affirmation assisted them in dealing with any sample negative comments that may be seen on the social media platforms. 5. Role-playing with ignoring technique: Testing of "mock" bullying or other situations to allow the child to rehearse ways of blocking out the unpleasant comments while reinforcing the positive messages within oneself. (a) Set the scene: Reconstructively, recreationally, or realistically depict typical situations where such remarks may be made. (b) Practice ignoring: Explain to the child that they need to say things like "that is their point of view" or "I do not have to listen to that" and then go on with the activity. (c) Reinforce positivity: In the power point presentation, incorporate an activity called "feeling droopy." after the role-play, ask the child how he or she felt and explain to the child that we need to stay positive.

(continued)

Table 6.8 (continued)

Technique	Home-based activities	Description
Desensitizing the stuttering situations	Desensitizing with strangers	1. Shopping trips: Further, let them practice in requesting for certain items preferably in a shop such as a grocery store or a mall. 2. Friendly greetings: It removes any possibility of the child, for instance, ignoring neighbors or even delivery personnel. 3. Community events: Go out in public places and start with the process of formally meeting people. 4. Library visits: This can be practiced in ways such as asking the librarian for assistance in finding books. 5. Pet walks: Talk to other pet owners who can be encountered while walking the pet around parks.
	Desensitizing phone calls	1. Mock phone calls: Simulate a phone conversation where you have to make conversation with a family member or a friend. 2. Ordering food: Particularly, the ability to order food from a favorite restaurant over the phone should be rehearsed. 3. Customer service: Dial customer service numbers to make inquiries about a particular product or a service. 4. Relatives chat: Make a phone call with relatives who are from other parts of the country or just from the other state at least once a week. 5. Telephone pictionary: Ask someone to draw something on paper and the other person to draw the same figure but with their eyes closed and listen to a description that the first person is giving to them over the phone.
	Desensitizing at family functions	1. Event preparation: Calm down and improvise possible situations that may be encountered at a family party. 2. Photo sharing: Ensure the child is around and engage him/her to discuss pictures of families with several students. 3. Cultural celebrations: Join a cultural or religious occasion and urge the child to explain the customs. 4. Home gatherings: Small family dinner can be arranged to meet and greet other people in a safe environment to eradicate social anxiety. 5. Family bingo: Make a bingo card using the regular family function tasks (for instance, greeting a relative, presenting one's school project).

(continued)

Table 6.8 (continued)

Technique	Home-based activities	Description
Desensitizing the stuttering situations	Desensitizing to new words	1. Word jar: Choose five new words from a jar and incorporate them into sentences that can be used in the course of the day. 2. Flash cards: Teach them with flash cards and new words; engage the child with it in low-stress activities. 3. Word association games: Engage in word games where a child can relate new words with the familiar ones. 4. Daily word challenge: Start a "word of the day" and try to use that word in conversation as often as possible. 5. Reading together: Select books that will present words the child is not familiar with and ask them to read and explain their meanings and how they are used.
Modifications	Budget planning activity	Let the child be part of developing the family's financial budget. As one is guiding the child when it comes to the priorities and expenses, he/she should make sure that they employ cancellation, pull-out, and preparatory set technique as he/she explains the reasoning. Cancellation: This is found in situations where the child stutters on the requested expense item; they stop, think, and then smoothly provide it. Pull-out: In stammering, the child becomes fluent right from the middle of the word or phrase in order to complete it. Preparatory set: The child expects that during their speaking, the upcoming words will be difficult and set themselves up to encounter them easily.
	Recipe instruction activity	Let the child recite, in order, a favorite or desired recipe using speech techniques. Cancellation: If they stumble and say something like "hmm st-starch, umm for stirring," then they consciously say the same thing fluently. Pull-out: Guide the child out of any stutters with the description while ensuring that it is smooth. Preparatory set: Prior to reading, the child gets himself or herself ready for the hard words that are going to be encountered.
	Family debate activity	Have a mock controversy on the type of food to prepare and what should be prepared this week such as "why my favorite meal should be cooked this week." Cancellation: If the child stutters while presenting the argument, they let the child correct themselves and say the phrase fluently. Pull-out: In the debate, if they get into a stutter, they will know how to gracefully exit from it. Preparatory set: When making a point, the child bluntly alerts themselves to areas that may contain difficult words.

(continued)

Table 6.8 (continued)

Technique	Home-based activities	Description
Modifications	Shopping list creation activity	Sit down and make a list of all the goods you need. Decide which products are more important. Cancellation: For instance, if the child stutters on an item's name, the child becomes silent, contemplates, then repeats the same item in a fluent manner. Pull-out: Explain to them to use pull-outs whenever they have a stutter on the names of items. Preparatory set: Much in the same way a child might crouch before releasing a ball, a child prepares to utter what they know will be a difficult word to say.
	Homework help activity	Encourage the child to ask questions about a particular subject and then help by answering the questions that the child cannot answer. Cancellation: When they are not sure of an answer they give, they lose words, rethink, and restate the emerging word flawlessly. Pull-out: Suggesting the students to ease out of the stutters during explanations. Preparatory set: Before doing these, the child expects some words that are difficult to pronounce, and he or she prepares to breeze through them.
Voluntary stuttering	Story time with shared voluntary stuttering	In families with such children, they both deliberately stammer on some selected words during family reading time. For example, when one is reading a bedtime story, both can stammer at the word "cat" each time it is mentioned. Gradually, the parent starts minimizing their stuttering which will eventually prompt the child to continue on his or her own. Voluntary stuttering must be dropped as the child becomes more comfortable in order to concentrate on reading fluently.
	Role-playing conversations with family	Perform simulated parenting incidences in which the parent and the child participate in voluntary stuttering of some words. For example, one can pretend to be ordering food in a restaurant, and both can repeat the word "menu" and "order" when stuttering, though the parent fades out when the kid gains confidence. Gradually move to the practice of these scenarios while not stuttering, where the speech fluency should be as natural as possible.
	Cohosting a cooking show	Let the child and a family member perform a pretend cooking show, where both intentionally stutter on words like "ingredient" and "recipe." then gradually over time, the family member decreases his/her stutter while allowing the child to continue on their own. Subsequently, proceed to an actual culinary task, where the child describes how they prepared the dish, focusing on clear and smooth enunciation without stammering.

(continued)

Table 6.8 (continued)

Technique	Home-based activities	Description
Voluntary stuttering	Simulated phone calls	Teach the child and the parent how to engage in pretend conversations on the phone and deliberately use voluntary stuttering. For example, in a pretend phone call where one of them has to pretend to order pizza, both of them can "stutter" when saying "pizza" or "delivery." the parent then stops stuttering as the child becomes comfortable. Passages from mimicking the actual phone calls with a focus on proper flow of the conversation tone.
	Collaborative shopping list discussion	Make a shopping list with voluntary stuttering and explain to each other the purpose of every item to be bought. The parent stutters on "milk" and "bread" while the child does the same at some other point in the conversation. Gradually, the parent becomes less of a stutterer, thus enabling the child to be more in charge. On the last stage, it is recommended to practice the given shopping list in a manner that resembles normal conversation where the emphasis should be made on the fluidity of speech throughout the process.
Pausing and chunking	Family dinner conversations	During the family dinner, encourage everybody to pause and chunk their speaking during conversations. During dinner, the parent and the child engage in dialogue with talking turns; the parent talks while the child listens and vice versa with the purpose of performing temporal breaks between the ideas as well as between the words. For example, when they are talking about the events which happened during the day, they take a few seconds to speak again. The parent gradually fades out over time while steering the child to speak and reducing the occurrences of hesitating with unnatural cueing just the way the child is going to produce a continuous conversation.
	Neighborhood walk and talk	Go for a walk in the area and try to pause and chuck in conversation with the people encountered along the way. Neighbors are also greeted and using different sentences and short pauses between them; the child is encouraged to talk. For example, while discussing the events of the day, they take a break for some time after each or any statement to be made. During the second phase of the treatment, the parent withdraws, and the child provides focused conversation, and the parent prompts fluent speech only.

(continued)

Table 6.8 (continued)

Technique	Home-based activities	Description
Pausing and chunking	Phone conversations with relatives	In order to incorporate better pausing and chunking, make practice phone calls with relatives. Bring each of the immediate family members and set up a weekly phone conference with the parents and the child, where they both have to take turns speaking, and count to 10 before they speak. For instance, while speaking to the grandparents, the child breaks the conversation to include news about their week. Slowly, the parent stops interjecting, and the child keeps on talking on their own, keeping the flow of thoughts smooth.
	Role-playing with strangers	Role-plays and act out encounters with people one does not know. Teach the child and the parent to act out situations in which it may be necessary to speak to strangers, for instance, to ask for directions or order a meal. Both stop and use subheadings during the role-play. For example, while faking their request for directions—Can speak in a manner where after each sentence, there will be a brief moment of silence. In the process, the parent gradually steps down his/her intervention with the child performing such interactions independently and approach fluency.
	Family function speeches	Speak for a few minutes at the family events. It is helpful to prepare a brief presentation, a speech for a family occasion, and make the child practice pausing and chunking. For instance, they may discuss where they went on their summer holidays, but do it in segments, making pauses between each segment of that story. In the course of the event, the parent and the child rehearse the performance, and the role of the parent is diminished step by step. Finally, the child is required to make the speech on their own, the key points being fluency and confidence.

Step 5: Preparing for Variability in Stuttering

It is true that for children, especially preschoolers and school going children, stuttering is often accompanied by very noticeable changes in speech fluency. There are circumstances which may enhance or reduce stuttering or even make it appear or cease completely. To parents, it is important to grasp these differences so as to know how to support the child adequately and ensure that they have a favorable channel of communication. These factors are:

1. *Emotional states*: The feelings of children are in a way directly related to their fluency disorders. Stress, especially stress that comes with excitement, anger, fear, or even sadness, can worsen the stuttering. For instance, in families, when they are celebrating or even quarrelling, children are likely to stutter. On the other hand, when children are

relaxed and comfortable, for instance, during play in which there is little talking or at night when they are going to sleep, their speech may be less disrupted.

2. *Communication pressure*: Stuttering may also be enhanced by the pressure to convey a message. It could arise when at a family dinner having to narrate their day at school or work or when presenting in front of their kin. At the same time, when having a chat with the closest relatives at home, for example, there is usually less stuttering.
3. *Fatigue*: Stress and fatigue play a big role in worsening the speech fluency of a person who stutters. Listening, speaking, understanding, and writing are best done when the child is well rested, for instance, after a busy day at school or after playing. This can help in managing the variability, by making sure that the child is well rested and has a regular sleep schedule.
4. *Rapid speech*: This is especially so when children try to speak fast in an effort to match with fast-speaking individuals or when they get agitated. One should advise the child to speak slowly and not rush when they are speaking to minimize stuttering.
5. *Competitive speaking environments*: Stuttering may be worsened by family situations that make the child feel the need to compete for their turn to speak, for example, during dinner conversations or when playing with the siblings. The pressure comes from having to speak up and not being able to say something without the other child interrupting. A good solution is to establish a turn-taking system, to give each child a chance to speak without the other child interfering.
6. *Anxiety and stress*: Stress and anxiety which may be in relation to speaking or any other factor can tend to make one stutter. It can also be seen in a child before a large family gathering like a wedding or just when a child is transitioning to a new house. Creating a comfortable environment for the student may help to reduce the level of their anxiety and in turn their speech difficulty.
7. *Changes in routines or environments*: Stressors can include changes in the child's environment or schedule, and these can result in a child stuttering more. Some of the events that can influence speech include joining a new school, changing houses, or disturbance in the family. In some ways, it is advisable to try as much as possible to be normal, to have as much routine and structure as possible to deal with stuttering.
8. *Linguistic challenges*: Some of the activities that may worsen stuttering include narrating an elaborate story or learning new words. It is also possible to use simpler speech during the interactions and increasingly introduce new words to overcome these problems.
9. *Health and physical well-being*: Stress, pain, or any physical ailment that can in any way affect the individual can further flare up stuttering. A child who has a cold or is unwell or uncomfortable may present more stuttering. The child's physical welfare being taken care of enhances the child's speaking capabilities.
10. *Social interactions*: The kind of interactions that take place in homes also has a great influence. Having family members who are more tolerant and who do not hurry the child can help the child to be less stressed about speaking and, as a result, he or she will stutter less. On the other hand, there are interactions that relate to peer pressure or negative incidences, and these also have the opposite effect.

Step 6: Implementing Relaxation Exercises in Daily Routine

Parents should assist children who stutter through relaxation and mindfulness activities within the home environment. It can help to manage anxiety, increase self-awareness, and thus improve the quality of life. Here's how parents can support and guide their children in using these methods, which can also be implemented in school during yoga or physical training sessions:

- *Introduce relaxation exercises*: The parents can therefore begin to educate their children on simple relaxation techniques. Some of the ways that can be employed are deep breathing exercises, progressive muscle relaxation, or guided imagery. When these exercises are included into the daily routine, parents establish a healthy and positive environment at home.
- *Provide dedicated time*: It is critical to create some schedules in the day to perform relaxation exercises and mindful practices. This can be done in the morning, after school, or just before retiring for the day. Ensure that children opt in voluntarily and ensure that the environment set is one that is conducive to these practices.
- *Teach breathing techniques*: Certain breathing exercises, for example, diaphragmatic breathing, can assist a child to control speech and minimize stress connected with stammering. The parents can also model for the children how to breathe in the right manner and tell them to take deep breaths when they are angry or when they want to speak fluently.
- *Incorporate mindfulness activities*: It is possible to use mindfulness practices like mindful listening, body scan, or mindful eating to foster children's awareness of the present moment. Practicing short mindfulness activities with your child helps the child learn to watch his or her thoughts and feelings without criticizing them. This practice assists children in developing self-compassion and feelings of relaxation which leads to better communication and language development. Such activities as relaxation and breathing exercises and awareness of the self and the world can play a big role in the home environment for children who stutter. These techniques not only have the benefit of reducing anxiety and tension but also increasing the awareness of the self, the ability to modulate emotions, and improving general health. Few such relaxation techniques are described below:

A. *Mindfulness and Stuttering: A Journey of Awareness and Acceptance*

Mindfulness as a therapeutic strategy for stuttering is based on meditation procedures which are originated from Buddhist traditions. Jon Kabat-Zinn, doing much of the foundational work in the field of mindfulness, introduced mindfulness to the west through the Mindfulness-Based Stress Reduction (MBSR) in the late 1970s. Kabat-Zinn did not develop mindfulness for stuttering, but it was the first program of its kind to explore the use of mindfulness for various conditions, including speech impairments.

In the field of stuttering, scholars such as Dr. Hugh-John McIntyre, a speech-language pathologist/communication disorders clinician and mindfulness practitioner, has applied mindfulness in speech therapy. They have been able to show how mindfulness can be of great value to people with a stutter since it aids in controlling one's thoughts regarding speech.

Stuttering is the incomplete or interrupted flow of speech, and mindfulness, which is the act of being conscious of the present moment, has the potential of being highly therapeutic for such individuals. It entails watching thoughts, emotions, and the way people express themselves without prejudice. This practice allows people to gain insight into the mechanisms of their stammering, as well as the patterns of their speaking and listening environment, which fosters reasonable self-esteem. The following are the steps for this:

(a) *Observing stuttering behaviors*: Mindfulness entails a way of observing stuttering without prejudice. This is very useful for the realization of personal speech patterns and tendencies.
(b) *Noticing listener responses*: It assists people to understand the reaction of other people to their stuttering, thus offering a better understanding of interpersonal communication.
(c) *Minimizing judgment*: People are trained to notice their stuttering without evaluating it as positive or negative and, therefore, improve their attitude toward themselves.
(d) *Addressing secondary symptoms*: Mindfulness enables the awareness of the other behaviors that are closely related to stuttering like avoiding, thus making the person face and deal with these symptoms.
(e) *Developing realistic self-esteem*: It encourages the recognition of the fact that one is a responsible person and that one's reactions are determined by a number of factors. Thus, it encourages understanding and a balanced view of oneself.

Practicing Mindfulness in Daily Life

The mindfulness tasks can be practiced through sitting meditation and being mindful during the various activities that one does in the day.

(a) *Formal meditation*: This entails concentrating on a particular object for a particular duration, for instance, on the breath, observing the mind and bringing it back to the object of focus.
(b) *Mindful daily activities*: Simplify activities and make them more intentional; when you are eating, exercising, or even talking to someone, be present and focused on the present.
   - *Mindful speaking techniques*: As for the Zen meditation practices, it is possible to use rhythmic counting, mindful conversation, and other techniques in the group. These practices are all about different aspects of speaking and listening with emphasis on nonjudgmental approach. Such environments allow the student to practice different speech techniques, including how to deal with cases of being stuck for words in a safe space.

B. *Zen Meditation and Stuttering*

The specific manner of employing Zen meditation for stuttering cannot be linked to any particular person as it forms part of the general use of mindfulness and meditation in speech therapy. Zazen is a practice derived from Zen Buddhism, and it is based on mindfulness of the present moment and acceptance without criticism or evaluation. This approach was incorporated into stuttering therapy as a comprehensive view of the relation between the mind and the body in speech production.

The principles of Zen, most of all, mindfulness, acceptance, and focused attention, are quite relevant to the needs of the stutterers. These principles help in controlling stress and the emotions that are involved with stuttering, hence helping in achieving a more relaxing and conscious attitude toward speaking. Integrating Zen into stuttering therapy, there is a combination of the eastern tradition and the western approach to treatment of speech disorders. This integration signals the increasing importance being assigned to mental and emotional aspects of communication disorders and the potential of such interventions in health promotion and maintenance.

Zen meditation is the process of sitting with a certain posture, more often in silence, and watching the thoughts, feelings, and sensations that emerge and pass through without generating any form of association or aversion. The aim is not to let the thoughts, or the experiences, disappear but to just watch them. Thus, with regard to stuttering, Zen meditation has much to teach us. This concept tells people to accept the moment for what it is, which can be quite inspiring for people with stuttering. This approach helps to maintain a passive attitude toward the episodes of stuttering, which helps one to observe his or her speech behavior in an unbiased manner. It can result in an improved knowledge of the causes and the behaviors associated with the stuttering problem.

Also, Zen practices include the use of breathing exercises that can help in controlling the physical part of stuttering. Deep breathing makes it easier to manage stress and anxiety that are known to be some of the causes of stuttering. From Zen meditation, one can gain composure and concentration in speaking and, thereby, feel that they have the reins in their hands.

Zen meditation focuses on the acceptance of things as they are and people being in the moment, which is quite effective. It helps people with stuttering to embrace the fact that they stutter and that it is a part of their present life, not something that has to be corrected. This acceptance is an important process in the minimization of the emotional and psychological consequences of stuttering, in the development of a more positive self-concept, and in the improvement of communication. The steps include:

(a) *Establish a daily practice*: To establish a routine, choose a particular period of the day, and if possible, in a calm area, to practice Zen meditation.
(b) *Comfortable posture*: To meditate, one should find a comfortable position which should not be too comfortable; one may sit on a cushion on the floor or a chair and should not slouch since this will make one sleepy.
(c) *Focus on breath*: Slowly bring your awareness to your breathing, without attempting to change it in any manner. This facilitates developing concentration and relaxation.
(d) *Observe thoughts nonjudgmentally*: Just observe the thoughts and/or feelings that come up during meditation without engaging with them. This is useful in the formation of self-reflection of one's inner speech and responses.

(e) *Apply mindfulness to speaking*: Start applying the mindfulness that you have learned from meditation into actual speaking situations in a gradual manner beginning from the least stressful contexts to the most.

C. *Yoga and Stuttering*

Yoga as a treatment for stuttering is derived from general use of yoga when it comes to treating people with different complex disorders, and treatment of stuttering is also considered to have a link with the mind and body. Yoga is a practice that is believed to have originated from India and involves physical exercises like postures, breathing exercise, and meditation. Thus, all of these components help to enhance the quality of life and relaxation. From the development of yoga, there has been the use of the principles in speech therapy, especially for children with stuttering.

It can be assumed that the inclusion of yoga into stuttering therapy stemmed from the understanding that breath control, muscle relaxation, and mental relaxation, as practiced in yoga, could help persons who stutter. These principles are very handy in easing the tension and the language fear that is associated with stuttering, which makes it more of a mindful approach to speaking. Indeed, this combination of so-called oriental practices with western approaches to speech therapy gives a complete picture of speech disorders and shows how much impact the mental and emotional status of patients has on speaking practice.

Yoga can be described as a physical exercise which consists of certain postures (asanas) besides certain forms of breathing patterns known as pranayama and meditation. These practices together aim at achieving physical ease, mental focusing, and psychological well-being.

Regarding the application of yoga in the context of stuttering, it can be said that the practice of Yogasana has the following advantages: It encourages a person to pay attention to the breath and the body and to keep it relaxed and this in itself helps in lessening the amount of tension and anxiety that is felt when a person stutters. When the stutterer has practiced yoga, they become more mindful and aware of their body which will ensure they are more knowledgeable on when to speak, and how to speak, that is if they had wanted to avoid speaking in a certain way or avoided speaking fluently due to the stuttering episodes.

Being accepting and nonjudgmental in yoga practice may further promote a positive self-image among the stuttering people. This is because cases where one feels that they must modify their stutter are the ones that have the most damaging emotional effects, and removal of such feelings would improve communication.

While they are young, it is suggested to establish a routine practice of yoga in the morning at a calm location. Regularity is significant to build up the advantages of yoga to manage stammering. Some poses are most effective when practiced by children who stutter. These asanas help promote relaxation, improve breath control, and reduce physical tension. Some examples include:

(a) *Mountain pose* (*Tadasana*): Bergen's second pose, Tadasana or mountain pose, assists in general toning and separating of the component parts of the body in order to render them more reliable.

(b) *Child's pose* (*Balasana*): This pose helps to calm the body and at the same time stretch out the back and shoulder region where people generally have stiff muscles.
(c) *Bridge pose* (*Setu Bandhasana*): This backbend assists in chest expansion and improving respiratory muscles while relaxing the upper body muscles.
(d) *Cat-cow pose* (*Marjaryasana-Bitilasana*): They also assist in stretching the spinal column as well as facilitating the coordinated breathing pattern and thereby lessening the general tension in the body.
(e) *Corpse pose* (*Savasana*): This is the final relaxation position that needs to be maintained for the accomplishment of the benefits of the practice apart from deep relaxation.
(f) *Lion pose* (*Simhasana*): This is a facet of stretching in which specific muscles of the face and tongue are stretched, and it may benefit students who have problem in articulating their speech.
(g) *Saying "Om"* (*chanting*): Recitation of Om can help in modulation of voice and control of breath which can help in calming of the mind and bringing concentration.
(h) *Neck stretches* (*Jalandhara Bandha*): The most effective exercises are gentle neck stretches, which will allow lessening the tension in the area of the neck and throat, which is usually a problem for people with this speech disorder.

Parents should teach children to use the elements of yoga, for example, to breathe and calm down before speaking in everyday situations. Practice should begin in environments where there are low stakes involved and then progress to environments that involve higher stakes.

Step 7: Family-Based Therapy Programs to Manage Stuttering at Home
Family-based therapy programs are especially important in the management of stuttering because their implementation means the involvement of family members into the therapeutic process. These programs are meant to encourage a home environment that will enable a child who stutters to practice and develop their speech fluency skills that are learned in school. The parents and other family members are involved in these programs so that the child is continuously encouraged as this is very vital in the management of stuttering.

1. *The Lidcombe Program*

This is a classic example of a family-centered program that engages the parents to participate actively in the speech therapy of the child. Through a focus on social goals and COMM-education, it enhances the skills of both therapists and families. Family-based therapy emphasizes building strong alliances between families and therapists, simultaneously fostering the child's communication development and confidence.

The Lidcombe Program named after its creators, speech therapists Mark Onslow and Ann Packman, was designed in the beginning of the 1990s as a behavioral therapy approach suitable for early childhood. The program is also highly distinctive in that it requires heavy parental investment. The goal here is to help the child speak fluently in his or her daily environment. Steps involved in the Lidcombe Program are:

A. *Parental Training*
   1. Training by speech therapists: Parents are supervised by the speech therapists on how best to put into practice the Lidcombe Program.
   2. Maintaining normalcy: The specific use of verbal contingencies does not alter the child's general speech and family life but rather adds interactions.

B. *Verbal Contingencies*
   1. Structured sessions: All parents are instructed on how to interact with their children during formal therapy sessions as well as in everyday life when their child stutters or does not stutter.
   2. Initial scores: Orientation of the patient in rating assignment is done at the initial time of therapy.
   3. Identifying stuttering: Parents learn the signs of stuttering and what type of stuttering it is for the child.
   4. Encouragement and praise: Parents use individual and encouraging comments only when the child is speaking fluently and effortlessly.
   5. Fostering self-evaluation: Children are expected to assess their own speaking rates throughout given minutes or hours, thus being self-monitored.

C. *Treatment Goals*
   1. The main purpose is to make the stuttering as low as possible.
   2. The emphasis is on how this lower level of stuttering can be sustained in the long run.

D. *Severity Rating (SR) Scale*

1. Self-observation of the severity is done using the SR scale and the assessment is carried out on a scale of 0 (no stuttering) to 9 (very severe stuttering).

E. *Weekly Sessions with Speech Therapists*

1. Both parent and the child see the speech therapist on a weekly basis, for 45–60 minutes each, to ensure correct application of the treatment plan.

Treatment Scenarios

- Daily conversations: In the course of eating, especially during dinner, a parent might commend a child for speaking well, hence promoting positive speaking behaviors.
- SR training utilization: A parent may hear a story the child has produced and give an SR score and then compare it with the speech therapist.
- Promoting self-evaluation: After a period of rather extended and seamless speaking, a parent could then turn to the child and request the child to speak more clearly, which helps to increase the child's self-consciousness about the act of speaking.

Implementation of Lidcombe in School

While family-based therapy programs are structured mainly for home use, it is possible to coordinate the programs' application in schools in order to meet the needs of children who stutter. Fortunately, parents are able to recommend these strategies to teachers and school counsellors so that concepts of programs such as the Lidcombe Program are practiced at home as well as in school. Thus, parents and educators as well should form a united team focusing on the child's needs and being able to support him/her in developing effective communication as well as strong self-esteem. This can be done in the following ways:

- *Positive reinforcement in the classroom*: Let the child speak and encourage one another; as teachers observe the fluency the child is capable of, they should encourage and acknowledge the child. This form of encouragement even assists in boosting the child's morale and plays a significant role in encouraging the child into practicing more fluent speech.
- *Structured speech sessions*: This requires the independence of time for the structured speech sessions where children are able to practice fluent speech without any pressure. These can be placed into various streams of concern and/or be at certain times within the day where the child can consistently be working on his or her speech.
- *Collaboration with parents*: Frequent communication with parents must be kept in order to keep the atmosphere at home and school clients congenial. The teachers should communicate the observations made to each other and coordinate themselves as to how to assist the child to gain better speech. This partnership plays the role of assisting in the formation of a combined strategy for addressing the case of stuttering, which gives encouragement to the child.
- *Creating a safe space*: It is therefore important that students be made to understand that there should be tolerance in the class. Teachers' ought to create platforms where all learners feel comfortable to express themselves without being mocked. Such an environment most certainly can reduce anxiety and pressure connected to speaking and thus would make those children who stutter to speak more fluently.

When the Lidcombe Program and other supportive steps are applied in the classroom, the children who stutter will be more confident in their communication skills. There are no contraindications of this comprehensive approach to intervention since it not only focuses on concerns of the child's speech but also creates a safe environment that enables learning. In this way, parents contribute to their child's success by recommending these strategies to teachers and school counsellors so the child continues to get constant support in all spheres of life.

2. *RESTART DCM Program*

The Reassembling Phoneme Sequences for Articulatory Reorganization Treatment-Dynamic Core Pathway (RESTART DCM) approach was developed to empower children who stutter by helping them modify their speech patterns for enhanced fluency. This method is highly based on the research and practice concerned with the modification of the actual sound production to minimize stuttering. It is expedient for such children who may exhibit only mild to moderate tension or difficulty in speaking.

The RESTART DCM method was introduced by a group of speech-language pathologists and scientists who realized that there is no effective unidimensional approach for the clients suffering from stuttering that would focus on reflexive and psychological factors. Combining ideas borrowed from various therapeutic schools, they developed a comprehensive conception that is built around the principle of differentiation, implying the development of special techniques that would be used for each child depending on his or her communication disorder characteristics.

In this procedure, the parents are involved in increasing the chances of success in the RESTART DCM approach. For incorporation of the principles into practice, the parents came up with ways by which they can assist their children develop confidence and, hence, be more comfortable in their interactions.

Key Aspects of RESTART DCM Are

(a) *Understanding individual capacities*: The initial step is to do a general and individualized communication development profile for your child. These assessments therefore become the basis of individual management of stammering.
(b) *Analyzing communication demands*: Know the kind of pressure different speaking situations cause to the child whether in social, school, or home context. This also enables the development of strategies that are suitable and efficient for the organization.
(c) *Developing personalized strategies*: Create individual approaches which will correspond to child's capacities and demands of various conditions to improve the quality of communication.
(d) *Focus on holistic development*: It also encompass self-perception, feelings, and attitudes as well as the manner of speaking and the errors that characterize the stutters. These are confidence building, reduction of anxiety, as well as general effectiveness in interpersonal communication.
(e) *Collaborative approach*: Be supportive and report any positive change by working with the child's speech therapist as parents can role model these strategies to the child.

The Application of RESTART DCM Can Be Done in Various Situations

- During family meals: Suggest to the child, when talking in the family, to speak at a slow rate, soft voicing at the start of the word, and gradual changes of phonemes. Praise them for the attempts and smoothness as well as the anticipated errors.
- In social gatherings: Support the child in using the techniques learned from the RESTART DCM to overcome stuttering during social settings. If they are unlikely to do so, then it is advisable to work more on their strength and conform to the requirement of the social setting.
- After-school activities and studying: If a child needs assistance with homework or studying, arrange for an environment that the child will be relaxed to practice on his/her speech drills.

3. *Palin Parent-Child Interaction: Promoting Communication Independence*

The Palin Parent-Child Interaction (PCI) therapy, used in the Michael Palin Centre for Stammering in London as an innovative therapeutic strategy, focuses on enhancing communication patterns within the parent-child relationship. It is most helpful in a child who gets stressed or stutters during the speech so that they are made comfortable to speak well. Palin PCI also seeks to engage the parent as well as the child so as to ensure that the process is handled in an environment that is relaxing and stress free so as to allow for proper communication.

Comprehensive Approach: Customized Support for Each Child A comprehensive, child-focused approach includes adaptable techniques designed to meet each child's unique needs. This strategy is beneficial for children with varying levels of speech tension or fluency challenges, enabling the development of personalized treatment plans. In this approach, children collaborate with parents and speech-language pathologists to explore supportive methods, which can enhance fluency and confidence. By personalizing support, parents are empowered to help their children manage their stuttering experience while simultaneously fostering self-assurance.

Such a "customized" approach may therefore enable parents to support their children in coping with their individual stuttering experience while at the same time building up their confidence.

Operant Conditioning Therapy: Shaping Fluency Through Rewards Operant conditioning therapy proposes to use differential contingencies whereby rewards are sought to be established for fluent speech as opposed to stuttered speech. In the context of this technique, it is possible to provide a home exercise in which a reward plan will enhance fluency. For instance, parents can emulate the reward system in that the children try to use standard fluent language when speaking and receive stickers or other minor forms of reward each time they do it. It helps children to work toward enhanced oral and written communication at the same time making it fun to avail.

Desensitization and Gradual Exposure: Reducing Anxiety and Promoting Confidence Desensitization and gradual exposure refer to the gradual process of exposing children to speaking situations that are difficult for them and being supportive in order to minimize anxiety and gradually build up the child's self-esteem. Parents should ensure they set an example at home of how children should be treated by providing an environment that welcomes free speech. Through offering occasions to communicate and perform, increasing their frequency, and gradually increasing the difficulty level of interactions, parents foster children's coping abilities and confidence.

Reducing Rate of Speech: Encouraging Clarity and Fluency Through Pausing and Chunking The approach of reducing the speaking pace should be added to the list of helpful techniques that improve the aspects of clarity and fluency. Closely, parents can manage to teach their children how to breathe in between phrases and parcel their words into comprehensible segments. This in turn enables the child to be more fluent in expressing their ideas in a more deliberate and ensured manner, hence minimizing the stammering acts. Talking slowly helps children improve their speaking and does not make them feel that they are being controlled.

Promoting Acceptance and Reducing Tension: Creating a Positive Mindset Acceptance and relaxation are prominent factors in any therapy for stuttering. Parents have a significant contribution to offer to facilitate the kid's feeling of being worthy to be valued in society. Explaining stuttering to peers and friends, telling success stories of people who struggled with precise difficulty and succeeded, appreciating attempts that people make while speaking, etc., may also decrease pressure and stress. Parents should foster self-esteem through the communication of the values that children should choose to be themselves as they are, without being defined by the efficiency or fluency of their language.

6.22.5 What NOT TO DO as Parents When Managing Children with Stuttering

It is quite natural for parents to feel differently at various times, ranging from helplessness to anxiety, especially when it comes to thinking about their child's future and well-being. All these issues, however, can be addressed, and if tackled correctly, they will offer no cause for concern. To foster proper self-esteem and a positive attitude in a child with stuttering, not only toward speech fluency but also toward life, parents must avoid various pitfalls:

1. *Forcing a child for therapy*: Parents should note that there is no ideal time when kids should begin therapy. Stuttering therapy typically begins around 6 months after the onset of stuttering, but parents should seek an early intervention if the risk factors exist, or if stuttering interferes with the child's life. At the same time, therapy should focus on a child's participation. It is therefore suggested that parents wait for the child to come up with the desire to go for therapy. The worst thing one can do is to compel the child to change the way of speaking or to constantly prompt the child to utilize lessons learned through therapy.
2. *Do not ignore the stuttering*: Articles of Stuttering Association highlight that stuttering should not be shameful. Children and young people who have learned of their stuttering must be encouraged to discuss it with their parents, if they want to, or if they show signs of distress regarding their speech.

3. *Do not rush the speech*: Parents also should not be in a hurry or let something come in between them when they are talking. It is important not to allow the child to think that the speed of speaking is more important than the words they say.
4. *Do not shy from seeking professional guidance*: Parents should not shy off from seeking assistance from professionals. It is thus important not to assume that the child will just grow out of stuttering without any support.
5. *Do not interrupt during speech even if stuttering*: Teachers should refrain from finishing the words of the child or interrupting them while they speak. This could lead to increased pressure and anxiety levels, issues that make it worse to stutter.
6. *Do not impose high expectations*: Parents should not have high expectations of the child in particular situations or expect the child to speak perfectly. High expectations may put pressure on them and make the child feel stressed and nervous, consequently increasing the frequency of the stuttering.
7. *Do not rush the speech*: Parents should avoid speaking in this manner because children learn much of their communication from their parents. A slow speaking rate should be used, and the child should occasionally be allowed to pause to ensure them that there is no hurry.
8. *Do not limit your support*: In parents, they should not display anger or disappointment whether the child stutters or not. Conditional support from the parents negatively impacts a child's self-esteem and confidence level. It is important that parents should not leave their child to struggle alone or be unaware of the case of the stuttering. Inadequate participation results in ignorance of some aspects of the child's experience and requirements.
9. *Do not expect immediate improvement*: Parents should not expect such outcomes to happen in a day's work. This may result in pressure and frustration in stuttering management since impatience is likely to affect the management process.
10. *Do not be inflexible with changes in speech relationships*: Parents should not oppose the natural evolution that takes place in a child's relation to speech as they develop. Inflexibility can only stand in the child's way and slow their development as well as their ability to adjust to new situations.
11. *Do not keep routine and unengaging speech drills*: These exercises should not be made boring or nerve-jangling to the child. More importantly, the activities should be stimulating in nature especially for the young kids in their tender ages. Besides, parents should not fail to monitor their child's progress in therapy. When things are not monitored, it is hard to appreciate the corresponding milestones and also manage the corresponding challenges adequately. Parents also should not let go of the speech therapist even after all the therapy sessions are over. They need frequent contact to discuss patient's progress and other advice that may be of help with the child's treatment.
12. *Do not shy away from support networks*: Leaving from the issue of accuracy, it is important for parents not to shy away from associating with people. One can obtain useful information and support from other parents as well as from the children themselves, which is quite vital.

6.22.6 What Therapy Techniques TO AVOID as Parents

When parents hear their child stammer, they feel a wave of emotions such as despair, remorse, and fear of the child's future experiences and encounters. They may be worried about their social life and career, which can be quite a source of anxiety. Sometimes, it is as useful to know what not to do as it is to know what to do in a particular situation.

Stuttering is a subtype of fluency disorder that is not related to the physical strength of a person. The exercises meant to strengthen the muscles of the face are therefore useless and may only frustrate the child. Just as trying too hard does not make one speak fluently; it rather tends to make one's speech more broken.

SLPs and research support tasks that are meant to repattern speech, not strengthen muscles. Stuttering activities that are well developed assist children to cope with and accept their speech. But there are some practices which are more dangerous than useful despite the fact that they are performed with good intentions. Here are techniques parents should avoid:

1. *Skip the straw*: Sipping through a straw may be helpful in minimizing spills but lacks any scientific evidence as a tool in enhancing speech delivery. No matter how big or how small, or what shape it is, a straw cannot be considered a treatment for stuttering.
2. *Dutch jaw-strengthening routines*: The exercises that are undertaken with a view to strengthening the facial muscles or enhancing the flexibility of the jaw do not in any way affect the stuttering as it is a neurologically based disorder and not a musculoskeletal one.
3. *Avoid the AEIOU drill*: In an attempt to get a 3-year-old to repeat vowels, one is likely to end up frustrated and the task in itself can be quite conceptual. Speech exercises should in no way interfere with a child's communication and should not be annoying to the child.
4. *Stop constant corrections*: Kids do not have a negative perception of stuttering unless they are made to feel that there is something wrong with it. Prolonged instructions to the child to "try again" will make the child aware of their speech problems and they may become reluctant to speak.
5. *Postpone rhythmic speech techniques*: Syllable-timed speech is useful for older children as for younger children who are still in the process of constructing sentences, it may hamper their learning process.
6. *Avoid word avoidance*: This makes children afraid of hard words and hence discourages them from attempting to read them. Rather, they should be made to confront these words, and they should be helped to build strength and confidence.
7. *Eliminate "calm down" commands*: It is right to say that emotions should be freely expressed. It is unhelpful to tell a child not to show excitement or frustration as it may worsen fluency. It should be okay for them to speak sans inhibition, with stutters and all.

It is therefore equally important to know the things that one should not do when supporting a child who stutters. It is therefore important to understand that every child that has stuttering has his/her own unique experience. Although some paths may hold a clear direction to the right path, some others may hold difficulty. It is the role of the parents to direct, to encourage, and to be with their child to facilitate the process of achieving the goal of correct and fluent use of language with lots of forbearance, tolerance, and love.

References

Abramovitz A, Goyeneche C, Cánchica A, Burgues T, Sucupira E. Botulinum toxin application in the facial muscles for the treatment of stuttering. J Laryngology and Voice. 2017;7(1):14–7. https://doi.org/10.4103/jlv.JLV_6_17.

Azrin NH, Nunn RG. A rapid method of eliminating stuttering by a regulated breathing approach. Behav Res Ther. 1974;12(3):279–86.

Bloodstein O, Bernstein Ratner N. A handbook on stuttering. 6th ed. Delmar Cengage Learning; 2008.

Bothe AK. Evidence-based treatment of stuttering: empirical bases and clinical applications. 1st ed. Psychology Press; 2004. https://doi.org/10.4324/9781410610522.

Bunton K. Resonance and voice quality in stuttering therapy. J Speech Lang Hear Res. 2018;61(4):1025–34. https://doi.org/10.1044/2018_JSLHR-S-17-0120.

Chesters DW, Möttönen R, Watkins KE. Investigating the neuroanatomy of stuttering using functional neuroimaging. Brain Lang. 2018;175–176:14–21. https://doi.org/10.1016/j.bandl.2018.06.004.

Craig A, Tran Y. Chronic and social anxiety in people who stutter. Adv Psychiatr Treat. 2005;12:63–68. https://doi.org/10.1192/apt.12.1.63.

Craig A, Hancock K, Tran Y, Craig M. Anxiety levels in people who stutter: a randomized population study. J Speech Lang Hear Res. 2003;46(5):1197–206. https://doi.org/10.1044/1092-4388(2003/093).

Fraser J. The stuttering foundation: resources for clinicians and clients. Semin Speech Lang. 2010;31(4):272–5.

Guitar B. Stuttering: an integrated approach to its nature and treatment. 4th ed. Lippincott Williams & Wilkins; 2014.

Höbler F. Differences in implicit motor learning between adults who do and do not stutter. Neuropsychologia. 2022;172:108342. https://doi.org/10.1016/j.neuropsychologia.2022.108342

Ingham RJ, Kilgo M, Ingham JC, Moglia R, Belknap H, Sanchez T. Evaluation of a stuttering treatment based on reduction of short phonation intervals. J Speech Lang Hear Res. 2001;44(6):1229–44.

Kent RD. Nonspeech oral movements and oral motor disorders: a narrative review. Am J Speech Lang Pathol. 2015;24(4):763–89. https://doi.org/10.1044/2015_AJSLP-14-0179.

Ladouceur R, Saint-Laurent L. Stuttering: a multidimensional treatment and evaluation package. J Fluen Disord. 1986;11(2):93–103.

Liu J, Yu F, Feng C, Li S. The pausing strategies in Chinese preschool children's narratives. J Speech Lang Hear Res. 2022;66(2):431–43. https://doi.org/10.1044/2022_JSLHR-21-00542.

Manning WH, DiLollo A. Clinical decision making in fluency disorders (5th ed.). Plural Publishing. 2025.

Onslow M, O'Brian S. Management of childhood stuttering. J Paediatr Child Health. 2013;49(2):E112–5.

Onslow M, Packman A. The lidcombe program of early stuttering intervention: a clinician's guide. Singular Publishing Group. 1999.

Reardon-Reeves NA, Yaruss JS. School-age stuttering therapy: a practical guide. Stuttering Therapy Resources, Inc; 2013.

Sheehan JG. Stuttering: research and therapy. Harper & Row; 1970.

Smith LF, Smith JK. The nature and growth of aesthetic fluency. In: New directions in aesthetics, creativity and the arts. 1st ed. Routledge; 2020. p. 12. https://doi.org/10.4324/9781315224084.

Smith A, Weber C. How does a stuttering event come to pass? Evidence from neuroimaging studies. J Speech Lang Hear Res. 2017;60(3):327–41. https://doi.org/10.1044/2017_JSLHR-S-16-0211.

SpeechIRL. Speech therapy for stuttering. 2023. Retrieved from https://www.speechirl.com/

Van Borsel J. The efficacy of light articulatory contacts in stuttering treatment. Fluency Disfluency Speech. 2018;34(3):78–89. https://doi.org/10.1016/j.jcomdis.2018.01.005.

Van Lieshout P, Boyle JB, Harms M. The impact of early life adversity on language development: a review. J Dev Orig Health Dis. 2020;11(4):410–4. https://doi.org/10.1017/S2040174419000692.

Van Riper C. The nature of stuttering. Prentice-Hall; 1982.

Williamson DA, Epstein LH, Coburn C. Multiple baseline analysis of the regulated breathing procedure for the treatment of stuttering. J Fluen Disord. 1981;6(4):327–39.

Yairi E, Seery CH. Stuttering: foundations and clinical applications. 2nd ed. Pearson; 2015.

Yaruss JS. Evaluating treatment outcomes for adults who stutter. J Commun Disord. 2001;34(1–2):163–82.

Yaruss JS. It's (almost) NEVER breathing in stuttering therapy! Stuttering Therapy Resources. Retrieved from Stuttering Therapy Resources; 2021.

Yaruss JS, Reardon-Reeves NA. Early childhood stuttering therapy: a practical guide. Stuttering Therapy Resources, Inc; 2007.

Yaruss JS, Reardon-Reeves NA. Stuttering and the school-age child: practical ideas for treating children in schools. Stuttering Therapy Resources; 2013.

Yaruss JS, Coleman C, Hammer D. Treating preschool children who stutter: description and preliminary evaluation of a family-focused treatment approach. Lang Speech Hear Serv Sch. 2006;37(2):118–36.

Zhao Y, Wu X, Cheng Y. Examining factors and mechanisms of reading comprehension and reading fluency: longitudinal evidence for Chinese children from grade 1 to grade 6. Learn Individ Differ. 2021;85:102467. https://doi.org/10.1016/j.lindif.2024.102467.

Zocchi L, Estenne M, Johnston S, Del Ferro L, Ward ME, Macklem PT. Respiratory muscle incoordination in stuttering speech. Am Rev Respir Dis. 1990;141(6):1510–5. https://doi.org/10.1164/ajrccm/141.6.1510.

Role of AI in the Management of Stuttering

7

Abstract

This chapter explores the integration of artificial intelligence (AI) in stuttering management, offering a fresh perspective on how technology enhances therapy and daily communication. It introduces AI's role in modern life and its potential to revolutionize speech therapy through tools such as speech recognition systems, real-time feedback applications, and virtual speech therapists. Emphasizing the latest research, the chapter illustrates how AI enables personalized therapy, adaptive learning, and effective progress tracking.

Practical implementation strategies are discussed for both school and home settings, focusing on how parents and teachers can collaborate with professionals to promote the generalization of therapy skills beyond clinical environments. Management techniques include interactive games, virtual reality experiences, and individualized learning plans that encourage fluent communication in real-world situations.

Keywords

Artificial intelligence · Apps for stuttering · Real-time speech therapy · Online learning
Ethical considerations

Artificial intelligence (AI) is a form of computer science that is rapidly finding its way into our day-to-day lives and making things easier and more effective. Today, artificial intelligence is imperceptibly acting as a part of our lives, usually without drawing attention to itself. AI is enhancing the rate of innovation in various fields such as healthcare and entertainment. It is improving performance, informing outcomes, and designing improved interactions for businesses and consumers. Several industries and sectors have adopted the use of AI and have therefore opened new endless possibilities.

R. Kaur, *Navigating Childhood Stuttering*,
https://doi.org/10.1007/978-981-96-6206-7_7

To parents and teachers, the knowledge of AI may provide new opportunities to help children, especially those who have speech issues, such as stuttering. Coping and treating stammering can be quite daunting, but with the current developments in the field of AI, there is new hope. This chapter seeks to explain how parents and teachers can use AI to assist people with stammering in speaking and improve their lives.

7.1 What Is AI?

AI is a subfield of computer science that aims at developing intelligent systems that are capable of solving problems that would otherwise require human intervention. These tasks are learning from experience, language comprehension, pattern recognition, and decision-making. Unlike the conventional programs that run with predefined procedures, AI systems can learn and iteratively enhance their own performance.

Let us understand the basics of what AI actually means; it is essentially technology that enables computers to learn and reason on their own, just like humans do. While traditional computer applications are designed with a clear set of rules to follow, AI can learn and change, analyze information, identify patterns in it, and even grow wiser with time.

AI is the simulation of human intelligence processes by machine or the ability of a machine to perform tasks that would have otherwise been done by a human. It is worth pointing out that the aim of AI is to design machines that can emulate the human thought process.

7.2 Everyday Examples of AI

AI is ubiquitous today, though it can be quite invisible at times. Here are some common examples:

1. *Smartphones*
   - *Voice Assistants*: Apple's Siri, Google Assistant for Android, and Amazon's Alexa are some of the examples of Voice assistants that are AI-enabled. Some of the things that they can do include setting reminders, sending messages, answering questions, and even controlling the smart home devices through voice commands.
   - *Predictive Text and Autocorrect*: It can predict our choice of words based on an analysis of our preferences. For example, it learned from my typing habits that when I type "thn," it means "then" and autocorrects it for me when I am typing.
2. *Streaming Services*
   - *Recommendation Systems*: Companies such as Netflix, Spotify, or YouTube use AI algorithms to offer recommendations for movies, TV shows, music, or videos that the user could be interested in, based on their previous watch or listen choices. This assists in finding content specific to the user's preference.

3. *Online Shopping*
   - *Personalized Shopping Experience*: Companies like Amazon and other online retailers employ the use of AI to suggest products that you may be interested in, depending on your browsing history, the products that you have purchased, and products that other customers have bought.
4. *Social Media*
   - *Content Filtering*: Popular social media platforms such as Facebook, Instagram, and Twitter employ the use of AI to display posts that a user is most likely to be interested in. It investigates users' activity, the likes, comments, and shares, to determine which content to display on the feed for maximum engagement.
   - *Photo Tagging*: When photos are uploaded, AI can identify faces and can suggest tags for friends.
5. *Navigation and Travel*
   - *GPS and Maps*: Google Maps and Waze are some of the apps that utilize the application of AI in traffic management, offering traffic updates, the best routes to use, and time of arrival.
   - *Ride-Sharing Apps*: Apps like Uber and Lyft use artificial intelligence to help you find your driver, charge you a fare, and regulate prices based on demand.
6. *Home Automation*
   - *Smart Home Devices*: Nest thermostats, for example, can learn the user's temperature preferences and set the temperature on their own. Some lights can automatically switch on and off as you use the room or are present in the room.
7. *Customer Service*
   - *Chatbots*: Most of the websites employ chatbots that are driven by artificial intelligence to attend to consumers' complaints and queries. These bots can answer several questions, ranging from the order tracking to problem-solving.

7.3 The Role of AI in Stuttering Management: Latest Research and Developments

There is no doubt that AI has become a large part of most areas of the world, including the field of speech therapy. The use of applications and tools can help children who stutter get individualized, convenient, and efficient assistance. Such tools employ the following features to understand the learner's speech, provide feedback, and monitor the learner's performance. Recent research and developments have introduced innovative tools and techniques that can aid in the management of stuttering:

1. *AI-Powered Speech Recognition and Analysis*

The current state of AI technology has given birth to improved speech recognition systems that can recognize and differentiate stuttering. Having compared the results of the auditory analysis of audio recordings with the results of the visual analysis, these systems can identify repetitions, prolongations, and blocks that are important for speech therapists. This approach to the assessment makes it easier to address the needs of each child during therapy sessions, hence making the therapy more effective.

The application of AI in speech recognition and analysis has brought a lot of change in the field of speech therapy, especially in the management of stuttering. These systems incorporate complex algorithms and machine learning to analyze and discern speech patterns. Below is the detailed analysis of the technologies mentioned, recent findings, and their application for the management of stuttering.

7.4 Latest Research and Developments

Studies on AI-based speech recognition and analysis have been on the rise, and many of them have pointed to its usefulness in the management of stuttering. Here are some key developments:

- Researchers from the University of Toronto have created a deep learning model for real-time classification of stuttering events. The model had a high level of classification with regard to various forms of stuttering, making it useful in therapy sessions (King et al. 2023).
- Research has it that using AI in speech recognition to provide therapy support is beneficial. For instance, the Fluency Coach app employs artificial intelligence to listen to speech and give feedback to the speaker to aid fluent speech, with the option to track the progress (Patel et al. 2022).
- Some of the most recent work has been directed toward the combination of visual and auditory feedback in speech analysis. Multimodal systems offer a better way of understanding speech patterns as they incorporate both the audio part of the speech and the visual information, including lip movements and facial expressions (Huang et al. 2021).
- Speech Analytics Platforms: Services such as Google Speech-to-Text and IBM's Watson Speech to Text have been improved to help speech therapists identify stutters.

2. *Real-Time Feedback Systems*

Real-time feedback systems for stuttering management are meant to give the individual simultaneous feedback as he or she is talking. It employs the recently developed AI technologies to recognize speech in real-time and identify stuttering occurrences, and provide feedback to the speaker. These tools are useful in that they give users a real-time indication of their speech and thus assist in modifying their behavior during the speech therapy session.

Another strength of using AI in speech therapy is the possibility of giving feedback immediately. Such an application can listen to a child as he or she speaks and give feedback on the child's speech as soon as the child speaks. This immediate feedback enables children to be conscious of how they speak, which is a vital part of the process as it helps them monitor themselves. Feedback is something that can be given to an individual as they speak, in order to assist them in being more conscious of their speech and thus modify the way that they are speaking.

7.5 Latest Research and Developments

Real-time feedback in the management of stuttering has been under research for some time now. Here are some of the latest studies and developments:

- Study: In the work of Patel et al. (2022), they assessed the utility of smartphone applications for providing immediate feedback on the fluency of speech in people who stutter. The research revealed that those users who engaged with such applications had a marked enhancement in their speech articulation in 3 months.
- A recent work by Zhao et al. (2022) was conducted on wearable devices that included microphones and vibration motors, which give haptic feedback. The research also showed that, when haptic and auditory cues were used together, they greatly assisted the users in controlling their stuttering.
- A study done in the year 2023 by King et al. (2023) tried to understand the feasibility of using deep learning models to identify and label real-time occurrence of stuttering. It was effective and had a high accuracy rate and was incorporated into a feedback mechanism that gave immediate adjustments.
- Huang et al. (2021) investigated the application of auditory and visual feedback to improve the interaction experience of the user. These systems also employ facial identification and movement detection, as well as voice recognition.
- Fluency Coach: This application was developed at the University of Toronto, and it is based on the technology of AI, which helps to analyze speech and provide the user with real-time feedback that will help the user to practice fluent speech in various situations.
- SpeechMon: An application that utilizes AI to give users real-time feedback on their speech, allowing the users to track and modify their speech delivery.

3. *Virtual Speech Therapists*

Virtual speech therapists are designed to mimic a human speech therapist, and they are AI-based interfaces. The services offered include one-on-one speech therapy sessions through digital devices, including smartphones, tablets, and computers. It employs natural language processing (NLP), machine learning, and speech recognition to provide the user with specific stretches, feedback, and monitoring of their progress for people who have speech issues such as stuttering. Using AI, virtual therapists can mimic normal conversations that may be of interest to children, which helps the children with speech developmental problems practice in a controlled environment. Such virtual therapists can change the level of complexity of the tasks depending on the child's progress and give specific feedback. This flexibility enhances the aspect of making therapy less boring and thus less frightening to children.

Virtual speech therapists are a relatively new area of research, and there are many current studies and innovations that can help improve their quality. Here are some of the latest developments:

- A 2023 study by Zhang et al. (2024) examined the ways to enhance the performance of the state-of-the-art deep learning models and NLP methods in enhancing the quality of speech recognition and the assessment of virtual speech therapists.
- Current research by Smith et al. (2022) involved the creation of adaptive learning systems that modify the therapy set of exercises depending on the user's advancement and accomplishment.
- A work by Martinez et al. (2022) focused on the application of AI for recognizing emotions and stress in patients during speech therapy.
- Among the most recent works, the study of Brown and Smith (2023) focused on the employment of VR environments for the development of effective speech therapy scenarios.
- Virtual therapists employ AI to create conversational situations, thus giving the patient a safe environment to practice speech. Sophie: A virtual therapist created by the Massachusetts Institute of Technology is capable of understanding and responding to the users and offers speech exercises and feedback.

4. *Progress Tracking and Data Analytics*

Modern speech therapy for stuttering cannot do without progress tracking and data analytics in the process. These technologies use sophisticated algorithms and data analysis to track and analyze a user's speech patterns and progress over time, and thus, assist in guiding and assessing the progress of therapy sessions. AI tools can capture and interpret a child's speech over time and come up with an analysis of the progress. This information can be passed to the parents, teachers, and speech therapists, so they can also assist in the management. These tools are of benefit in the identification of trends and patterns so that therapy plans can be altered accordingly, and goals can be set that are more achievable. AI tools can gather and interpret speech data of a child over time, giving a detailed account of their development and assisting in the formulation of therapy plans.

The tracking and data analytics for research in progress for stuttering management have produced several new methods and technologies. Here are some of the latest studies and developments:

- Johnson et al. (2022) focused on real-time data analytics platforms that help to monitor the course of the process and provide feedback in the course of the therapy. All these platforms leverage cloud to compute and analyze speech in real time.
- A study done by Patel et al. (2022) sought to explore the effectiveness of gamification in tracking systems for work progress. The study used elements of game design, including achievements, levels, and rewards within the tracking process.
- In a 2022 study, Lee and Lee (2022) focused on the possibility of using wearable devices in combination with tracking systems. Wrist-worn devices with microphones and accelerometers always record speech and motion.
- Liu et al. (2022) did a study on the application of predictive analytics for anticipating the results of therapies with the help of past records. The study applied machine learning algorithms for making a prognosis and finding out determiners of favorable therapy outcomes.
- Voice Analyzer: Stanford University developed this tool, and it incorporates AI to determine speech patterns of the child, and it comes with analytics of fluency, hence providing the parent or teacher with a clear view of the child's progress.

7.6 AI-Powered Speech Therapy Applications

Among the state-of-the-art techniques in the treatment of stammering, AI-based speech therapy applications are among the most promising. Some of these apps offer individualized exercises and immediate feedback to make speech practice convenient and efficient.

New age speech therapy applications that use artificial intelligence are changing the way stuttering and other speech disorders are diagnosed, managed, and treated. These applications use AI to offer customized, engaging and effective therapies that can be received at any location. These applications leverage AI technologies to provide personalized, interactive, and efficient therapy solutions that can be accessed from anywhere. AI-powered speech therapy applications are revolutionizing the way speech disorders, such as stuttering, are managed and treated. Here's an in-depth look at these applications:

7.6.1 How AI-Powered Speech Therapy Applications Work

- *User Interaction*: It is important to note that the application's interface is availed to the users through a handy and familiar device like a mobile phone, tablet, or a computer. The interaction is generally through voice or text entry.
- *Speech Recognition*: The interface of the application is based on the recognition of the user's speech with the help of AI-based speech recognition technology that provides accurate transcription of the user's speech. This technology can capture the types of stuttering including repetition, prolongation, and blocking.

- *Personalized Therapy Plans*: In light of the initial evaluation and constant monitoring, the application establishes individualized treatment regimens that are in tune with the user's spoken output and development.
- *Real-Time Feedback*: In the process of therapy exercises, the application gives feedback to the user immediately. This feedback can be visual, auditory, or textual kind of feedback. It helps users to correct their mistakes on the go.
- *Progress Tracking*: The application tracks the development of the user, recording the data of speech activities and achievements. Strict report and presentation are made to follow the progress at different intervals.
- *Adaptive Learning*: The application employs the use of machine learning algorithms in the provision of therapy exercises by adjusting the exercises according to the progress and the performance of the user, thus making the exercises challenging yet manageable.

7.7 Notable Applications

AI-Powered Speech Recognition and Analysis

1. *Stamurai*

   Stamurai is an automated speech therapy application that features exercises that are designed for the user and then monitors the user's improvement. It has a feature to assist in fluency and speech drills.
   - Stamurai Official Website: https://stammer.ai/
   - Stamurai for iOS
   - Stamurai for Android
2. *Speech Blubs*

   Speech Blubs is a speech therapy application that is not limited to stuttering but is an application that contains AI speech therapy with the voice-activated interface and videos for children. It consists of activities that may help children who stutter.
   - The official website of Speech Blubs: https://speechblubs.com/
   - Speech Blubs for iPhone
   - Speech Blubs for Android
3. *Stutter Stars: Stuttering Help*

   Stutter Stars: Stuttering Help is a generalized app developed for use by those who stutter. This app presents a number of tools and materials, which are designed to help users to enhance fluency and confidence and to provide support for people with stuttering.

   Benefits:
   - Interactive Exercises: It has activities that are aimed at enhancing the fluency of the speech of the user and it provides the user with a platform to practice speaking in a safe environment.

- Progress Tracking: The app has a mechanism that records the progress of a user and thus helps the user to have the motivation and knowledge of the changes they are making.
- Supportive Community: The app provides the user with a platform where they can meet other people with the same condition and share their experiences, tips, and moral support.
- Tailored Content: The content and the exercises are specific to each client so that the assistance offered will be useful to him or her.

4. *BeneTalk*

BeneTalk is a wearable device and a mobile application that is designed for people who stutter to enhance their speech with the help of real-time feedback and tasks. BeneTalk is intended for embedding in daily use to help in stuttering treatment without attracting much attention to it.

Benefits:

- Real-Time Feedback: BeneTalk gives an instant reaction to the speaking habits, which will assist the users to modify their speech and be conscious of how they are speaking.
- Personalized Training: The app provides exercises to the user according to his/her speech and that enhances the fluency of speech.
- Portable and Discreet: Since it is a wearable device, BeneTalk can be used by patients to practice and enhance their speech at any time and in any place without attracting undue attention from other people around them.
- Long-Term Tracking: BeneTalk has a record of user's progress to encourage them and make them aware of their changes.

5. *Speechtools: DAF PRO*

This is a highly effective app that applies the technique of delayed auditory feedback (DAF) to support people who struggle to speak without stutters. DAF is a widely used technique in which the patient hears their voice with a delay, which slows down the speech and prevents the outburst of speech.

Benefits:

- Proven Technique: DAF has been seen to be very helpful in the management of stuttering as it helps in slowing down the rate of speech, hence making it easier for one to speak fluently.
- Customizable Settings: DAF PRO gives the users the ability to control the delay and feedback depending on what they want, hence giving them the freedom they need.
- Portable Solution: DAF PRO can be downloaded as an application that can be installed on a mobile device to allow for portable practice and improvement of speech.

- Versatile Use: This app can be applied in different conditions. It is possible to apply it during the therapy sessions or in the course of the day, which means that it is a rather convenient tool for the management of stuttering.

6. *Speechify*

   Speechify is an AI-powered tool that is used to help people work on their speech and presentations, especially for those who have a stutter.

   Key Features:

   - *Speech Analysis*: Looks at different aspects of speech, such as the flow, the speed, and even the way the words are delivered.
   - *Real-Time Feedback*: Gives real-time feedback on the speech performance, thus allowing the user to correct errors made in real time.
   - *Personalized Coaching*: Provide individual and goal-oriented suggestions and techniques according to the patient's speech.
   - *Practice Scenarios*: Offers a range of practice topics, including speaking in front of an audience, interactions in personal life, and professional settings.

   Benefits:

   - Helps in improving speech and its fluency through a set format.
   - Offers an opportunity to rehearse actual life speaking scenarios.
   - Gives users a detailed analysis of certain aspects of their speech to enhance.

7. *Orai*

   Orai is an application for the improvement of public speaking and communication that is based on practice and feedback. It is designed for the single user as well as the corporate training environment.

   Key Features:

   - *Speech Recognition*: Leverages on the latest speech recognition technology to transcribe speech in real-time.
   - *Feedback and Tips*: This gives real-time feedback on aspects of speech, which include the use of filler words, pace, and energy levels.
   - *Practice Modules*: Each of the following areas of practice is covered: impromptu speaking, storytelling, and presentation skills.
   - *Progress Reports*: Creates detailed progress reports in order to show how the conditions have been changing over time.

   Benefits:

   - Aids in the elimination or reduction of habitual words and enhances the intelligibility of spoken language.
   - Improves, in general, communication skills since it is constant practice.
   - Offers information that can be used by the users in order to become more confident speakers.

8. *Elsa Speak*

   Elsa Speak is an application that has been developed to assist the users in improving their English pronunciation. The students of the English language often employ it to improve fluency and comprehensible speech.

   Key Features:

   - Pronunciation Analysis: Relates to the user's speech and is able to determine where the user is going wrong in his/her pronunciation.
   - Real-Time Feedback: Gives immediate result of correct pronunciation and also gives suggestions on how to correct it.
   - Personalized Lessons: It provides lessons tailored for the user's native language and their particular difficulties with pronunciation.
   - Speech Games: Comes with speech activities, such as games, to ensure that learning is enjoyable.

   Benefits:

   - Aids in enhancing the user's pronunciation of the English language.
   - Offers a special form of learning that addresses the learner's requirements.
   - Holds the users' attention with light and entertaining activities to practice the contents learned.

9. *Real-Time Feedback Tools*

   Feedback tools that are real time employ the use of AI to assess speech as it is being made and provide recommendations for the same. These tools can be embedded into wearables or mobile applications for easy access at all times.

   - Smart Earbuds: Smart devices that give the speaker a hint in the form of a sound to slow down and regulate their speech.

7.8 Stuttering Management Using AI in Educational Settings

The use of technology in the form of artificial intelligence in the development of educational software is revolutionizing the academic experience of the students and the teaching and learning process.

Therefore, in the context of stuttering, AI-based educational materials can be highly helpful for both learners and tutors. Special educational programs developed with the use of artificial intelligence can help teachers create individual lessons and activities for students who have stammering.

Applications of speech recognition and analysis powered by AI can be very useful, especially for teachers in a class with students who stutter. These tools could be used to facilitate learning goals per learner, give instant feedback, and use fun quizzes and activities. Here's how these applications can be integrated into educational settings:

1. *Classroom Support*
   - Integration: It is possible to use the AI-based speech therapy tools as an additional educational resource in the classroom and help the students who stutter.
   - Benefits: These tools can assist the student to rehearse speech in a protected way and support the techniques that he or she had learnt in traditional speech therapy.
2. *Individualized Learning Plans*
   - Personalization: The use of AI application can help in designing unique learning programs that are suited for individual students and their performance.
   - Benefits: It is advantageous in a way that every student gets the aid they require to enhance their speech fluency.
3. *Monitoring and Analysis*
   - It can help track the development of patients who are taking speech therapy to help the therapist, parents, and teachers.
   - Speech Analytics Platforms: These platforms focus on the analysis of speech patterns and produce a detailed report about fluency; this helps in the identification of the most suitable strategies for use as well as those that are not very effective.
   - Data Visualization: AI can help to show graphs and charts of progress, thus making it easier to comprehend and illustrate the advancement.
4. *Home Practice*
   - Continuity: The use of these applications is possible at home to maintain the consistency of practice between therapy sessions.
   - Benefits: In addition, constant and repetitive exercises and drills may cause student to achieve better performance on their speech and increase their self-confidence.
5. *Teacher Training*
   - Professional Development: The following applications can be adopted by teachers for their own professional improvement, so as to have a better understanding of children who stutter.
   - Benefits: Stuttering is a condition that can be explained and understood, and by raising awareness on the condition, the learning institutions can embrace people who stutter.
6. *Interactive and Engaging Tools*

   There are a number of learning tools and activities that can be used in order to enhance speech practice, and these can be made more engaging with the use of game elements and artificial intelligence, particularly for children.

   Examples
   - *Speech Therapy Games*: It is the games that are created in order to make speech fluency exercising more fun and engaging.
   - *Virtual Reality (VR) Environments*: Virtual situations that enable individuals to rehearse their speech in one way or another to ensure that the anxiety level is low while the confidence is high.

7.9 Stuttering Management Using AI in Home Settings

The use of AI extends to offering some of the helpful resources and tools that parents can employ when at home to assist in the speech development of their child.

7.9.1 Tools

- *Guided Exercises*: Special therapeutic procedures used for practice in order to focus on the aspect of speech fluency.
- *Parental Support Apps*: Apps that provide tips, tactics, and support actively and passively from other parents and professionals.
- *Enhancing Communication Devices*: For people using an Augmentative and Alternative Communication (AAC) device, AI can enhance the predictive level and speech output, thus enhancing the ability of communication.

7.9.2 AI Implementation at Home

To effectively integrate AI tools into the management of stuttering, parents and teachers can follow these practical guidelines:

- *Daily Practice*: Parents must engage children in speech therapy programs with daily encouragement to use apps based on artificial intelligence. It is also to the benefit of the patient to engage in the consistent practice of these techniques to enforce them with what is learned during the therapy sessions.
- *Interactive Games*: Some of the AI features used in the practice comprise of gamification to make speech practice fun. Parents may employ the above games with a view of using them to motivate children to work harder. It is important to have access to the child's progress data and share this information with the speech therapist so as to make sure the therapy goals are still on target.
- *Inclusive Environment*: Some of the AI solutions, such as Fluency Coach and SpeechEasy, can be employed by parents to support their child with fluency. When used in activities, such as when reading or when rehearsing presentations, a parent fosters confidence in their children's speaking. The part of the parent, therefore, is to simply help the child to use these tools and make them comfortable enough to practice daily.
- *Collaborative Efforts*: Mothers and fathers also have a significant role of easing transitions from therapy to home setting with AI tools such as BeneTalk and Stamurai. Some of these tools enable the tracking of the development of the child in real time and can be shared with the speech therapist involved. Parents are to always ensure that they are supervising the usage of these tools by their children and remain in touch with the therapists rendering the therapy to make sure that it is being given frequently and to a good standard.

- *Peer Support*: AI use which include BeneTalk and Fluency Friends can be used to enhance group interaction and peer support in order to support children who stutter when they are placed in a group. Thus, parents can help a child to turn to these tools during social interactions, which will provide them with the necessary extent of confidence and, at the same time, minimize the communicative barriers. The entire primary responsibility of the parent here is to affirm and endorse the positive experiences of the child in such social processes and nudge them to continue using such tools.

7.10 Addressing Challenges and Ethical Considerations

- *Privacy and Security*: Parents have no recourse to guarantee that the prosthesis, whether it be Stamurai or SpeechEasy, is fail-safe, aesthetically friendly, and safe in terms of privacy laws. There is a concern that parents should read and comprehend the provisions on data protection to protect their child's information.
- *Accessibility and Equity*: It is for this reason that some families may not be in a position to secure the latest available AI instruments. Parents should look for an item that is cheap or available and, if necessary, campaign for that item. Such tools as Speak Up can be one of the possible choices for parents wanting to find cheap tools. Parents can also engage other organizations to make sure that a child has the required technology for his or her needs.
- *Human Touch*: Despite this, they are special tools that can be an important channel of communication but cannot replace person-to-person contact in the process of therapy. It must be the parents' responsibility to make sure that such tools enhance rather than take over parental care and support. For parents, it might be vital to aim for employing AI as an assistive tool while still being as close to the child as possible and building relationships without AI.

In the best way and with an active participation in their child's stuttering treatment, parents can do much in favorable way for their child's fluency and confidence.

7.11 Conclusion

AI in management of stuttering offers a frontier that parents and teachers need to embrace for effectively helping the child. This way, with the help of AI tools, it will be possible to offer individual, efficient, and meaningful support for those who stutter, so that they can express themselves better and with less difficulties. To conclude, it is important to always stay informed of the technologies created and do our best to integrate and learn about the development of artificial intelligence for the best of everyone.

In the right perspective, AI can be the friend that helps people to speak fluently and confidently as they should.

The incorporation of AI in the administration and therapy of stammering has plenty of promise. With the help of AI tools, parents and teachers will be able to address the problem of stammering better and with much more effectiveness than that is now possible, that will help individuals with stammering to acquire better communication skills and gain the necessary confidence. Because technology is under constant development, one can be hopeful that more and more sophisticated and effective interventions for the treatment of stammering will be developed giving a fighting chance to the stuttering individuals.

References

Brown K, Smith J. The role of quantitative finance in financial market analysis and decision-making. Financ Anal J. 2023;78(1):44–60. https://www.scirp.org

Huang YT, Blomquist C, Newman RS, Edwards J. Children with cochlear implants use semantic prediction to facilitate spoken word recognition. J Speech Lang Hear Res. 2021;64(5):1636–49. https://hesp.umd.edu

Johnson M, Lee W, Chen S. Navigating the online landscape: strategies for language learning in the post-pandemic era. Lang Educ Res. 2022;17(3):201–23. https://files.eric.ed.gov

King C, Wambaugh J, Maas E. A comparison of sound production treatment and metrical pacing therapy for apraxia of speech: a single-case experimental design. Am J Speech Lang Pathol. 2023;32(5S):2493–511. https://asha.figshare.com

Lee W, Lee J. Embracing technology: exploring language learning adaptations in the post-pandemic era. J Appl Linguist. 2022;45(2):123–45. https://files.eric.ed.gov

Liu J, Yu F, Feng C, Li S. The pausing strategies in Chinese preschool children's narratives. J Speech Lang Hear Res. 2022;66(2):431–43. https://doi.org/10.1044/2022_JSLHR-21-00542.

Martinez R, Smith J, Johnson L. Exploring mental health and well-being among university faculty members. J Ment Health Well Being High Educ. 2022;14(3):215–30. https://campusmentalhealth.ca

Patel P, Bhil D, Vaja M, Pathak S, Dogra P, Ranawat N, Mangla K. The clinical spectrum of paediatric mesial temporal sclerosis: a case series. NeuroQuantology. 2022;20(6):4363–6. https://www.researchgate.net

Smith DM, Gillett NP, Simpson IR, Athanasiadis PJ, Baehr J, Bethke I, Bilge TA, Bonnet R, Boucher O, Findell KL, Gastineau G, Gualdi S, Hermanson L, Leung LR, Mignot J, Müller WA, Osprey S, Otterå OH, Persad GG, Scaife AA, Schmidt GA, Shiogama H, Sutton RT, Swingedouw D, Yang S, Zhou T, Zhang L. Attribution of multi-annual to decadal changes in the climate system: the Large Ensemble Single Forcing Model Intercomparison Project (LESFMIP). Am J Hum Genet. 2022;109(5):1–14. https://pubs.giss.nasa.gov

Zhang M, Tang E, Ding H, Zhang Y. Artificial intelligence and the future of communication sciences and disorders: A bibliometric and visualization analysis [Preprint]. Preprints.org. 2024. https://doi.org/10.20944/preprints202401.2235.v1.

Zhao Y, Guo Y, Zhang Y, Liu X. Association between the COVID-19 pandemic and the risk for adverse development in children aged 0–6: a systematic review and meta-analysis. BMC Public Health. 2022;22(1):1451. https://bmcpublichealth.biomedcentral.com

Relapse of Stuttering 8

Abstract

This chapter examines the phenomenon of relapse in stuttering, focusing on its causes, management, and prevention within a concise framework. Relapse depends on contributing factors like psychological triggers (stress, low self-esteem), environmental influences (social pressures, lack of support), and physiological aspects (neurological changes, developmental shifts). Adolescence is identified as a high-risk period for relapse. The chapter discusses Starkweather's holistic approach to relapse, emphasizing the importance of addressing emotional factors alongside speech techniques. The chapter offers practical relapse prevention strategies, including continued therapy, family involvement, mindfulness, and healthy lifestyle habits. Parents and teachers are guided on reinforcing speech strategies, fostering supportive environments, and collaborating with speech therapists.

Cultural considerations, including myths about stuttering in India, are discussed to reduce stigma and promote understanding. By providing actionable solutions and encouraging collaboration among caregivers, educators, and individuals who stutter, this chapter aims to maintain fluency gains and support long-term communication confidence.

Keywords

Relapse in stuttering · Stuttering prevention · Psychological triggers · Cultural considerations · Fluency maintenance

R. Kaur, *Navigating Childhood Stuttering*,
https://doi.org/10.1007/978-981-96-6206-7_8

8.1 Understanding Relapse

Relapse in stuttering refers to the ability of a child, an adolescent or an adult who has made improvement or has developed fluency to start stuttering again. Guitar (2006) defined relapse in stuttering as the regression of severe stuttering after the completion of a structured speech therapy. Following the works of Yaruss and Quesal (2006), relapse in stuttering is the recurrence of stuttering behaviors that were initially reduced or eliminated in the frequency and intensity following a speech therapy program. Among patients, relapse is very often attributed to stress, fatigue, or other situational pressures (Bloodstein and Bernstein Ratner 2008).

8.2 Why Relapse Occurs in Stuttering

Stuttering exacerbation may stem from several factors to do with psychological factors, environmental factors, and physiological factors. Relapse is frequent due to noncompliance with the treatment or when the pressure of the environment increases (Smith and Weber 2017). Learning these factors will enable the design of measures that may assist in preventing or dealing with the likelihood of relapse.

A. *Psychological Factors*
   1. *Stress and Anxiety*: Stress and anxiety are two of the most significant psychological factors that lead to the relapse of the patient. Stress or anxiety can be a major factor that causes one to start stuttering. For instance, a child who has attained fluency may experience a setback when put under pressure, for instance, when presenting before an audience, writing an examination, or going through a major life event (Bloodstein and Bernstein Ratner 2008).
   2. *Self-Perception and Confidence*: Stigma, negative attitude toward stuttering, and reduced self-confidence of the individuals can also have an important impact. It has been established that low self-esteem and negative perception of oneself will make the person fear stuttering, and this compounds the risk of relapse. It is fairly uncommon for the person to develop what is known as anticipatory anxiety, a fear of stuttering that can lead to the person stuttering more often since they expect it (Yaruss and Quesal 2006).
   3. *Cognitive Load*: The process of keeping up with the flow may demand a lot of cognitive resources, and when an individual is cognitively exhausted or stressed, they may struggle to effectively apply the strategies that were learnt in therapy. This leads to cognitive overload, which may cause a temporary or chronic return to stuttering (Smith and Weber 2017).

B. *Environmental Factors*
   1. *Lack of Support*: The amount of support from the family and friends, teachers, and other people around the child can predispose them to relapse or not. Unsupportive

or even hostile feedback, such as a lack of encouragement, can break an individual's confidence and fluency (Guitar 2006).

2. *Changes in Environment*: Relocation, change of school, or job is not easy and can lead to a relapse of the individual's substance abuse problem. These alterations can challenge the existing patterns and mechanisms of everyday life and thus hinder fluency (Van Riper 1982).
3. *Social Pressures*: It is also important to note that social pressure and interaction can also lead to relapse. The desire not to stutter can lead to even more tension and stress during conversation, and this can worsen the stuttering (Yaruss and Quesal 2006).

C. *Physiological Factors*

1. *Neurological Factors*: Stuttering is considered a neurological disorder, and the changes in neurology may lead to the recurrence of the problem. For example, tiredness, sickness, or alteration in the dosage of drugs may impact the brain's ability to control speech (Smith and Weber 2017). In the study conducted by Smith et al. (2014), the authors sought to explore the neurological substrates of stuttering relapse. They found that alterations in neurological activity, for instance, due to tiredness or sickness, may lead to relapse. The study highlighted the significance of the physical well-being of a person, as well as neurological aspects, in treating stuttering.
2. *Developmental Changes*: To children and adolescents, the period of growth and development can be a hindrance to fluent speech. These are organic factors, such as hormonal changes that occur during puberty that may impact on neuro motor mechanisms that are used in speech production and lead to a temporary deterioration of the speech disorder (Bloodstein and Bernstein Ratner 2008).
3. *Lapses in Treatment*: If speech therapy is stopped completely or made less frequent, there is a high chance of relapse. As with many other skills, it is often a continuous process, and to preserve the fluency, there is a need for more practice; otherwise, the stuttering behaviors may reemerge (Guitar 2006). Craig and Tran (2005) used a longitudinal design in which they followed up people who had received intensive speech and language therapy. They established that a large number of patients experienced recurrence of the disorder within 1 year after ending the treatment. The findings of the study also showed that there is a need to have follow-up sessions in order to ensure that the learners retain the fluency gained. Ingham et al. (2001) in their study examined the efficacy of CBT in relapse prevention. Their research showed that the patients who underwent CBT together with speech and language therapy had a lower rate of relapse than those who only received speech and language therapy. This, therefore, points to the fact that addressing the psychological factors of stuttering may well lead to better long-term gains in fluency.

8.3 Starkweather's Perspective on Relapse

Dr C Woodruff Starkweather offers a new look at relapse in stuttering. He described it commonly as the return of stuttering after some time of change following treatment. In the past, it has been viewed as a deterioration or a slide that occurs during the course of treatment. Dr Starkweather also presents a different view on this subject, which is rather more complex than the one described above.

Dr Starkweather, who has a great deal of experience in stuttering therapy and has worked with various types of therapeutic methods, often observed what is known as relapse, that is, the return of stuttering after a certain period of stuttering-free speech. But he pointed out that this was not simply a reversal, but rather a manifestation of more complex problems.

8.3.1 Starkweather's Holistic Approach to Stuttering Therapy

According to Starkweather, the treatment should not be limited to the change of speech patterns. From his clinical practice in non-avoidance therapy, fluency shaping, and integrating the approach, he supports a multifaceted treatment that targets the emotional and psychological aspects of the disorder.

8.3.2 The Limitations of Traditional Therapies

Starkweather and other researchers have pointed out that traditional fluency shaping and non-avoidance therapies often result in what is viewed as relapse. These therapies, while helpful for changing the patterns of speech, do not always help to cure the causes of stuttering, which are the concealed psychological problems and conflicts, known as "unfinished business."

8.3.3 Unfinished Business: The Emotional Dimensions of Stuttering

Unfinished business is a key idea in Starkweather's thinking. He further submits that stuttering for many people is bound with the emotional and traumatic experiences of their speech. For example, a child who was made fun of for stuttering in the classroom will experience adverse psychological effects even in their adulthood. Such therapies very well may help a child or adult stutter less and feel more confident, but they don't heal the roots of the problem—the emotional pain. Therefore, when a person finds himself or herself in a situation that elicits these feelings, the stuttering may be brought back, giving the appearance of a relapse.

8.3.4 Integrating Experiential Techniques in Therapy

Starkweather believes that the therapies that include experiential methods for the mentioned emotional aspects can result in a more meaningful and sustainable positive changes in the clients who stutter. This approach not only includes altering one's speech but also altering one's connection with stuttering and oneself. It is about treating the psychological syndrome of stuttering and promoting recovery and positive outlooks. In the real world, this could include methods that help people face and regulate feelings related to stuttering and reform their experience of the condition. Therapy strategies may include awareness of self, being conscious, and management of feelings that are associated with stuttering.

Starkweather's approach is valuable since he acknowledges that stuttering is not merely a speech ailment but a multifaceted phenomenon that involves behavior, feelings, and thoughts. It is for this reason that effective therapy must go beyond the various dimensions and aspects described above in its aim to help people to enhance their ability to communicate and understand themselves.

For instance, a case might be of a young adult who was a victim of bullying in the course of their education because of their stuttering. Traditional fluency shaping was somewhat effective in reducing stuttering for some time, but stuttering recurred as soon as the speaker faced stress. Drawing from Starkweather's model, the therapy encompassed mindfulness, self-reflection, and narrative therapy to help the patient work through past traumas. In the course of the therapy, this person not only enhanced his/her fluency but also self-efficacy and the coping resources, which helped to prevent the relapse.

8.4 General Tips to Prevent Relapse

It is therefore important to identify the factors that cause the relapse of stuttering so as to come up with ways of managing it. Here are some approaches to help prevent and manage relapse:

1. *Ongoing Speech Therapy*: Having speech therapy sessions on a regular basis will help to strengthen the techniques and strategies achieved to deal with stuttering. Such therapists continue the treatment and modify the therapy regimen if needed to meet new difficulties (Yaruss and Quesal 2006). For instance, if a child has mastered a particular speech strategy but is unable to implement it, the speech therapist can provide new tasks or alter the previous ones in order to make the child regain control. Regular sessions also provide a setup in which progress can be measured and celebrated, and this is very important for the morale of the student.
2. *Support Groups*: One can get a feeling of belonging and people to share with when they join support groups. Group treatment also allows the client to be with others who have the same difficulties of stuttering, thus decreasing the feelings of isolation, and with the sharing of tips on how to prevent relapse (Van Riper 1982). According to Manning

(2010), the subjects who engaged in support groups had a lower relapse rate than those who did not engage in them. For example, a teenager might like to hear how other people deal with stuttering at school or with friends, gain new ways of dealing with it, and not feel so isolated. They can also form friendships and networks that they are able to seek emotional support from, apart from the support groups.

3. *Family Involvement*: Involving the family in the therapy process can thus assist in preparing the home environment for the child. Family members can be taught how to encourage positive behaviors and mitigate the stress and anxiety that comes with stuttering (Manning and DiLollo 2017). For instance, parents can engage in speech therapy, give encouragement to the child, and make sure that the child feels comfortable to speak. Other members of the family, especially the siblings, can help by not mocking the affected person, being tolerant and compassionate, and joining the affected person in activities he or she likes to do. Involvement of family guarantees that the child gets support even after sessions and between sessions, which is crucial for the child's improvement.
4. *Mindfulness and Relaxation*: Some of the strategies that can assist in stress management and hence prevent relapse include mindfulness, deep breathing, and progressive muscle relaxation. These strategies assist people in being relaxed and attentive; hence, they are able to use speech strategies effectively (Smith and Weber 2017). For example, taking slow and long breaths when preparing to make a speech in class can assist the speaker in the reduction of anxiety and help increase the flow of speech. Some of the mindfulness exercises include meditation or yoga. These can be done at any time of the day to ensure that one is emotionally balanced and not stressed.
5. *Cognitive Behavioral Therapy*: CBT can assist people to recognize and change undesirable thought processes and learn how to manage anxiety and stress. It is therefore important that people who stutter change their perception towards their stuttering so as to minimize the effect of stress on their speech (Guitar 2006). Packman and Onslow (1998) underlined the importance of including stress management in the program of stuttering treatment. For instance, a child can be taught to dispute negative thoughts, such as "I always stutter when talking in class," and come up with constructive, realistic thoughts, such as "I will use the strategies I learned to speak fluently." CBT can also help in acquiring problem-solving skills and relaxation skills that may be helpful in different situations.
6. *Healthy Lifestyle Choices*: Some of the ways include exercising regularly, getting enough sleep, and taking balanced meals, as these help in improving health status and minimize the chances of falling back into drug or alcohol use. Physical health is linked to mental and neurological health, which influences speech and language (Bloodstein and Bernstein Ratner 2008). For instance, exercise can help to combat stress and increase one's mood, while enough sleep will ensure that the brain and the body are as active as they can be. The diet should therefore contain all the nutrients required by the body for the optimum health and functioning of the nervous system. Promoting good habits can assist children and young people who stutter to manage their lives in a way that minimizes the physical and emotional factors, which precipitate stuttering.

7. *Consistent Routines*: It is important to set up habits, as this will help one have a schedule and feel less stressed. Such rituals can make people feel less anxious and more confident and, therefore, support fluency (Yaruss and Quesal 2006). For instance, a child may require strict rules on when to do homework, when to play, and when to sleep to avoid the ambiguity that leads to stress. Integrating speech techniques in these routines can help to guarantee that the child is always enhancing their skills. Lack of any significant variation in environment and routines gives the child a sense of order and knowing what to expect next, which is helpful to fluency.

8.5 Preventing Relapse by Educating Parents

Stuttering is a disabling condition that hinders the child in effective communication and unleashes a blow to their self-esteem. Even though a lot of attention is paid to speech therapy and other interventions, the home environment is also very important in the child's development. As the child's first teachers and caretakers, parents have the potential of shaping the speech patterns of their child together with their emotional health. It is essential to make parents understand how they can make their child's environment at home a supportive one so that the child does not relapse into stuttering.

Stuttering can be very different at different times, depending on the situation and who is around. At home, family interaction, the presence of figures of authority, and the environment can affect both the frequency and the severity of stuttering. To lessen these factors, parents should apply certain parenting strategies that will facilitate a good environment.

8.6 Strategies for Preventing Relapse at Home

1. *Create a Relaxed and Supportive Environment*
   - *Encourage Open Communication*: Ensure that your child is free to express himself or herself without the fear of being judged. This includes promoting and accepting discussion of stuttering and letting your child know that it is all right to stutter. This will also help to relieve the fear and make speaking a more pleasant experience.
   - *Model Calm and Patient Behavior*: Bearing these in mind, one can also notice that children usually copy their parents. Icing on the cake is that you can also free your child from anxiety when talking to you by mimicking nonaggressive and patient communication. For example, do not interrupt them or complete their thoughts. Allow them to have their say and provide them with the necessary time to do so.
   - *Reduce Communication Pressure*: Help the child to feel comfortable by not forcing him or her to articulate well. Let them speak at their own speed without imposing the pressure of high expectations of what they should say. Motivate them to continue their practice and not to pay much attention to the smoothness of their speech.

For instance, Sarah observed that Ben, her son, had a speech difficulty, especially when he was in the company of the entire family during dinner time. Hence, she chose to spend some quality time with Ben during the day since she realized that she only got to talk to him when things were a bit calm. She also informed her family about the condition and asked them not to interrupt people with speech disorder. Gradually, Ben relieved his tension in the course of speaking at dinner, and the stuttering became less severe.

2. *Address Emotional and Psychological Factors*
   - *Monitor Stress Levels*: You also need to observe for signs of stress or anxiety in the child. Some of the trigger factors that make stuttering worse include when one is angry, being in a critical discussion, or when they are under pressure. Teach your child other ways to handle stress, for instance, through breathing exercises or other relaxation techniques like meditation.
   - *Encourage Positive Self-Esteem*: Turn your attention to your child's talents and victories. Describe to them the things that interest them and which they can do well; this will improve their morale and overall mood.
   - *Provide Emotional Support*: Provide comfort to your child as young as possible. Acknowledge what they are saying and make them feel that they are being heard. Inform them that they do not have to face this alone and that you are with them in their process.

     For instance, Mark, who was a high school student, discovered that his stuttering became severe during the examination time. His parents helped him to discover how to cope with stress in a child-friendly way, including the use of breathing and relaxation techniques. They also comforted him and made him talk about his feelings and told him that it was fine to stutter. These strategies assisted Mark in controlling stress and, to a certain extent, minimizing stuttering during exams.
3. *Involve the Entire Family*
   - *Educate Family Members*: It is crucial to educate all the family members about the child's stuttering and what actions they should take in relation to the child. Inform them on the need to be patient and not to get angry when a child stutters. This is because family members are likely to have a common understanding of the issues that are likely to cause discomfort in the house.
   - *Promote Positive Interactions*: Spend time with the family, with the purpose of improving the interaction between the family members. It can be through games, telling stories, and family conversations, where your child can be encouraged to speak in a safe environment.
   - *Address Authoritative Dynamics*: If there are parental figures whose presence can enhance the possibility of stuttering, then the focus should be on enhancing the communication structures. Inform these family members to embrace the child and be more tolerant, thus taking pressure off the child.
4. *Consistent Reinforcement of Speech Techniques*
   - *Practice Techniques Learned in Therapy*: Help your child to practice speech techniques that he or she exercises in the process of speech therapy. Try to use these

strategies during the regular interactions with your child and teach the child to do the same. Encouragement and repetition can also be used to make sure that these skills become more ingrained in a person.
  - *Create Opportunities for Practice*: Ensure your child uses speech techniques in different environments to enhance them. This may mean reading to them, telling them stories, or being involved in family conversations. Ensure that the tasks become more challenging as your child gains more confidence doing the tasks.
5. *Collaboration with Speech Therapists*
  - *Maintain Regular Communication*: It is recommended that you maintain constant communication with your child's speech therapist. Share your child's achievements, difficulties, and concerns that you may be having. This way, you are going to be on the right track as to what the therapist wants you to achieve and how you will do it.
  - *Follow Through with Recommendations*: Follow the speech therapist's recommendations on what to do. This may involve particular activities that need to be performed, ways of interacting with the child, or alterations to the environment of the home. Establishing good coordination between home and therapy can do wonders for your child's improvement.

    For instance, Emma's parents used to talk with her speech therapist regarding the techniques that Emma had grasped. They used these techniques in their day-to-day lives, for instance, when reading to their children before they sleep or during family discussions. Over time, Emma's speech therapy continued to emphasize these techniques. Gradually, she became confident in her speech, and the stuttering reduced.
6. *Managing Situational Triggers*
  - *Prepare for Stressful Situations*: Assist your child to build up his/her confidence in dealing with stressful events, for instance, speaking in public, class assignments, or family events. They must also engage in speech drills and be given assurance prior to these occasions, so that they can be confident.
  - *Develop Coping Strategies*: Make sure that your child knows how to manage their anxiety as well as stress in order to avoid being overwhelmed. Such strategies as focusing on breathing, using imagination, and saying certain phrases to oneself can assist the child in controlling emotions and thus prevent stutters.
  - *Encourage Open Discussions*: Make sure that your child has a place where he or she can share how he or she feels about certain events that have happened to him or her. Suggest to them to express how they feel about it or the things that they have undergone as a stutterer. This can assist the individual in the management of emotions and also decrease the effects of stress on the language system.
7. *Promote a Healthy Lifestyle*
  - *Ensure Adequate Rest*: Make sure your child gets enough sleep. Stuttering may be worsened by fatigue, which means that a person should try to sleep at the same time every day.

- *Encourage Physical Activity*: Physical activity is known to have stress-relieving properties and is a good way of enhancing one's health. Ensure your child engages in sports or other activities that they like to do to be active.
- *Provide a Balanced Diet*: A balanced diet promotes good health and might also lead to improved neurological performance, which can be useful in improving one's speech.

To help a child with fluency, parents can employ various techniques that include lowering the communication pressure, tackling emotional issues, ensuring the whole family is involved, enhancing speech techniques, working with speech therapists, managing specific triggers, and encouraging healthy living. It may also contribute to the formation of a healthy environment that would enable children who stutter to grow and learn how to be more assertive in their interactions with others.

8.7 Preventing Relapse by Educating Teachers

Teachers are the key persons in the classroom and can greatly impact the communication experiences of students who stutter. It is thus possible to identify some practices that can be implemented to better help students manage their relapses and continue their learning process toward fluency and confidence.

1. *Reinforce Speech Therapy Techniques*: Consult with the speech therapists in order to make sure that the correct speech practices are regularly used in the classroom. Explain to the students how such methods can be used frequently so that fluency can be sustained and the rates of relapse prevented. Appreciate the student's achievements in implementing these techniques on their own. For instance, if a student is working the "easy onset" technique, where they begin their speech with a softer sound to minimize tension, teachers can simply tell the student to apply the same technique when making contributions during class or when presenting some information. In addition, try to give the students a chance to apply the learned speech techniques in nonthreatening conditions. For instance, in the morning meeting or any class discussion, set time for the student to make contributions using the techniques. Rejoice with them, for instance, when the student uses a particular technique to answer a question in front of the class and encourage them.
2. *Foster an Inclusive Classroom Environment*: Develop a class environment in which students would not be judged by their speech and would not be made fun of for having certain speech disorders. Discourage people from avoiding the subject of stuttering and clear any myths that may give people the fear of stammering. For instance, one may read a book or watch a video on stuttering and then lead the class into a discussion. Get the students to engage in the class and ask questions and express themselves. This can do much to explain stuttering and lessen the fear and prejudice that may surround it.

3. *Introduce Role Models*: Get people who stutter to come in and speak to the class. This can include successful adults who stutter or older students with good management of their stuttering. Listening to the stories of their peers could make the students feel that they are not alone and thus increase their level of acceptance.
4. *Educate Teachers and Peers*: Organize professional development sessions for teachers to learn about stuttering and effective strategies to support students who stutter. For instance, a workshop that can contain practical tasks, such as simulation of a situation in which a teacher has to interact with a student who stutters. Establish policies that are likely to enhance people's ability to appreciate others. For instance, the students who do not stutter should be made to undertake an activity where they get to speak like someone who stutters. This can be done by getting them to read the materials aloud and then deliberately pause and restore a word. Ask the student to explain how it felt and hence make a connection/empathize with the fellow classmates who stutter.
5. *Encourage Self-Advocacy*: Educate them on how to tell their needs. For example, when the student acts out a situation in which he or she requests additional time in class to complete a task or when he or she explains to a new teacher the ways in which he or she prefers to communicate. It is important to get students to take baby steps in the direction of self-advocacy. For example, a student can begin by telling their classmates about the stuttering and gradually do it in front of a large number of people. Affirm their efforts as well as the progress they have made in order to motivate them.
6. *Monitor Stress Levels*: Make sure to be aware of the stress or anxiety symptoms that can be seen in the patient. For instance, if a learner acts anxious before an examination or a performance, try to talk to them, alone. Reassure them and remind the person about the ways in which one can relax.
7. *Incorporate Relaxation Techniques*: Practicing mindfulness techniques in day-to-day life should be adopted. For example, students can begin the day with some meditation or deep breathing, or visualization exercises, for about 5 minutes. This can help in the prevention of stress in the class as well as maintaining a serene environment. This can be done by teachers every morning after the assembly time or before the commencement of classes.
8. *Promote Positive Communication Practices*: Promote active listening in your classroom by following these behaviors; this will help to teach your students to be active listeners. For instance, when a student is explaining something, ensure that you are making eye contact with the student, using gestures like nodding, and letting them complete their statement without making an attempt to contribute in the middle of the student's talk. This is a good demonstration for other students to emulate. Some activities that can be used are those that encourage taking turns and patience. For example, when in a group, one can use a stick or any other item to show who has the privilege of making the next contribution during the group's discussions. This makes sure that every learner is given the opportunity to express themselves without being interrupted by others.

9. *Set Realistic Goals*: Help the students and the parents come up with realistic goals and objectives they are to achieve. For instance, if a student is uncomfortable with oral presentations, the initial goals could be to make a presentation to a few people or even to record a presentation and make a video presentation at home. If the student is able to grasp the concept fairly easily, slowly make the problems more challenging.
10. *Celebrate Progress*: Celebrate the little achievements on the way. For instance, if a student can speak clearly in class and has done it well, then take time to appreciate the effort and growth. This can help give them more confidence and motivation to continue in their tasks.

8.8 Relapse During Teenage

Stuttering is known to reappear or get more severe during teenage years. This is quite frustrating and may lead to stress for both teenagers and parents. Stuttering is characterized by a series of changes that may occur during adolescence, and many factors may cause the onset of stuttering. These could be:

1. *Hormonal Changes*: Puberty hormones may also alter neuro-centric activities such as speech in one way or the other. Such changes may even worsen a stutter that had earlier improved.
2. *Emotional and Social Stress*: There are many challenges that have affected teenagers, including social and academic challenges. Such factors as the desire to conform and the fear of being mocked may worsen the fluency disorder. Stress factors such as speaking in public, being social, or taking tests can lead to a breakdown in fluent speech.
3. *Neurological Development*: The teenage brain is still under development, and this is especially so in the areas of self-control and executive functions. These neurological changes may impact the speech and the flow of speech for a while.
4. *Self-Consciousness*: As the teenagers gain more and more self-identity, they are also able to discern what they say. This increased sensitization can become cyclical and leads to more stuttering as the individual becomes more anxious about stuttering.
5. *Increased Communication Demands*: Having a teenage life, they need to communicate more often and on a higher level. The demands of passing messages across and the nature of interactions among teenage individuals make it easier to notice a person who stutters.
6. *Changes in Social Dynamics*: The changes in the processes of communication among teenagers and the rising concerns of peer acceptance put more pressure on young people to speak fluently and may cause more stuttering.
7. *Identity Formation*: Teens are in the middle of the process of identity development. The result is that those who stutter may have varying degrees of how much they incorporate stuttering into their identity or how much they see it as an impairment, and this affects the stuttering rate.

8. *Underlying Medical Conditions*: Quite often, the appearance of new diseases or the adverse effects of medications in teenagers can affect the speech flow.

8.9 Preventing the Recurrence of Stuttering During Adolescence

In a bid to reduce the chances of stuttering being worsened during teenage years, some measures can be taken. Here are some tips for preventing the recurrence of stuttering in adolescence:

1. *Consistent Speech Therapy*: Stuttering management should not stop even if there is progress, as it will help in keeping up with the fluency skills and ways of handling the times of high severity of stuttering. If there are any indications that the child is experiencing any emotional problems associated with stuttering, then one may have to seek counselling or therapy that can help deal with these feelings.
2. *Stress Management Techniques*: Encourage young people to engage in activities such as mindfulness, yoga, or meditation that can assist in reducing stress, which is a common companion of stuttering.
3. *Positive Communication Environments*: Promote positive communication with the teen at home, without feeling hurried, and make the teen feel validated.
4. *Encourage Social Support*: Encourage young people to interact with their peers who stutter through support group or social media platforms. It also helps in reducing the feeling of loneliness and gives one an idea of how to handle such a situation.
5. *Promote Self-Confidence*: Involve teens in activities that would make them have a sense of accomplishment and self-esteem. It is for this reason that positive experiences can assist in constructing a positive self-experience that is not determined by the ability to speak.
6. *Open Dialogue*: Encourage and also help the teens to be as open and truthful with their peers about their stuttering as possible. Be there for them and be a listener, without passing judgment on what they have to say.
7. *Educational Advocacy*: Help the school to provide conditions that will reduce the stress of speaking in public, for example, during presentation or reading tasks.
8. *Monitor Changes in Medication*: It is useful to find out if there are any possible side effects that involve speech in case the teen is on medication. All worries should be discussed with doctors and other healthcare professionals.
9. *Healthy Lifestyle Choices*: Exhibit good physical hygiene by taking regular exercise, sleeping well, and taking balanced meals. Positive physical health may also affect the emotional condition and the speech.
10. *Empowerment Through Knowledge*: Inform teenagers about stuttering so that they know that it is a part of them but does not make them who they are.
11. *Speech Practice*: Remind the teens to use speech techniques that were learned during the therapy so that they can retain the fluency learnt.

12. *Avoid Negative Reinforcement*: Avoid overemphasizing the instances of stammering. Rather, try to listen to the words that the teen is putting out there.
13. *Self-Expression Through Alternative Means*: In case of severe difficulties with speech, one should try to encourage other kinds of communication, for example, writing, painting, or music, which will also help the student to develop creativity.

8.10 Understanding Myths on Stuttering for Prevention of Relapse

Despite being relatively common, many myths and misconceptions persist about stuttering, which is actually a widespread phenomenon. Such myths can partly explain the stigma and misconceptions that people who stutter go through in society. It is high time to refute these myths to change the approach towards people who stutter and provide accurate information about stuttering.

Myth 1: Stuttering Is Caused by Nervousness or Anxiety
Of the many myths that are often told about stuttering, one of the most widely believed is that it is simply the result of overly nervous or anxious behavior. Although anxiety worsens the fluency disorder, it doesn't originate because of it. Stuttering is a highly disaggregated variety of communication disorder that has neurological, genetic, and environmental causes. The literature has established that the structure and function of the brain are different between people who stutter and those who do not (Smith and Weber 2017). Stuttering is not caused by anxiety though it may be provoked or made worse by the condition.

Myth 2: People Who Stutter Are Less Intelligent
One more falsehood is that the stuttering patient is not as smart as other people who do not have such a problem. This misconception could be a result of the fact that people who stutter may have trouble in expressing themselves verbally. Nevertheless, stuttering has nothing to do with intelligence. The facts are that people who stutter are not, in any way, less competent or less intelligent than people who do not stutter. Some of the successful people in society and in the workplace, such as scientists, writers, and people in the public domain, have had stuttering disorders (Bloodstein and Bernstein Ratner 2008).

Myth 3: Stuttering Can Be Cured Quickly
Some individuals think that stuttering has a fast solution through therapy or other techniques, which is incorrect. Although with the aid of speech therapy and other therapies,

individuals can improve their fluency and learn how to deal with their stutter, there is no such thing as a total cure. Most people who stutter have the condition throughout their lifetime, and the aim of treatment is mostly to control the fluency rather than cure the stuttering. Thus, regular practice and further encouragement are key to significant changes (Guitar 2014).

Myth 4: Stuttering Is a Psychological Problem

Many a time, people have thought that stuttering is a psychological problem resulting from an emotional problem or improper upbringing. Although psychological factors are known to play a role in stuttering, it has been found that stuttering has neurological and genetic roots. Research has also described structural variation in the speech and language areas in the brain of people who stutter (Chang et al. 2008). Stress and anxiety are known to trigger stuttering, but they are not the cause of it.

Myth 5: People Who Stutter Can Control It If They Try Hard Enough

A widely held assumption is that individuals who stutter can readily suppress their speech if they wish to do so. This stereotype about individuals who stutter may cause them a lot of frustration and make them feel that they are not good enough. Although there are some methods that might be useful for enhancing fluency, stuttering is not a condition that can be regulated by the force of one's personality. It is a chronic illness that demands special treatment and help. Simply telling people to "try harder" is counterproductive and unhelpful, and it is wrong (Yaruss and Reardon-Reeves 2007).

Myth 6: Stuttering Is a Sign of Weakness

Stuttering is often viewed as something that is negative and that denotes human vulnerability or frailty. This myth sustains the prejudice that people who stutter face in their day-to-day lives. In fact, it is a neurological disorder that has nothing to do with one's character or will to overcome it. People who stutter are known to work hard and face all the challenges that come with the fluency disorder and succeed in their pursuits (Van Riper 1982).

Myth 7: Only Children Stutter

Stuttering can start in childhood, but this does not mean that it is only confined to the young. Some people still stutter in their adulthood since most of those who stutter as children tend to do so well into adulthood. This stereotype that only children stutter can result in little or no help and compassion for the adults who stutter. This is because stuttering is not limited to children and young students, and there should be assistance and information for all (Yairi and Ambrose 2005).

Myth 8: Bad Parenting Causes Stuttering
Others have suggested that stuttering is caused by poor parenting or an unfavorable home environment. This myth can be quite damaging because it puts a lot of attention on the parents, which may lead to stress and even guilt. Stuttering has been found to be unrelated to the child's upbringing and the functioning of the family. However, it is important to note that making fun of a person in the home or having a negative home environment does lead to the development of stuttering as some people may think. Genetic and neurological factors are said to be the main cause of stuttering than the motor learning factors (Bloodstein and Bernstein Ratner 2008).

Myth 9: Bilingualism Causes Stuttering
It is a widely held view that children who are brought up bilingual become stutterers. However, research does not validate such a claim. Bilingual children do not necessarily stutter, although children who stutter may display barriers in both of their languages. Stuttering in bilingual children is no different from that in monolingual children, and the main factors that cause the disorder are still neurological and genetic (Byrd et al. 2018).

Myth 10: Stuttering Will Go Away on Its Own
Another myth is that the child will grow out of the stuttering without any form of help. Although some children will eventually grow out of their stuttering, most do not. It is therefore important that early intervention is made in order to control stuttering and therefore have a good prognosis. Stuttering can be helped by speech therapy in children as they are taught the ways and means of dealing with it and at the same time enhancing their communication (Yairi and Ambrose 2005).

8.11 Myths About Stuttering in India

In India, cultural beliefs and societal attitudes contribute to unique myths and misconceptions about stuttering. These myths can impact how individuals who stutter are perceived and treated within their communities. Addressing these myths is essential for promoting understanding and support for people who stutter in India.

Myth 1: Stuttering Is a Result of Karma or Supernatural Forces
One of the most widespread myths in India is that stuttering is an outcome of an individual's sins or the work of evil spirits. There are those who think that stuttering is a curse for some sins committed in the previous life, or that it is a result of a spirit attack. This myth can result in people who stutter being discriminated against. Hence, those who have a stutter are less likely to seek medical or therapeutic help. Stuttering has been found to be a neurological disorder that has genetic and environmental causes and is not because of any witchcraft.

Myth 2: Herbal Remedies and Traditional Practices Can Cure Stuttering
People in India still believe in the healing power of herbs and the old ways of curing the disorder of stuttering. Sometimes, some parents may try to cure their children's stuttering by using herbs, ceremonies, or visiting a traditional faith healer. Although these practices may give the immediate illusion of a solution and may help the individual feel better about himself or herself for a short period of time, there is no scientific evidence that these practices are useful in the treatment of stuttering. The current best practices in stuttering management are speech therapy and other evidence-based interventions.

Myth 3: Stuttering Reflects Poor Upbringing
There is a common belief in many Indian families that stuttering is a result of a child's poor upbringing or a lack of proper parenting. Parents of the affected child may be made to feel that they are to blame for the child's stuttering, and this results into guilt and shame. This myth can make families not seek professional help and support. Stuttering has been found not to be a result of parents' parenting styles but rather by genetic and neurological factors. Stuttering can be controlled in a supportive environment, but that does not mean that it causes it.

Myth 4: People Who Stutter Cannot Succeed in Life
There are many misconceptions in India that people who stutter cannot be successful in their academic, career, or even social life. This belief can restrict the chances of people who stutter and lead to low self-esteem. Some of the world's most successful people, ranging from actors to politicians to business tycoons, have been stutterers, which clearly shows that stuttering cannot be used to measure one's potential for success. Famous Indians like Hrithik Roshan, a famous Bollywood actor, has shared his story of stuttering, thus going against this stereotype.

Myth 5: Stuttering Is a Sign of Weakness or Lack of Intelligence
Stuttering is a common problem in India, but this affliction often causes them to be called weak or even stupid. This leads to prejudice and makes them feel lonely in society due to people avoiding them. One has to understand that there is no link between stuttering and the level of intelligence of an individual. It is also important to note that people who stutter are equally as intelligent and competent as those who do not. Campaigns and awareness programs are important in the fight against this myth to foster change for improved inclusion.

Myth 6: Stuttering Can Be Outgrown Without Intervention
Stuttering is considered by many people in India to be a condition that will go away without any need for treatment. Although some children may 1 day grow out of stuttering, many do not, and the earlier the help is sought, the better. Abasi (2022) also reveals that speech therapy offers ways and means to help individuals enhance their fluency and communication. If no action is taken, then the child will continue with the stuttering, and this might even make it worse and, hence, difficult to deal with later on.

Myth 7: Women Who Stutter Are Less Likely to Get Married

Some people in India, for instance, think that ladies who stutter cannot easily get married. This can lead to the isolation of women with stuttering in public, which in turn affects their confidence and future opportunities. These perceptions must be questioned, and the community should be made to know that stuttering does not, in any way, affect one's value or desirability. These attitudes can be changed through awareness campaigns and education and hence make the society more tolerant.

Myth 8: Bilingualism Causes Stuttering

There is also a belief in India, which is a multilingual country, that by speaking two languages, the child may develop a stammer. But the findings of many studies indicate that bilingualism does not lead to stuttering.

References

Abasi CH. The science behind stuttering: Reducing stigma and public misconceptions (Honors thesis). University of Texas at Arlington. 2022. https://mavmatrix.uta.edu/honors_spring2022/56.

Bloodstein O, Bernstein Ratner N. A handbook on stuttering. 6th ed. Clifton Park: Delmar Cengage Learning; 2008.

Byrd CT. Assessing bilingual children: Are their disfluencies indicative of stuttering or the by-product of navigating two languages? Semin Speech Lang. 2018;39(4):324–32. https://doi.org/10.1055/s-0038-1667161.

Chang S-E, Erickson KI, Ambrose NG, Hasegawa-Johnson MA, Ludlow CL. Brain anatomy differences in childhood stuttering. NeuroImage. 2008;39(3):1333–44. https://doi.org/10.1016/j.neuroimage.2007.09.067.

Craig A, Tran Y. Chronic and social anxiety in people who stutter. Adv Psychiatr Treat. 2005;12:63–8. https://doi.org/10.1192/apt.12.1.63.

Guitar B. Stuttering: an integrated approach to its nature and treatment. 3rd ed. Lippincott Williams & Wilkins; 2006. https://openlibrary.org/books/OL17888460M/Stuttering

Guitar B. Stuttering: An integrated approach to its nature and treatment (4th ed.). Lippincott Williams & Wilkins. 2014.

Ingham RJ, Kilgo M, Ingham JC, Moglia R, Belknap H, Sanchez T. Evaluation of a stuttering treatment based on reduction of short phonation intervals. J Speech Lang Hear Res. 2001;44(6):1229–44.

Manning WH. Clinical decision making in fluency disorders. 3rd ed. Clifton Park: Delmar Cengage Learning; 2010.

Manning WH, DiLollo A. Clinical decision making in fluency disorders. 4th ed. San Diego: Plural Publishing; 2017.

Packman A, Onslow M. The handbook of speech production. 1st ed. San Diego: Singular Publishing Group; 1998.

Smith A, Weber C. How stuttering develops: the multifactorial dynamic pathways theory. J Speech Lang Hear Res. 2017;60(9):2483–505. https://doi.org/10.1044/2017_JSLHR-S-16-0343.

Smith A, Goffman L, Sasisekaran J, Weber-Fox C. Language and motor abilities of preschool children who stutter: evidence from behavioral and kinematic indices of nonword repetition performance. J Fluen Disord. 2014;41:22–40. https://doi.org/10.1016/j.jfludis.2014.05.003.

Van Riper C. The nature of stuttering. Englewood Cliffs: Prentice-Hall; 1982.

Yairi E, Ambrose NG. Early childhood stuttering: for clinicians by clinicians. Austin: Pro-Ed; 2005.
Yaruss JS, Reardon-Reeves NA. Early childhood stuttering therapy: a practical guide. McKinney: Stuttering Therapy Resources, Inc.; 2007.
Yaruss JS, Quesal RW. Overall assessment of the speaker's experience of stuttering (OASES): Documenting multiple outcomes in stuttering treatment. J. Fluency Disord. 2006;31(2):90–115.

I Am Proud of Who I Am Inspiring Stories of People with Stuttering

9

Abstract

This chapter celebrates the resilience, determination, and success of individuals who have stuttered yet achieved remarkable accomplishments across various fields. By sharing real-life stories of globally renowned figures alongside everyday heroes, the chapter highlights that stuttering does not define one's potential or limit success. These narratives emphasize the power of self-acceptance, perseverance, and the support of family, professionals, and self-help groups.

The chapter explores how individuals who stutter have transformed their challenges into strengths, utilizing speech therapy, mindfulness, creative outlets, and community involvement to build confidence and enhance communication. By highlighting real-life experiences and showcasing diverse personal journeys, the chapter inspires readers to embrace their identity and pursue their goals fearlessly.

Keywords

Inspirational stories · Self-acceptance · Public awareness · Societal attitudes Overcoming adversity

One of the most popular depictions of King George VI's problem of stuttering is seen in the movie *The King's Speech,* which was an Oscar winner. King George VI was born as Albert Frederick Arthur George, and he became the king in the year 1936 after his brother King Edward VIII gave up the throne. Even though he was a king, George VI had a dreadful speech impediment, a stutter that started in childhood, and made him a very reluctant public speaker. His ill health was such that he did not even like to deliver speeches, which formed a major part of royal engagements.

R. Kaur, *Navigating Childhood Stuttering*,
https://doi.org/10.1007/978-981-96-6206-7_9

To this challenge, he turned to Lionel Logue, an Australian speech and language therapist with a rather uncustomary approach. Elementary as they were, Logue's techniques were not conventional; they entailed physical activities and psychological tactics, and they worked. Working together, George VI began to get the confidence and the skill to make effective and powerful speeches. He was most frequently inspirational and dedicated during World War II wherein he provided consistent and anchor-like broadcasts to the British population during the worst days of the war.

The story of George VI is one of the perfect examples of how a man with a disability—in this case, a speech impediment—could become a king with the support and fight against adversity.

1. *Samuel L. Jackson*

   Samuel L. Jackson, a renowned actor in Hollywood, had a speech impediment of stuttering during his childhood. He found a way to cope with his stutter and act in several hits such as *Pulp Fiction* and *The Avengers*. Jackson's story also shows how the process of finding one's passion and channeling it as a way to help oneself can be a very valuable one. He promotes people to be themselves and not to give up even when the odds are against them.
2. *Emily Blunt*

   The British actor Emily Blunt had problems with her speech and used to stutter. It was during her high school that she was encouraged by one of her teachers to perform in a school play. In order to speak fluently, she chose to take different characters that led her to acting. Now, Blunt is famous for the roles in *The Devil Wears Prada, A Quiet Place,* and *Mary Poppins Returns*. It is for this reason that her story shows that artistic activities can be very effective in the management of speech impairments.
3. *James Earl Jones*

   Star Wars' *Darth Vader* and The Lion King's *Mufasa* voice actor, James Earl Jones, had a speech impediment in his childhood. Although Jones was a stutterer, he had an interest in poetry reading and acting. Now, this man has one of the most distinctive and powerful voices in the world today. These aspects make Jones's journey a clear example of how arts can help people with speech impairment.
4. *Tiger Woods*

   The famous golfer, Tiger Woods, also had a problem of stuttering in his childhood. With speech therapy and a lot of effort, he learned to overcome his speech impediment and is today one of golf's all-time greats. Wood's success story shows that everybody should be offered help at an early age and that people should follow their dreams despite all the difficulties.
5. *Nicole Kidman*

   Australian-born actor Nicole Kidman, who has received an Academy Award, has spoken of her stuttering in childhood. "To support her with her speaking difficulties, she was made to read out loud and even act." Some of the most popular films in which she has acted include *Moulin Rouge*! Despite starring in numerous films grossing over

$4 billion worldwide, Nicole Kidman describes herself as exceptionally shy, a trait intensified by her childhood stutter. She recalls struggling to speak, often urged to slow down and think about her words. While Kidman still battles shyness, she remains committed to not letting fear dictate her life, inspiring those in the stuttering community to confront their fears with resilience (Stuttering Foundation 2017).

6. *Joe Biden*

   Joseph R. Biden, the 46th president elect of United States of America, has been very vocal about his longtime battle with stuttering. When still young, Biden had a speech impediment, and this made him a target of bullies, and he felt lonely. Through hard work and commitment, he was able to acquire skills that would enable him to control the stuttering, for instance, speaking to a mirror. Biden's political career that led him to the presidency is a perfect example of how one can work through the adversities and finally succeed.

7. *Dilip Kumar: The Tragedy King's Triumph*

   It is an open secret that Dilip Kumar, the stalwart of Indian cinema, had a very difficult childhood and he had to bear the brunt of stammering. However, he never allowed for his speech impediment to be the defining moment of his life. Dilip Kumar struggled through his ordeals, and through hard work and commitment, he was able to build his career in the film industry. He once said that "stuttering has made me a good listener, a good observer, to understand what is not being said and hear the silence." This ability to use silence to his advantage while performing on stage earned him the nickname "Tragedy King." The life of Dilip Kumar is a story that tells us that it is not bad to be different; rather, it should be embraced as we are strong in our weaknesses.

8. *Mammootty: The Megastar of Malayalam Cinema*

   Mammootty, one of India's finest actors, faced a similar problem of stuttering in his childhood. But this did not stop him from pursuing his dreams. In its place, he adopted acting as a tool to vent and articulate his feelings as he wanted. Mammootty's commitment and his will to face all the barriers made him one of the biggest stars in the Malayalam film industry. Once, he stated that "stuttering was never a hurdle for me, it was a pedestal which paved my way to explore myself." Mammootty's experience shows that passion triumphs over the speech impediments.

9. *S. S. Rajamouli: The Visionary Filmmaker*

   S. S. Rajamouli, the great filmmaker who has directed some of the most spectacular films, stammered in his childhood. It is interesting to note that he had quite a struggle with self-confidence and at times speech impediments on his journey to becoming a filmmaker. But Rajamouli's passion for the story could not be suppressed and so he transformed his supposed shortcomings into advantages. A young boy once diagnosed with stuttering, today Rajamouli's message is "my disability did not hold me back; instead, it made me work harder and become a better communicator through visuals." Indeed, he has been a role model and has pushed boundaries to reshape the Indian film industry.

9.1 The Everyday Heroes

This rousing account does not end with celebrities. It is also important to note that many average individuals also undergo drastic changes and defeat the speech impediment of stuttering. Thus, it is evident that everyone can fulfill their dreams. The interviews presented in this paper show that stuttering does not have to be a hindrance and that with the help of personal motivation, confidence, and professional assistance, anyone can succeed. Let's delve into the inspirational stories of these common life heroes:

1. *Atul Singh*

   Atul, the current senior leader of a private company, developed stuttering in the tenth standard. The chief reason for this was the fear that he had since childhood, worsened by his father's tendency to get angry easily only added to it.

   Despite the problem of stuttering, Atul was able to live a normal college life. However, as he stepped into the professional world, the issue came to the fore. This was worse when he had to engage with other colleagues and seniors for work-related duties. He stammered more, especially when dealing with seniors.

   Atul continued to advance in his career and the problem of stuttering began to interfere with his communication at work. However, he would not give up and so he consulted the services of a professional speech therapist. Atul never gave up and was able to find a very good therapist who took the time to listen to him, and the two began an aggressive therapy program. In fact, his speech gradually improved in the following weeks. It granted him a new lease of confidence and hope that enabled him to be more comfortable with his peers and even his seniors.

   The therapist recommended daily tasks such as jaw and tongue exercises and to read out books with hard-to-enunciate words at different speeds. These practices proved to be helpful to him and he was, therefore, able to reduce stuttering to a very large extent. Atul does these exercises daily even after more than 10 years and has included other exercises that help him in his speech control. It has become vital for him to do, meditate, and practice positive affirmations. Meditation keeps his mind in check and reduces stress, whereas positive affirmations replace negative thoughts with positive ones, thereby making him more confident.

   Atul sits for meditation and affirmative thinking twice a day, in the morning and before retiring to bed. This morning routine builds a good strong basis for the day, and the night practice works at a subconscious level during deep sleep and is more effective at handling problems.

   Today, Atul has learned how to handle himself very well in as far as speech is concerned in any situation. He can present topics without difficulty, address groups of people, and engage in meetings to address concerns of the day. Atul's story is one of courage and the potential of human spirit and the help that professionals can provide for individuals with disability.

Atul thanks his speech therapist who has worked hard and helped him to get his life back and help him to achieve his potential at work. This story is a testimony that with the help of people and determination, it is possible to overcome any obstacles that are set in our way.

2. *Shilpa Agarwal (Retrieved from TISA, 2021)*

Shilpa Agarwal, a 30-year-old engineer from India, has come across a hurdle of stammering since her childhood. She is also one of the national coordinators of The Indian Stammering Association (TISA) and part of the core team of the Indian Women Who Stammer (IWWS) group where she works actively for stammering awareness and supporting people who stammer. She is also involved with 50 Million Voices as one of the leaders from India. In her spare time, she loves to walk, do some yoga, and meditate.

There were some peculiarities in Shilpa's experience of growing up as a woman who stutters. In social situations, her speech was a way of determining her level of intelligence. She was criticized by both people she met on the street and her close relatives. Trying every possible therapy and visiting several doctors in the small town in Haryana, India, where the family lived, her speech did not progress much. This led to a period of increased anxiety as she got ready to begin college, and she worried that she would make a fool of herself when speaking her name during the course of her study. To this end, she decided to mute herself as much as possible in the conversations, and when there was a delay or a break, she would simply chuckle it off. This approach enabled her to survive her 4 years in the university but with very low self-esteem.

The turning point came in 2013 when Shilpa got the chance of doing her master's in another city. In her own words, "Starting at a new college in a new city, with friends who didn't speak my language, I found a sense of comfort and connection with them which was truly beyond my stuttered words." It was also during this time that she got affiliated to TISA, which was a positive change in her life. Attending weekly group meetings and national conferences with other people who stammered gave her a support group to turn to and increased her self-confidence.

Among the events that Shilpa found most inspiring was the time she did a podcast with Pamela Mertz for the "Women Who Stutter—Our Stories" in 2014. It was her first time on a podcast, and she said that she felt liberated. This made her able to share her weaknesses and get people to understand her and also spread awareness on the issue of stammering.

Shilpa celebrated getting her master's degree with flying colors, getting a job and climbing the career ladder within 6 years. She never hesitated to talk about her speech, which in the process boosted her confidence. It was also through 50 Million Voices, an organization that seeks to change the world for people who stammer in their workplaces, that she expanded her experience. She was able to get valuable information from the practice interviews and tips from actual human resource recruiters of the company.

Looking at it now, Shilpa knows that that one decision—deciding to move to a new city, joining a self-help group, and speaking out about her speech—was the best she could have made. Such little actions have played a monumental role in her life in one way or another. Shilpa's story shows how important it is to never give up, to have people who stand by your side, and to be able to accept the weak side of one's character. This journey should not just be about the person in question, but it should also be about encouraging other people to go through it as well.

This rousing account does not stop at the celebrities. It is also important to note that many ordinary individuals also undergo drastic changes and get over stuttering; it just goes on to show that if one can get the required support, then he or she can achieve anything in life. It is inspiring to be reminded that stuttering does not have to hold one back, and with hard work, confidence, and a good therapist, everyone can achieve their goals.

3. *Naman: A Shy Stutterer to a Successful Inspiration (Retrieved from TISA)*

   Let's picture ourselves in the shoes of a young student, Naman, who has to answer to the roll call in the class. While others merely say, "Present, mam," he has a hard time, "Pppppresent, mam…." This first public attempt, which is usually made with fear and embarrassment, is known as the "first-time fluency" and is a rather frequent occurrence among people who stammer (PWS). The overt stammer is only the tip of the iceberg; the real issues are far more involved:

Shame Naman's experience with the condition started at a tender age. The first time he felt self-conscious about how he spoke was when his mother told him to "speak without tension on the stage." Eventually, people's attitudes and own beliefs formed a strong feeling of shame in him. Stuttering, however, is not a criminal offense; it is not a disease either, but it gives one a feeling of being unwanted. This shame, which stems from the anticipation of other people's disapproval, can be deep and long-lasting.

Anxiety In medical terms, anxiety is the persistent and excessive worry and fear, with some of the common physical symptoms being pale complexion, sweating, and increased breathing rate. Naman's anxiety associated with a stammer was realized after he experienced his first stammer during a roll call at the age of 12–14 years. Realizing that his stammer could make the teacher think that he was absent, he performed this task every day, which made him even more anxious about speaking.

Diversity This made Naman conscious of the fact that he stammers and awareness of this made him feel disabled as compared to his peers. In a childhood memory, he wrote an appeal to his mother saying, "Mom, please treat my stammering," but he never dared to submit it. A role-play at a TISA national conference, where participants were asked to think about a world where 99% of people stammered, helped to illustrate how norms are constructed and how they influence attitudes toward diversity. In such a world, the non-stammerers are the ones who are unusual, to say the least.

Analyzing his experience, Naman comes to understand that the rational concern of being penalized for an absence because of stuttering has spread into other areas of his life with no reason. Why is he so self-conscious to state his name, a word that he has to use daily? This shows the extent to which shame can be linked with stammering, something which is otherwise seen as a minor imperfection.

Nevertheless, Naman points out several benefits of the experience with stammering as a psychological phenomenon. This has made him have friends from TISA and Toastmasters who have motivated him emotionally and professionally. That is where he met his chartered accountant, financial advisor, and some of the friends whom he cherishes most. In an interview, Naman was complimented for giving well-organized answers, a trick he had learned to manage his stammer. This additional effort and prior arrangement that have been induced by the need to control his utterance have made him more professional and efficient. Naman's story offers valuable lessons for readers:

- *Embrace Vulnerabilities*: It is liberating to share one's weakness, and it also creates awareness of stammering to the public.
- *Seek Support*: Being a member of a support network such as TISA can be of emotional and professional advantage.
- *Find the Positives*: It is possible to find some positive in every challenge, including better planning and response to the situations in the future.

From the story, Naman's journey can be seen that one can be stammerer but still achieve success in life like others. Thus, he shares the message of self-acceptance, the role of a community, and the significance of hard work. It is a reminder that anybody, celebrities included, can rise above their problems and succeed.

Naman's story, along with those of King George VI, Samuel L. Jackson, Emily Blunt, James Earl Jones, Tiger Woods, Nicole Kidman, Joe Biden, Dilip Kumar, Mammootty, S. S. Rajamouli, and Hrithik Roshan, highlights a universal truth that stammering is not a hindrance to success, defining the ability of the person to achieve it. Thus, these narratives speak to the value of hope, the value of support structures, and the value of accepting one's circumstances.

It is therefore possible to experience a range of emotions in response to stammering, for example, embarrassment, fear, and feeling out of place. These feelings as depicted by Naman and other characters are a result of the society's prejudices and the opinions that the individuals have adopted. However, it is through these struggles that one is able to show a lot of personal development and some hidden benefits. Naman's engagement in organizations like TISA and Toastmasters is an example of how communities can be both emotionally and professionally helpful in assisting people to develop their confidence and get what they want. In addition, these stories can be a potent source that shows that people with stammering can be more connected and that more people should be informed about this issue. Such narratives where people come forward and talk about their lives with stammering help in de-stigmatization of the condition, just as Naman's story does.

In conclusion, the above discussed people show that stammering is only a form of barrier that does not hinder one from being inspired. This chapter has shown that with determination, support, and a positive attitude, anyone can conquer his or her hurdles in life. This narrative goes beyond the well-known, well-trodden path of celebrities and into the many ordinary people who, despite their stammering, are brave and dignified in the face of the world, and who show that anything is possible if approached in the right way, and that no obstacle is insurmountable.

Reference

The Stuttering Foundation. Stuttering Foundation: A non-profit organization helping those who stutter. 2017. https://www.stutteringhelp.org/.

Closing Reflections and Future Directions 10

Abstract

This concluding chapter synthesizes key insights and practical strategies discussed throughout the book, providing a holistic understanding of stuttering and its comprehensive management. It highlights the impact of stuttering on daily life and explores how these challenges can be addressed through therapy, along with the extended support of teachers and parents. The chapter also emphasizes ongoing research and future directions to further enhance the understanding and management of stuttering.

Keywords

Research insights · Future directions · Conclusion · Integration of technology, research, and innovation in stuttering

Stuttering is a speech disorder that is defined as a communication disorder that affects the fluency of speech where there are dysfluencies that may include repetitions of sounds, syllable, or words; prolongation of sounds; and involuntary pauses or blocks. These disturbances are known to happen more frequently when the person is stressed or anxious. Although the cause of stuttering is still not well understood, it is argued that there are genetic, neurological, and environmental causes.

Stuttering is a disorder that develops in childhood, during the period of 2–5 years of age. In this stage, children are in the process of increasing the number of words they use and learning the choreography of the mouth muscles in order to produce words effectively. Some children experience this phase of language acquisition with the incidence of stuttering. Research shows that about 5% of children will stutter for at least 6 months, and of these, three-fourths will recover by the time they are in late childhood, which means that 1% of children will stutter into adulthood.

R. Kaur, *Navigating Childhood Stuttering*,
https://doi.org/10.1007/978-981-96-6206-7_10

The neurological underpinnings of stuttering have been found in neuroimaging investigations that have revealed dysfunctions in the brains of people who stutter especially in the speech and motor networks. These differences can alter the way in which muscles involved in speaking work. Stuttering also has a genetic factor; the condition can be inherited as it is often observed that members of the same family stutter.

Environmental factors may include family environment and parental practices, and stress levels may affect the intensity as well as the duration of the stutters. It is, therefore, equally important for children who stutter to receive early intervention and supportive environments in a bid to maximize on the fluency of their speech.

10.1 Impact of Stuttering in Life

Stuttering can bring about a lot of changes in the emotional, social, and even academic aspect of the child's life. This makes the children to develop anxiety, shame, or even anger when they expect to stutter, and this makes them avoid speaking situations. This avoidance behavior may lead to the child avoiding classroom activities, social interaction, and extracurricular activities, thus making the child feel isolated and have low self-esteem. Children who stutter may also experience bullying by their fellow children, which only worsens their emotional state. This leads to anxiety and people avoiding situations that can further result in a cycle that is hard to get out of. In the long run, this may lead to poor academic performance of the child and generally a poor quality of life.

At school, children who stutter may not volunteer, ask questions, or answer questions in the class, or read aloud. Children who are affected can be passive and may not be able to learn actively and actively participate in the learning process. Such a child may not be able to put their ideas across, and the teachers may think the child is not intelligent or interested in what is being taught, thereby worsening the child's academic performance.

Stuttering children may also have difficulties in social relationships and be unable to form and sustain close friendships. The concern of being doubted or mocked by other people makes them isolate themselves, which in turn affects their skills in interpersonal relationships. This isolation can worsen the child's mood and increase their feelings of loneliness and depression and therefore hamper the child's ability to engage with other people.

10.2 Challenges of Implementing Therapy Techniques in Daily Life

To the best of our knowledge, while speech therapy has been proved to be very efficient in treating children who stutter, the skills acquired in the therapy session are seldom adapted to other situations. Among the major problems, there is the issue of generalization of the techniques mentioned above to real life. The sessions are usually organized in child-friendly environments where children get to work on pronunciation of words. However, communication can occur in any given day and is not usually in a controlled environment or with the use of prepared materials. Therefore, the children may not be able to use the strategies learned in day-to-day life.

This is another major challenge. It is recommended that therapy sessions take place on a weekly basis, but the use of the techniques should be done on a daily basis. It is the duty of parents and teachers to support these techniques. However, due to their tight schedules and little knowledge, this support may not be forthcoming. Some children may also be uncomfortable to perform speech techniques in the presence of their peers. Thus, they will not be able to practice it much outside the therapy session.

Additionally, the desire to produce perfect speech can cause the child to become anxious, and in turn, they may go back to the previous way of speech. This underlines the significance of a caring and tolerant perspective from parents, teachers, and fellow students. Reminding children of the importance of speech practice and praising their efforts, even when they are small, can help children feel more confident and willing to use the learned approaches in real life.

10.3 Practical Strategies and Techniques for Parents and Teachers

To avoid the recurrence and to guarantee that stuttering will not become a lifelong problem, the following practical measures and approaches should be continuously applied by parents and teachers. These strategies bring a link between the theory and practice, helping the application of speech therapy in daily life, instead of using it only within the therapy sessions. The following strategies are therefore crucial to be put in place. Speech therapy is a process in which children are taught on how to handle their stuttering and other speech disorders. However, such skills may not be well internalized in the child's communication use in all aspects of their daily life. It is in this aspect that parents and teachers come in handy.

Thus, children are free to practice their speech at home and in school because the environment is safe and does not ridicule them. This kind of environment allows them to practice the techniques they have learned from the therapy and therefore increase their rate of fluency. For example, parents and teachers can speak slowly and calmly to the child so that the child can observe and be more willing to try it out for themselves.

The daily scheduling of speech practice is also a very important strategy. It can range from basic tasks such as reading out, talking in the family, or even giving orders in a restaurant. These interactions can give the child many chances to use speech techniques in different settings and, therefore, apply the skills acquired during the therapy.

Praising the child is significant in encouraging him or her to do more and build his or her confidence. Praising the children and acknowledging their efforts help them to keep on using the speech methods they have learned. This reinforcement assists in the alleviation of fear that is normally related with speaking and therefore improves the confidence of the learner in their speech practice.

The child should also be involved in the therapy goals for the child to have ownership of the goals. It makes it easier for children to own their speech progress when they are a part of the process. The children are, therefore, encouraged and inspired to work toward their achievements, challenges, as well as their goals.

Having frequent contact with the speech therapists helps the parents and teachers to be on the same page with the therapy plan for the child. Therapists can help advice on how to go about practicing the child's speech more often at home and even at school. In the lack of these practical strategies, the techniques learned in speech therapy are likely to be abstract to the child's real life. The use of the strategies in this manner also serves to support the skills learned during therapy and thus leads to further and more permanent gains in the child's speech intelligibility.

Parents and teachers can help the children who stutter to a large extent by preparing for a conducive environment, encouraging regularity, and keeping the lines of communication open with the therapists.

10.4 Role of Speech Therapists, Parents, Teachers, and Society

Stuttering is therefore not just the concern of speech therapist, parents, teachers, and society in the management and possible cure of the condition. All groups are essential for the child and for the creation of an environment that will foster speech development.

Speech Therapists These professionals guide children on how to cope with their stuttering by offering them unique skills and knowledge. They do evaluations, design treatment plans, and provide information to people who do not stutter on how to communicate with someone who has the disorder. Speech therapists also have the role of educating parents and teachers on how best to assist the child in speech development at home and in school.

Parents It has also been found that since parents are the first and most important caregivers of the child, they exert much influence on the child's growth. Some of the responsibilities that they have is to ensure that the child has a conducive home environment, that the child practices regularly, and that the child is appreciated for his or her progress. Parents should also ensure that they stand for their child in matters to do with education and seek for more help and information from other parents and organizations.

Teachers Teachers are very important in the process of ensuring that all the learners are accepted in the class. They should be aware of the child's speech targets and ensure that they assist the child to have a voice in class. In order for teachers to create a good environment, they should encourage their colleagues to be tolerant and accept one another. They should also make sure that they incorporate speech-friendly activities in their lessons.

Society The society also has a part in diminishing the prejudice that is linked with stuttering to ensure that people who stutter regain their confidence and feel normal. These include social marketing campaigns in the public domain, inclusive policies at the workplace, and support for speech therapy services. Specifically, the following can be done: Carry out conversations about stuttering to enable people to appreciate that it is normal, and positive portrayal of people who stutter and especially in the media will also help in the fight against the social stigma.

In conclusion, managing stuttering requires a multidimensional approach that includes understanding the disorder, addressing its impact on daily life, overcoming challenges in implementing therapy, and employing practical strategies. Thus, parents and teachers can greatly help the child by fostering a positive climate and keeping up the child's practice. It therefore means that speech therapists, parents, teachers, and the society as a whole must come together to assist children who stutter in order to enable them to communicate effectively and lead fulfilling lives.

10.5 Future Directions in the Management of Childhood Stuttering: Insights for Parents and Teachers

1. *Early Intervention and Prevention*

   Time is of essence when it comes to the treatment of childhood stuttering. It has been established that early intervention is possible in preschoolers and is most effective if the treatment is initiated before the age of 6; it can help to minimize the severity of stuttering and prevent further development of the disorder in some cases. Chang et al. (2019) highlighted the need for early intervention, as the brain is most malleable during early childhood, and the child can easily be treated to change their speech and enhance fluency. Singer and Ludlow (2020) discovered in another research that if the condition is addressed early, the social and emotional effects of stuttering will be less severe and the chances of having anxiety disorders in the future will be low.
2. *Parental and Teacher Involvement*

   Usually, it is the parents and teachers who are the first to realize that there are changes in the child's speech and, therefore, they should be involved in the identification of the problem at an early stage. In a study undertaken by Langevin et al. (2015), the authors noted that there is evidence that suggests that parents who are knowledgeable on stuttering are more likely to seek early intervention services and this may result in better outcomes. Awareness programs about the training programs for parents and teachers should be carried out so that they can know how to handle the child and ensure that intervention is done immediately.
3. *Collaboration with Speech-Language Pathologists (SLPs)*

   The present study also emphasizes on the fact that collaboration between parents, teachers, and SLPs is crucial in identifying the best ways and means of intervening for children's language development.

The study by Winters and Byrd (2020) provides supports to the notion that SLPs should collaborate with educators and families to deliver interventions that meet the child's needs. This makes the therapy more productive and also guarantees that the child gets similar attention from other people he or she interacts with in other contexts.

4. *Tailored and Grounded Evidence Interventions*

   The management of stuttering in children should be based on an individual approach to treatment and regarding the child's peculiarities. New methods and techniques of assessment and psychotherapy make it possible to choose the most effective and efficient treatment with the possibility of its maintenance.

5. *Assessment and Diagnosis*

   Newer studies on neuroimaging as well as genetics have given a more explicit explanation for the occurrence of stuttering. For instance, Chang et al. (2019) showed that there are certain neuroanatomic markers in child's persistent stuttering, and these could be the focus of early intervention. Such results are useful in the designing of better diagnostic procedures that would enable the SLPs to come up with better and more specific treatment regimens.

6. *Tailored Therapy Programs*

   Some of the evidence-based programs that have been found to be useful in the treatment of childhood stuttering include the Lidcombe Program and the Social Cognitive Behavioral Therapy (SCBT).

   Leclercq et al. (2022) conducted a trial (TreatPaCS) that showed both of these programs work and that the choice of program should be made depending on the child's particular case, the degree of stuttering, and possible comorbidities. This work restates the notion that each child's case should be managed in a manner that takes into account all the features of their condition.

7. *Integration of Technology*

   Technological developments are now being used in the treatment of stuttering and are becoming crucial in the management of the condition. More and more, there are apps that give feedback, virtual reality for practicing speech in different situations, and teletherapy. As pointed out by McAllister (2016), the applications of these technologies not only increase the chances of receiving therapy but also ensure that the patients practice regularly, which is very important for the patient's recovery.

8. *Assistance to Parents and Teachers*

   Stuttering being a condition that requires management in children cannot be left for the children's parents and teachers to handle on their own. The future of stuttering management has been identified to be the training of parents and teachers, provision of resources, and collaborative practices.

   Parent Training Programs: It has been evidenced that parent-focused interventions are quite helpful in the management of childhood stuttering. For instance, research by Yairi and Ambrose (2013) showed that when parents engaged in the child's therapy, the child made more progress in fluency. Subsequent parent training programs will probably provide parents with wider information and tools, such as online lessons and parental groups, on how to establish a favorable home environment.

It is therefore important that parents as well as teachers take an active role in helping children who stutter in the classroom. Weidner et al. (2015) underlined the need for professional development of teachers concerning the identification of stuttering and related adjustments. Possible future research may focus on the enhancement of the training of teachers and the provision of school-based programs aimed at helping children who stutter.

Collaboration Between Home and School: The management of childhood stuttering is best done in the home and school setting. According to Blood and Blood (2004), when parents, teachers, and SLPs are in constant communication with each other, then the child is likely to receive more accurate and frequent help. New technologies of communication and progress control may be used in the future to help manage stuttering.

9. *Psychological and Emotional Dimensions*

The emotional and psychological factors of stuttering cannot be overlooked in the same way as the speech difficulty. The management of the future shall eventually incorporate these features to enhance the general standard of living.

Cognitive Behavioral Therapy: It has been found that CBT is useful in helping the patient to overcome the anxiety and negative thinking that is related to stuttering. In their meta-analysis of the effectiveness of CBT in the treatment of stuttering in children, Singer and Ludlow (2020) established that children who received CBT had significantly lower levels of anxiety and higher levels of self-esteem. Possible future developments may involve the increasing use of CBT in the treatment of stuttering, especially in the children who are likely to develop social anxiety.

Emotional Support for Families: Stuttering not only has psychological effects on the child but also affects the family in its whole. Briley et al. (2019) has pointed to the fact that family interventions that include parents and siblings require emotional support. Possible future services are family education and support groups for families dealing with stuttering.

Promoting Positive Attitudes Toward Stuttering: It is necessary to change the perception of society toward people who stutter to fight the prejudice and to accept them. I think raising awareness of the public and schools and organizations about the difficulties of stuttering and the need for supportive interaction can help a lot. According to research done by Langevin and his colleagues (2015), school-based peer education programs are beneficial in the reduction of bullying and the enhancement of empathy among children who have a classmate who stutters.

10. *Research and Innovation*

Continued study is important in the progression of the treatment of childhood stuttering. Subsequent studies will probably include genetic and neuroimaging investigations, follow-up data, and the creation of a multispecialty approach to treatment.

Genetic and Neurological Research: Some of the recent reviews including the one by Chang et al. (2019) have started pointing toward the specific genetic markers and neuroanatomical variations linked with stuttering. These results may result in an earlier detection of the disorder and specific treatment that can make a huge difference in the lives of these children who stutter.

Longitudinal Studies: Such kind of studies can be useful for comparison of the efficacy of various treatments and their impact in the long-term perspective. According to McAllister (2016), further longitudinal research will assist in optimizing treatments, understanding positive outcomes indicators, and enhance the strategies that may be useful in the lifetime treatment of stuttering.

Interdisciplinary Collaboration: Future research will be more and more interdisciplinary with the contribution of speech and language pathology, psychology, neurology, and genetics. This kind of approach will ensure that better and holistic treatment measures are developed since stuttering is a complex phenomenon.

10.6 Conclusion

The future of treatment and management of childhood stuttering is very promising with much hope for the young children who stutter. The main strategies that should be employed in order to deal with the difficulties associated with stuttering include an early onset of intervention, the application of individualized therapeutic techniques, the integration of technology, and the provision of substantial parental and pedagogical support. Focusing on the psychological and emotional side of stuttering in present and future developments will make sure that children get the best treatment possible and will not be afraid to speak out. Thus, by working together and further researching the issue, we can achieve a major progress in the treatment of childhood stuttering and its impact on the lives of children and their families.

References

Blood GW, Blood IM. Bullying in children and adolescents: a modifiable risk factor for stuttering. J Commun Disord. 2004;37(3):211–22. https://doi.org/10.1016/j.jcomdis.2003.09.002.

Briley PM, O'Dwyer N, Smith A. Investigating speech motor control in adults who stutter using a novel paradigm: speech cycling. J Speech Lang Hear Res. 2019;62(8):2756–72. https://doi.org/10.1044/2019_JSLHR-S-18-0434.

Chang S-E, Garnett EO, Etchell A, Chow HM. Functional and neuroanatomical bases of developmental stuttering: current insights. Neuroscientist. 2019;25(6):566–82. https://doi.org/10.1177/1073858418803594.

Leclercq. TreatPaCS, Treatment for preschool age children who stutter. 2022. Retrieved from https://treatpacs.be/.

Langevin M, Packman A, Onslow M. Peer responses to stuttering in the preschool setting. Am J Speech Lang Pathol. 2015;24(4):562–73. https://doi.org/10.1044/2015_AJSLP-14-0166.

McAllister J. Behavioural, emotional and social development of children who stutter. J Fluen Disord. 2016;50:23–32. https://doi.org/10.1016/j.jfludis.2016.09.003.

Singer CM, Ludlow CL. Clinical characteristics associated with stuttering persistence: a meta-analysis. J Speech Lang Hear Res. 2020;63(5):1493–508. https://doi.org/10.1044/2020_JSLHR-19-00256.

Weidner ME, St. Louis KO, Burgess ME, LeMasters SN. Attitudes toward stuttering of nonstuttering preschool and kindergarten children: a comparison using a standard instrument prototype. J Fluen Disord. 2015;44:74–87. https://doi.org/10.1016/j.jfludis.2015.01.001.

Winters KL, Byrd CT. The effects of self-disclosure on male and female perceptions of individuals who stutter. J Commun Disord. 2020;87:106029. https://doi.org/10.1016/j.jcomdis.2020.106029.

Yairi E, Ambrose NG. Epidemiology of stuttering: 21st century advances. J Fluen Disord. 2013;38(2):66–87. https://doi.org/10.1016/j.jfludis.2012.11.002.

GPSR Compliance

The European Union's (EU) General Product Safety Regulation (GPSR) is a set of rules that requires consumer products to be safe and our obligations to ensure this.

If you have any concerns about our products, you can contact us on ProductSafety@springernature.com

In case Publisher is established outside the EU, the EU authorized representative is:

Springer Nature Customer Service Center GmbH
Europaplatz 3
69115 Heidelberg, Germany

Batch number: 08645883

Printed by Printforce, the Netherlands